Pharmacology and Drug Development

Pharmacology and Drug Development

Edited by **Ned Burnett**

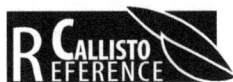

R CALLISTO REFERENCE

New York

Published by Callisto Reference,
106 Park Avenue, Suite 200,
New York, NY 10016, USA
www.callistoreference.com

Pharmacology and Drug Development
Edited by Ned Burnett

International Standard Book Number: 978-1-63239-745-4 (Hardback)

Printed in the United States of America.

Contents

Preface

It is often said that books are a boon to mankind. They document every progress and pass on the knowledge from one generation to the other. They play a crucial role in our lives. Thus I was both excited and nervous while editing this book. I was pleased by the thought of being able to make a mark but I was also nervous to do it right because the future of students depends upon it. Hence, I took a few months to research further into the discipline, revise my knowledge and also explore some more aspects. Post this process, I began with the editing of this book.

Pharmacology is the science of drug action and drug delivery. It studies the interaction of drugs whether natural or artificial with the biological systems. It also deals with discovery, research and characterization of chemicals that have the capability of curing a disease. It studies drug synthesis and design, molecular and cellular mechanisms, interactions, toxicology, etc. The objective of this book is to give a comprehensive overview of the different areas of pharmacology and drug development. Also included in this book is a detailed explanation of the various concepts and applications of pharmacology and drug development. With state-of-the-art inputs by acclaimed experts of this field, this book targets students, professionals, pharmacologists and anyone else interested in this field.

I thank my publisher with all my heart for considering me worthy of this unparalleled opportunity and for showing unwavering faith in my skills. I would also like to thank the editorial team who worked closely with me at every step and contributed immensely towards the successful completion of this book. Last but not the least, I wish to thank my friends and colleagues for their support.

Editor

Knowledge, Perception and Attitude of Pharmacists, Nurses and Doctors about Home-Care Medical Devices in Sharjah and Ajman, UAE

Hafsa Tayyab Mustafa[1], Abduelmula R. Abduelkarem[2*]

[1]AME GLOBAL FZE, Sharjah, United Arab Emirates
[2]College of Pharmacy, University of Sharjah, Sharjah, United Arab Emirates
Email: hafsatm01@hotmail.com, *aabdelkarim@sharjah.ac.ae

Abstract

Background: Medical Equipments are designed to aid in the diagnosis; monitoring or treatment of medical conditions. Upgrades in technology also help continuously educate healthcare professionals. Where previously the use of devices like "mercury sphygmomanometers" is common place, they are now being replaced by either aneroid or "mercury-free" devices. It indicates the development of technology in this area. However, trends show that healthcare professionals still seem to trust "old school" equipment a lot more. Thus, it would be motivating to see why healthcare professionals have such engraved perceptions regarding medical equipment and to be able to investigate their knowledge about current medical devices and what their thoughts are on new technology available in this area. Objectives: This research is designed with an aim to gauge perception and knowledge of targeted HCPs on the risks, benefits, issues, usage and perception on the difference between older medical equipment and the newer ones with state of the art technology available in the market. Methods: A cross-sectional study using a 34 item questionnaire was used to survey a convenient sample of nurses, pharmacists and doctors across community practices in Ajman and Sharjah, UAE. Conclusion: Discouraging HCP's from a long standing bias towards certain brands may lead towards better therapeutic outcomes for patients. Also, comments from HCP's prove that HCP's in these Emirates really do care for their patients and overall improvement of the health care industry.

Keywords

Knowledge, Perception, Medical Device, Healthcare Professionals, Healthcare Industry

---

*Corresponding author.

1. Introduction

The Food and Drug Administration, Center for Devices and Radiological Health (FDA, CDRH) defines home care/use medical devices as a medical device intended for users in a non-clinical or transitory environment, is managed partly or wholly by the user, requires adequate labeling for use, and may require training by the licensed health care provider in order to be used safely and effectively [1]. In simpler terms, home care medical device refers to those devices that a patient purchases to take home for either their chronic illness or to monitor conditions, such as fever, weight gain, and blood pressure monitoring. Home-use medical devices fall within an area where medical devices overlap consumer products [2].

It is also easy to state that the healthcare industry occupies a large part of the world from an economical aspect considering global revenue for makers of medical equipment and supplies is about \$340 billion [3]. A major portion of the markets include the US, Japan, Germany, France, and Italy [3].

Furthermore, patient-centered in-home care for individuals with diabetes, heart disease, and other chronic conditions is ideal for most patients. Indeed, home care is often seen as less costly and more patient-friendly [4]. Now, technology is advancing to meet the challenge with medical devices in the home that quickly and easily link to electronic health provider records [5]. It is critical not only to collect the data from these devices, but to seamlessly provide that information through common practices between nursing services, doctors, hospitals, pharmacies, insurance companies, and other care providers [5]. According to the World Health Organization, there are 1 billion overweight adults, 860 million chronic disease patients, and 600 million people over age 60 worldwide. Records show that chronic disease management consumes up to 85% of total healthcare spending, displaying a larger portion of the healthcare spending and the necessity of these devices for the improvement of quality in life amongst patients [5]. Furthermore, the growth of technology in home care means that lay people with varying levels of technical skills and education become direct users of health technology [6]. Hence, the only people gauging patient feedback in regards to these devices, are healthcare professionals.

On the other hand, the presence of these devices is economically more beneficial to patients since, for example, devices like blood pressure cuffs, pulse oximeters, and glucose meters are available for less than the cost of a single doctor's visit. Other possible requirements for chronic care monitoring can include a weight scale, fitness equipment, a pedometer, a pressure switch on a bed that monitors sleep, or motion sensors to monitor activity in a house [5]. These products also provide important information about a patient's health [5].

Previously conducted researches have focused on both the risks and benefits of using medical equipment along with medicines, but this does not truly give light to the perceptions of HCP's regarding medical equipment at least in the Gulf Region. Consequently, the rationale of this present study was to explore the Knowledge, perception and attitude about medical devices amongst Healthcare professionals (HCP's), nurses, pharmacists and physicians (who are majorly in contact with medical devices and are usually the ones that show their patients how to use them) in Sharjah and Ajman, United Arab Emirates. The objectives were to investigate an in depth perspective of HCP's on their experience; to gauge their satisfaction with current technology; elicit their opinion and attitude with medical devices.

2. Method

A cross-sectional study using a 34 item questionnaire was used to survey a convenient sample of nurses, pharmacists and doctors across community practices in Ajman and Sharjah, UAE.

A questionnaire was first designed to retrieve data from the expected sample pool. The questionnaire covered sections on the pools' demographics, their performance and experience, overall satisfaction with the available technology of medical devices and opinions and attitudes. For most questions, the respondents were asked to rate their response using the options "strongly agree", "agree", "Undecided", "disagree" and "strongly disagree". There are many examples in literature to support the use of a five-choice (Likert) scale. There was also a section inviting comments at the end of questionnaire. (A copy of the questionnaire is available in the **Appendix I**).

The poor response rate expected from using postal service for the distribution of questionnaires necessitated face to face visits to the pharmacies, hospitals and clinics. In order to increase the response rate, the non-respondents were reminded by telephone and a personal visit to complete the form, which was then collected in a week's time. However, due to the reluctance of many of the pharmacists, nurses, and doctors approached, a sample of only 89/200 participants from throughout Ajman and Sharjah responded and completed the survey during the study period.

There is no requirement to obtain ethical approval for such a study in the UAE, however, before every participant was interviewed, informed consent was obtained from them. They were educated about their anonymity on participation in the study, and that their responses would be used for educational purposes. The study was carried out over a period of five months (January to May, 2013).

2.1. Validity and Reliability Testing

The validity of an instrument is the extent to which it actually measures what it is designed to measure [7]. Evidence of validity may be gained through observation, expert lay judgment, and empirical inquiry. To ensure the face validity of the series of questions prepared for this study, the questionnaire was submitted to a group of 5 individuals from different parts of the medical field; two community pharmacists, a doctor, a nurse and a general manager who works in the medical device industry. All of their views and comments were considered and incorporated into the final version of the questionnaire. To assess test-retest reliability, the questionnaire was sent on two separate occasions to 5 individuals randomly chosen in an area of study interest. The second response was elicited three weeks after the initial test. No problems were highlighted, and test-retest reliability was calculated using Spearman's correlation coefficient (r). The rho value was 0.87, which implies an acceptable level of test re-test reliability. The alpha coefficient was 0.71; indicating that all of the items included make a valid contribution to the overall score.

2.2. Data Analysis

The participants' responses were encoded and the data were analyzed using Statistical Package for the Social Sciences (SPSS, version 20.0, Chicago, IL, US).

When analyzing the data, the responses from the five-point scale were reduced to three categories: strongly agree/agree, Undecided, and strongly disagree/disagree. This enables more reader comprehensible confidence intervals for the relative proportions to be calculated.

Descriptive analysis was used to calculate the proportion of each group of respondents who agreed/disagreed with each statement in the questionnaire. Also, Chi Square test was used to identify any significant difference among the participants' responses regarding certain statements or questions in the questionnaire with a significant level of p value of <0.05.

3. Results

A total of 89 of the 200 questionnaires were returned, giving a response rate of 44.5 percent over the study period of five months [January to May, 2013]. Some of the HCPs who declined to take part in the study interestingly said or wrote comments on the questionnaire. These included: *"sorry, I am very busy"*, *"it will take a long time to solve"*, *"I am not interested in solving questionnaires"*, and *"please go ask someone else to help you"*.

3.1. Demographics

Of the 89 returned questionnaires, more than half 47 (52.8%) were pharmacists, 25 (28.1%) were nurses and 17 (19.1%) were physicians. Fifty five (61.8%) of the respondents were female. The majority 78 (87.6%) of the sample pooled were in the age range from 20 years to 50 years and less than half 41 (46.1%) were in the experience bracket of 1 - 10 years during the time of the study. The nationality of HCPs under investigation comprised (59, 66.3%) and (12, 13.5%) from Eastern Asia and Arabs originating from Africa respectively. **Table 1** describes the characteristics of our study population.

The frequency of occupation of 55 female HCPs included in the study was eight physicians, twenty five pharmacists, and twenty two nurses. In contrast, 34 male respondents comprised 9 physicians, 22 pharmacists, and 3 nurses. The differences in gender distribution according to their occupation were statistically significant (p = 0.006). **Table 2** summarizes the proportion and significance difference of HCPs' gender, years of experience and their field of practice (occupation).

3.2. Evaluating Performance/Experience

The majority of the respondents (82, 92.1%) either strongly agreed or agreed on the statement "I understood

Table 1. Healthcare professionals' demographic information (n = 89).

Demographic characteristic	n(f)	%
Age		
• 20 - 30	27	30.3
• 31 - 40	32	35.9
• 41 - 50	19	21.3
• 51 - 60	10	11.3
• 61 - 65	1	1.2
Occupation		
• Nurse	25	28.1
• Pharmacist	47	52.8
• Physician	17	19.1
Experience		
• 1 - 10	41	46.1
• 11 - 20	28	31.5
• 21 - 30	15	16.9
• 31 - 40	5	5.5
Nationality according to region:		
• Eastern Asia	59	66.3
• Iraq and GCC countries	10	11.3
• Arab countries in Africa	12	13.4
• Arab countries in Middle East	8	9.0
Gender		
• Female	55	61.8
• Male	34	38.2
Emirate		
• Sharjah	47	52.8
• Ajman	42	47.2

Table 2. Proportion and significance difference of HCPs' gender, years of experience in their fields of practice.

	Physicians n (%)	Pharmacists n (%)	Nurses n (%)	p-value
Gender:				
Male	9 (26.5)	22 (64.7)	3 (8.8)	0.01
Female	8 (14.5)	25 (45.5)	22 (40.0)	
Years of Experience:				
1 - 10 Years	3 (7.3)	29 (70.7)	9 (22.0)	
11 - 20 Years	6 (21.4)	14 (50.0)	8 (28.6)	
21 - 30 Years	6 (40.0)	3 (20.0)	6 (40.0)	0.01
31 - 40 Years	2 (50.0)	0 (0)	2 (50.0)	
Above 40 Years	0 (0)	1(100)	0 (0)	

p value (p < 0.05), 95% Confidence interval for single proportion (%) of respondents who either strongly agreed or agreed with the each statement.

what is meant by 'home-care' medical devices". Almost three quarter 66 (74.2%) of studied sample either agreed or strongly agreed that they interact with medical devices on an everyday basis. However, more than three quarter 69 (77.5%) and 70 (78.7%) reported that they either agreed or strongly agreed on the statement "I understand how to functionally use these devices" and the statement "I show my patient how to use these devices" respectively.

Interestingly, a high proportion 74 (83.1%) of the sample pooled either agreed or strongly agreed with the statement "I recommend that device that has trust worthy certificates". On the other hand, 70 (78.7%) and 72 (80.9%) reported that they believe that the devices are reliable machines and it is safe to be used to monitor patients' condition respectively (**Table 3**).

3.3. Satisfaction with Available Technology

Majority of the respondents (73, 82%) Strongly agreed/agreed with the statement that they are "satisfied with the

Table 3. Participants' perception on performance/experience with medical devices.

Statement	Strongly agree/agree n (%) (95% CI)	Undecided n (%)	Strongly disagree/disagree n (%)	p-Value
I understand what is meant by home care devices				
Physicians	15 (88.2)	2 (11.8)	0 (0)	
Pharmacists	45 (95.7)	2 (4.3)	0 (0)	0.43
Nurses	22 (88.0)	2 (8.0)	1 (4.0)	
Total (95% CI)	82 (92.1) (86.5 - 97.7)	6 (6.7)	1 (1.1%)	
I interact with them on every day bases				
Physicians	11 (64.7)	5 (29.4)	1 (5.9)	
Pharmacists	39 (83.0)	4 (8.5)	4 (8.5)	0.11
Nurses	16 (64.0)	8 (32.0)	1 (4.0)	
Total (95% CI)	66 (74.2) (65.1 - 83.2)	17 (19.1)	6 (6.7)	
I understand how to functionally use these devices				
Physicians	11 (64.7)	5 (29.4)	1 (5.9)	
Pharmacists	39 (83.0)	6 (12.8)	2 (4.3)	0.62
Nurses	19 (76.0)	5 (20.0)	1 (4.0)	
Total (95% CI)	69 (77.5) (68.9 - 86.2)	16 (18.0)	4 (4.5)	
I show my patient how to use these devices				
Physicians	12 (70.6)	4 (23.5)	1 (5.9)	
Pharmacists	40 (85.1)	4 (8.5)	3 (6.4)	0.18
Nurses	18 (72.0)	7 (28.0)	0 (0)	
Total (95% CI)	70 (78.7) (70.2 - 87.1)	15 (16.9)	4 (4.5)	
As HCP, believe these devices are safe for my patient				
Physicians	15 (88.2)	2 (11.8)	0 (0)	
Pharmacists	39 (83.0)	8 (17.0)	0 (0)	0.37
Nurses	18 (72.0)	7 (28.0)	0 (0)	
Total (95% CI)	72 (80.9) (72.8 - 89.0)	17 (19.1)	0 (0)	
HC devices are reliable machines for monitoring my patients' condition				
Physicians	13 (76.5)	4 (23.5)	0 (0)	
Pharmacists	38 (80.9)	9 (19.1)	0 (0)	0.87
Nurses	19 (76.0)	6 (24.0)	0 (0)	
Total (95% CI)	70 (78.7) (70.2 - 87.1)	19 (21.3)	0 (0)	
I recommend the device that has trust worthy certificates				
Physicians	14 (82.4)	2 (11.8)	1 (5.9)	0.49
Pharmacists	40 (85.1)	4 (8.4)	3 (6.4)	
Nurses	20 (80.0)	5 (20.0)	0 (0)	
Total (95% CI)	74 (83.1) (75.4 - 90.8)	11 (12.4)	4 (4.5)	

p value (p < 0.05), 95% Confidence interval for single proportion (%) of respondents who either strongly agreed or agreed with the each statement.

technology available in Home care medical devices now days". When asked if there was "an improvement in technology of home care medical devices now compared to 10 years ago", more than three quarter of the respondents (80, 89.9%) agreed.

Interestingly, only a little more than half (59.6%) stated that "medical representatives introduced them to new technologies". More than half of them 69 (77.5%) of them relied on patient feedback about the devices other than advertisements. Surprisingly, about a quarter of the respondents (25, 28.1%) were undecided to the statement that "they understood the functions of different technologies available in these medical devices".

Respondents seemed divided in their opinion about the statement "I face more and more issues with home care medical devices due to newer technology" as only half of them (50, 56.2%) agreed to it. Sixty five of the respondents believed that it would be "beneficial for their patients if they were more involved in the design and overall output of these devices". An interesting pattern was noticed when respondents were asked if they preferred more "computerized devices" where a little more than half (55 (61.8%)) of the respondents agreed (**Table 4(a)** and **Table 4(b)**).

3.4. Opinions/Attitudes

About three quarter of the respondents (70, 78.7%) Strongly agreed/agreed that "having home care medical de-

Table 4. (a) Participants' perception on satisfaction of technology in medical devices. (b) Participants' perception on satisfaction of technology in medical devices.

(a)

Statement	Strongly agree/agree n (%) (95% CI)	Undecided n (%)	Strongly disagree/disagree n (%)	p-Value
I am satisfied with the technology available now days				
Physicians	12 (70.6)	4 (23.5)	1 (5.9)	
Pharmacist	38 (80.9)	7 (14.9)	2 (4.3)	0.47
Nurses	23 (92.0)	2 (8.0)	0 (0)	
Total (95% CI)	73 (82.0) (74.1 - 89.9)	13 (14.6)	3 (3.4)	
There is definite improvement in the technology in devices now than 10 years ago				
Physicians	16 (94.1)	1 (5.9)	0 (0)	
Pharmacist	42 (89.4)	5 (10.6)	0 (0)	0.56
Nurses	22 (88.0)	2 (8.0)	1 (4.0)	
Total (95% CI)	80 (89.9) (83.7 - 96.1)	8 (9.0)	1 (1.1)	
The medical Representative always updates me about new technology				
Physicians	9 (52.9)	7 (41.2)	1 (5.9)	
Pharmacist	30 (63.8)	10 (21.3)	7 (14.9)	0.54
Nurses	14 (56.0)	8 (32.0)	3 (12.0)	
Total (95% CI)	53 (59.6) (49.4 - 69.7)	25 (28.1)	11 (12.4)	
Besides advertising, I rely on my patients' feedback about the product				
Physicians	13 (76.5)	4 (23.5)	0 (0)	
Pharmacist	41 (87.2)	4 (8.5)	2 (4.3)	0.02
Nurses	15 (60.0)	10 (40.0)	0 (0)	
Total (95% CI)	69 (77.5) (68.9 - 86.2)	18 (20.2)	2 (2.2)	

p value (p < 0.05), 95% Confidence interval for single proportion (%) of respondents who either strongly agreed or agreed with the each statement.

(b)

Statement	Strongly agree/agree n (%) (95% CI)	Undecided n (%)	Strongly disagree/disagree n (%)	p-Value
I understand the function of different technologies available				
Physicians	8 (47.1)	8 (47.1)	1 (5.9)	
Pharmacist	36 (76.6)	8 (17.0)	3 (6.4)	0.09
Nurses	13 (52.0)	9 (36)	3 (12.0)	
Total (95% CI)	57 (64) (54.1 - 73.9)	25 (28.1)	7 (7.9)	
I face more and more issues because of the technology				
Physicians	8 (47.1)	7 (41.2)	2 (11.8)	
Pharmacist	32 (68.1)	12 (25.5)	3 (6.4)	0.17
Nurses	10 (40.0)	13 (52.0)	2 (8.0)	
Total (95% CI)	50 (56.2) (45.9 - 66.4)	32 (36.0)	7 (7.9)	
It is beneficial for me to be involved in the design of the product				
Physicians	12 (70.6)	3 (17.6)	2 (11.8)	
Pharmacist	35 (74.5)	9 (19.1)	3 (6.4)	0.93
Nurses	18 (72.0)	4 (16)	3 (12.0)	
Total (95% CI)	65 (73.0) (63.9 - 82.2)	16 (18)	8 (9.0)	
I prefer it when the device is more computerized				
Physicians	11 (64.7)	5 (29.4)	1 (5.9)	0.65
Pharmacist	31 (66)	10 (21.3)	6 (12.8)	
Nurses	13 (52)	9 (36)	3 (12)	
Total (95% CI)	55 (61.8) (51.8 - 71.8)	24 (27)	10 (11.2)	

p value (p < 0.05), 95% confidence interval for single proportion (%) of respondents who either strongly agreed or agreed with the each statement.

vices available to their patient, aid in patient assessment in the form of log books". Majority of the respondents, 78 (87.6%) strongly agreed/agreed with the statement "home care medical devices improve their patients' quality of life and overall health". Significantly, only half (44, 49.4%) the respondents believed that "they like to focus on a specific brand of medical equipment for their patients"; while in another questions seventy three (82%) believed that the "brand of the device does not matter but the quality and reliability of the product does".

Sixty one (68.5%) thought those "home care medical devices were economically profitable to their patients" while only half (50, 56.2%) that they were "*cost effective* to their patients". Less than half (49, 55.1%) thought their patients could "easily afford such items for their home use". 70 thought that the "home management industry has improved over the past 10 years". Also, 78 (87.6%) of the respondents strongly agreed/agreed that "calibrating the devices from time to time ensured their patients' safety". Meanwhile, a major proportion of the respondents (70, 78.6%) used home care medical devices within a span of *daily* to *few times a week* (**Table 5(a)**, **Table 5(b)**, and **Table 6**).

Table 5. (a) Participants' perception on opinions/attitudes about medical devices. (b) Participants' perception on opinions/attitudes about medical devices.

(a)

Statement	Strongly agree/agree n (%) (95% CI)	Undecided n (%)	Strongly disagree/disagree n (%)	p-Value
Being HCP, the homecare medical devices available to your patients aids in your patient assessment while being away in the form of "Log Books"				
Physicians	14 (82.4)	3 (17.6)	0 (0)	
Pharmacist	37 (78.7)	9 (19.1)	1 (2.1)	0.64
Nurses	19 (76.0)	4 (16.0)	2 (8.0)	
Total (95% CI)	70 (78.7) (70.2 - 87.1)	16 (18.0)	3 (3.4)	
I feel having such devices available to my patient has improved their quality of life and overall health				
Physicians	14 (82.4)	2 (11.8)	1 (5.9)	
Pharmacist	43 (91.5)	4 (8.5)	0 (0)	0.59
Nurses	21 (84.0)	3 (12.0)	1 (4.0)	
Total	78 (87.6) (80.8 - 94.4)	9 (10.1)	2 (2.2)	
I prefer to focus on a specific "brand" of medical devices for my patients				
Physicians	7 (41.2)	4 (23.5)	5 (29.4)	
Pharmacist	20 (42.6)	15 (31.9)	0 (0)	0.12
Nurses	17 (68.0)	6 (24.0)	0 (0)	
Total (95% CI)	44 (49.4) (39.1 - 59.7)	25 (28.1)	1 (1.1)	
The brand of the device does not matter but the quality and reliability of the product does				
Physicians	14 (82.4)	0 (0)	3 (17.6)	
Pharmacist	37 (78.7)	6 (12.8)	4 (8.5)	0.17
Nurses	22 (88.0)	0 (0)	3 (12.0)	
Total (95% CI)	73 (82) (74.1 - 89.9)	6 (6.7)	10 (11.2)	
Such home care medical devices are economically profitable for my patients as they can record data at home and don't have to visit the clinic as often				
Physicians	12 (70.6)	4 (23.5)	1 (5.9)	
Pharmacist	35 (74.5)	10 (21.3)	2 (4.3)	0.11
Nurses	14 (56)	5 (20)	6 (24)	
Total (95% CI)	61 (68.5) (58.9 - 78.1)	19 (21.3)	9 (10.1)	

p value (p < 0.05), 95% confidence interval for single proportion (%) of respondents who either strongly agreed or agreed with the each statement.

(b)

Statement	Strongly agree/agree n (%) (95% CI)	Undecided n (%)	Strongly disagree/disagree n (%)	p-Value
I feel the prices that many of the devices that are available in the market are cost effective				
Physicians	10 (58.8)	7 (41.2)	0 (0)	
Pharmacist	28 (59.6)	11 (23.4)	8 (17.0)	0.229
Nurses	12 (48.0)	7 (28.0)	6 (24.0)	
Total (95% CI)	50 (56.2) (45.9 - 66.4)	25 (28.1)	14 (15.7)	
My patient can easily afford such items for their home use				
Physicians	10 (58.8)	7 (41.2)	0 (0)	
Pharmacist	27 (57.4)	14 (29.8)	6 (12.8)	0.392
Nurses	12 (48.0)	8 (32.0)	5 (20.0)	
Total (95% CI)	49 (55.1) (44.8 - 65.3)	29 (32.6)	11 (12.4)	
Home management industry has improved over the past 10 years				
Physicians	15 (88.2)	1 (5.9)	1 (5.9)	
Pharmacist	36 (76.6)	11 (23.4)	0 (0)	
Nurses	19 (76.0)	6 (24.0)	0 (0)	0.157
Total (95% CI)	70 (78.7) (70.2 - 87.1)	18 (20.2)	1 (1.1)	
Calibrating the medical device from time to time is important to ensure my patients safety				
Physicians	15 (88.2)	1 (5.9)	1 (5.9)	
Pharmacist	43 (91.5)	4 (8.5)	0 (0)	
Nurses	20 (80.0)	5 (20.0)	0 (0)	0.139
Total (95% CI)	78 (87.6) (80.8 - 94.4)	10 (11.2)	1 (1.1)	

p value ($p < 0.05$), 95% confidence interval for single proportion (%) of respondents who either strongly agreed or agreed with the each statement.

Table 6. How often do the HCP's use medical devices with their patients?

	Once or more times a day n (%)	A few times a week n (%)	A few times a month n (%)	Hardly ever n (%)	Never n (%)	p-Value (95% CI)
Physician	7 (41.2)	6 (35.3)	2 (11.8)	2 (11.8)	0 (0)	
Pharmacist	15 (31.9)	22 (46.8)	7 (14.9)	2 (4.3)	1 (2.1)	0.37 (31.4 - 51.8)
Nurse	15 (60.0)	5 (20.0)	4 (16.0)	1 (4.0)	0 (0)	
Total	37 (41.6)	33 (37.1)	13 (14.6)	5 (5.6)	1 (1.1)	

p value ($p < 0.05$), 95% confidence interval for single proportion (%) of respondents who either strongly agreed or agreed with the each statement.

3.5. View Point

This was an optional comment section of the questionnaire where respondents were asked "if they would suggest a device be invented which was not already available in the market". Although most of the respondents chose to leave this section empty, 33 (37.1%) answered where some of the responses consisted of: "*cheap lipid profile devices*", "*digital BP devices for children*", "*accuracy in existing devices*", "*device calibrator*", "*improvement of Hault device*", "*a device that would let the person know he's about to have a heart attack*", "*hemoglobin and cholesterol kit*", "*non-invasive blood glucose testing*", "*simplified version of existing transdermal insulin device*", "*Bluetooth/wireless BP monitor*".

When the respondents were asked to "write any final comments regarding the topic", majority of the responses consisted of, "*Good project*", "*Good attempt*", "*your project has made me bring more attention to these services provided by the medical industry*", "*good survey*", "*well done*", "*well selected topic*", "*excellent topic to cover*", "*survey covered all major aspects of the topic*".

4. Discussion

The response rate received was 44.5%. It can be assumed that the slightly low response rate is either due to the fact that healthcare professionals in these two Emirates are really busy or just have a lack of interest in studies that promote healthcare. Suggesting activities that enhance this interest and promote the need to advance in the field of healthcare may prove to be beneficial for all HCP's involved in the industry. It was also noticed, while conducting the research, that it was easier to approach pharmacists compared to physicians or nurses perhaps due to their availability in the community area while the other two are either in hospitals and clinics and appointments are needed to meet them. It may also be that physicians have a lack of time to spare from outside their patients while nurses were slightly more willing to stop and inquire about the questionnaire.

It was interesting to see that majority of the respondents were from East Asia (59, 66.3%) which may be due to their increasing population in the country or since most of the respondents were pharmacists, East Asians are seen more in this profession. It was also seen that more females willingly responded to the questionnaire than men which can be attributed to the fact that women were usually more approachable and want to help.

The positive aspect derived from this study was that majority of the participants (75%) responded in a positive nature towards the questions, which shows that as HCP's they look for what is best for their patients. Only in three questions was an accepted, significant difference seen in answers (chi square test, p value < 0.05); "gender (p value = 0.006)" experience (p value = 0.014)" "besides advertisements, I rely on my patients feedback about the device (p value = 0.022)", which indicates that even in different professions, their thought process and ability to understand these devices was similar. Furthermore, the fact that close to a quarter (16, 18%) of the respondents were undecided if they "fully understood how to functionally use these devices" indicates that they either are confused about the devices or medical representatives are not fully telling them about these equipment. This coincides with similar findings in the study where more than half (53, 59.6%) said that the medical representative updates or informs them about new technology or newer ways of using the device. This lack in the system can be avoided by advising medical representatives to perhaps spend more time with the HCP's so that concepts of the devices are more clear or holding seminars with HCP's that show the use of different devices and lets them practice. Perhaps introducing CME programs that cover such topics for Healthcare professionals will prove to be beneficial. This will ensure that the information is being passed equally to all HCP's and by practicing they will be able to guide their patients more fruitfully.

Although safety was previously the primary concern (for the purchase of medical devices), there is now a growing demand for data on efficacy and cost effectiveness to enable this selectivity [8]. It was hence noticed that only a little more than half (49, 55.1%) of the respondents thought that their patients could afford these home care devices. This can also be construed from a different angle where it can be assumed that perhaps HCP's may be biased towards long standing brands that are quite high in prices and only recommend those products to their patients. The ultimate aim of any prescribed medical therapy is to achieve certain desired outcomes in the patients concerned. These desired outcomes are part and parcel of the objectives in the management of the diseases or conditions [9]. Consequently, when the patient goes to the pharmacy or drug store to purchase this device, the price proves to be a hindrance or turn off as the patient does not realize that the device could be an investment in their health. Hence, overall a recommended reduction in price or perhaps a better variety in price range can be suggested so that patient compliance may be improved. A different angle to this point is also the fact that there is great emphasis on multinational companies to make sales and provide bigger figures hence enforcing healthcare professionals to recommend more expensive devices. However, Companies will have to adapt their marketing campaigns since cost savings, done correctly, will benefit everyone [10].

Recent decades have witnessed major advances in medical technologies that have been responsible for earlier and more accurate diagnoses, more effective treatments, and the ability of people to live longer, healthier lives [8]. More than half (55, 61.8%) responded that they would like to see more computerized devices or even prefer them. This can be construed positively as it shows that HCP's are interested in improving technology that improves quality of life. This increase in computerized devices will perhaps make things easier for the patient where only "one touch" application may increase patient compliance to monitor their conditions. It will also help the contact and relation between patient and HCP to improve since features like "Bluetooth or wireless" programs in the device will make it easier for the physician or pharmacist to be more aware of their patients' conditions. On the other hand, one can argue that the use of more sophisticated machines will increase confusion amongst patients as they will not always come out with the same readings due to either human error or machine error.

The comments and the views received from the different HCP's indicates that they are willing to look further into the topic and that home care medical devices form an integral part of the health care industry. The fact that there were various suggestion to be included to the market of devices to be invented also shows that HCP's are looking for improvement in the industry and that they realize what is lacking in patient health in the form of devices.

5. Limitations of This Study

Despite the fact that self-administered questionnaires are often the only financially viable option when collecting information from a large population, it has been shown that this method of collecting data has some disadvantages. This was especially demonstrated when healthcare professionals did not spend enough time reading questions and considering them before answering. It was also seen that due to many constrains and limited period of time to conduct the study, it was not possible to approach a larger sample pool.

6. Future of the Study

It would be intriguing to study this area of the medical industry again by incorporate cultural aspects to questions which may affect the way HCP's from different cultures would give answers. Also, using a similar sample pool of pharmacists, physicians and nurses to be to compare answers in findings from other emirates, especially Abu Dhabi and Dubai would be interesting. One could gauge and see if perhaps city of practice may provide a change in responses.

7. Conclusion

This study has been able to explore the knowledge, perception and attitude of pharmacists, nurses and doctors about home-care medical devices in the Emirates of Sharjah and Ajman. It can also be suggested that the response rate may be improved by perhaps increase the study time dedicated to this study to more than five months. Discouraging HCP's from a long standing bias towards certain brands may lead towards better therapeutic outcomes for patients. Also, comments from HCP's prove that HCP's in these Emirates really do care for their patients and overall improvement of the health care industry.

References

[1]   FDA (2010) Improving Patient Safety by Reporting Problems with Medical Devices Used in the Home. http://www.fda.gov/MedicalDevices/Safety/MedSunMedicalProductSafetyNetwork/ucm205434.htm

[2]   University of Cambridge (Engineering Design Centre) (2003-2006) Good Design Process for Home-Use Medical Devices. https://www-edc.eng.cam.ac.uk/projects/homeusedevices/

[3]   Wood, L. (2012) Research and Markets: 2012 Report on the $85 Billion US Medical Equipment & Supplies Manufacturing Industry Featuring Baxter International Incorporated. Boston Scientific Corporation, Johnson & Johnson, Medtronic PLC. http://www.businesswire.com/news/home/20120215005994/en/Research-Markets-2012-Report-85-Billion-Medical%23.VJfCGsAA#.VPf-DnyUfX9

[4]   Parent, K. and Anderson, M. (2015) Developing a Home Care System by Design. *Healthcare Papers*, **1**, 46-52. http://www.ncbi.nlm.nih.gov/pubmed/12811172?dopt=Abstract&holding=f1000,f1000m,isrctn

[5]   Mfontanazza (2010) Medical Devices Come Home. http://www.mddionline.com/article/home-devices

[6]   Kaye, L.W. and Davitt, J. (1995) Importation of High Technology Services into the Home. In: Kaye, L.W., Ed., *New development in Home Care Services for the Elderly: Innovations in Policy, Program and Practice*, The Haworth Press, New York, 67-94.

[7]   Smith, F. (1997) Survey Research: (2) Survey Instruments, Reliability and Validity. *International Journal of Pharmacy Practice*, **5**, 2016-2226. http://dx.doi.org/10.1111/j.2042-7174.1997.tb00908.x

[8]   Ventola, C.L.V. (2014) Challenges in Evaluating and Standardizing Medical Devices in Health Care Facilities. *Pharmacy and Therapeutics Journal*, **33**, 348-359. http://www.ncbi.nlm.nih.gov/pmc/articles/PMC2683611/?report=classic

[9]   Jin, J.J., Sklar, G.E.S., Oh, V.M.S.O. and Li, S.C.L. (2014) Factors Affecting Therapeutic Compliance: A Review from the Patient's Perspective. *Therapeutics and Clinical Risk Management*, **4**, 269-286.

http://www.ncbi.nlm.nih.gov/pmc/articles/PMC2503662/

[10] Fisher, W. (2014) Weighing the Cost of Technology Advances in Medical Devices.
http://www.kevinmd.com/blog/2013/07/weighing-cost-technology-advances-medical-devices.html

Appendix I

Knowledge, Perception and Attitude of Pharmacists, Nurses and Doctors about Home-Care Medical Devices in Sharjah and Ajman, UAE

The objective of this study is to establish the knowledge and perception of medical devices amongst healthcare professionals (HCP's), which includes doctors, pharmacists and nurses in the Northern Emirates of the United Arab Emirates. The other objective is to get an in depth perspective of HCP's on their experience, satisfaction with current technology and their opinion and attitude with medical devices. In this questionnaire, the term "Home-Care medical equipment" includes a wide list of equipment that your patient may take home to aid in the treatment/of their chronic illness or other conditions. These devices include for example, blood pressure monitors, nebulizers, glucometers, pulse oximeters, thermometers, weighing scales, pregnancy test kits. This questionnaire is for a study conducted by Ms. Hafsa Tayyab, a Bachelor's of Pharmacy student at Ajman University of Science and Technology, Faculty of Pharmacy. This study is part of her dissertation for her final year in the program. It will be highly appreciated if you could answer this questionnaire on receiving it, as being part of the healthcare community in the UAE.

1) Demographics:

Age:

20-30 ☐   30-40 ☐   40-50 ☐   50-60 ☐   60-65 ☐   Other ☐

Gender:

Male ☐   Female ☐

Occupation:

Doctor ☐   Pharmacist ☐   Nurse ☐   Other ☐

Years of experience in the field:

1-10 years ☐   10-20 years ☐   20-30 years ☐   30-40 years ☐   other ☐

Specialization (If applicable): _____

Nationality: _____

City/Emirate: _____

2) Evaluating performance/experience:

Please choose only ONE answer by ticking √ in the appropriate box.

Statement	Strongly agree	Agree	Somewhat agree	Disagree	Strongly disagree
I understand what is meant by "home-care medical devices".					
I interact with "home-care" medical devices on an everyday basis.					
I understand how to functionally use most of these "home care medical devices".					
I show my patients how to use the medical device before they take it home to use on their own.					
As a healthcare professional, I think home-care medical equipment is safe for monitoring my patient's conditions.					
Home care medical devices are reliable machines for monitoring my patients' conditions.					
I only recommend that device to my patient which has a trust worthy certificate and attestation. (e.g. *CE mark*, *ISO*: 13485, etc.).					

3) Satisfaction with the available technology:

Please choose only ONE answer by ticking √ in the appropriate box.

Statement	Strongly agree	Agree	Somewhat agree	Disagree	Strongly disagree
I am satisfied with the technology in "Home care medical devices" available now days.					
There is a definite improvement in the technology of home care medical equipment available now than 10 years ago.					
Whenever a new technology is introduced in a medical device, the medical representative always updates me about it.					
Besides the advertising done for this new technology, I rely on my patients feedback about the device.					
I fully understand the function of different technologies *available* in different medical devices.					
Because of newer technology, I face more and more issues with this home care medical equipment (e.g. *data management, patient unable to use machine*).					
I think it would be beneficial for my patients if as a Healthcare Provider, I was more involved in the design and overall output of these "home care devices" as I understand what my patient needs.					
I prefer it when the medical device is more computerized (wireless, bluetooth) than simple.					

4) Opinions/attitudes questions:

Please choose only ONE answer by ticking √ in the appropriate box.

Statement	Strongly agree	Agree	Somewhat agree	Disagree	Strongly disagree
Being a Health care professional, having such "home care medical device" available to your patient, aids in your patient assessment while being away in the form of "Log Books".					
I feel having such equipment available to my patients has improved their quality of life and overall health.					
I prefer to focus on a specific "brand" of medical equipment for my patients.					
As a health care professional, the "brand" of the devices does not matter to me but the quality and reliability of the product does.					
Providing your patients with such "Home care devices" is more economically profitable for my patients as they can record their data at home and don't have to visit the Clinic as often.					
I feel the prices that many of these medical devices that are available in the market are cost effective to my patient.					
I feel my patient can easily afford such items for their home use.					
Home management industry has improved over the past 10 years.					
Calibrating the medical devices from time to time is important to ensure my patient's safety.					

How often do you use medical devices with your patient?

☐ Once or more times a day   ☐ Hardly ever
☐ A few times a week   ☐ Never
☐ A few times a month

5) Your view

a) What kind of other equipment/devices would you suggest and see invented in the future that you feel are lacking in the market right now and will help your patients?

_____
_____
_____

b) Do you have any final comments on this topic?

_____
_____
_____

2

Awareness, Knowledge, Perception and Attitude towards Prescription Medicines Abuse among Medicines Prescribers and Dispensers in Nnewi Nigeria

Prosper Obunikem Uchechukwu Adogu[1]*, Ifeoma A. Njelita[2], Nonye Bibiana Egenti[3], Chika Florence Ubajaka[4], Ifeoma A. Modebe[5]

[1]Consultant Public Health Physician (MBBS, FWACP, FMCPH), Department of Community Medicine, NAU/NAUTH, Nnewi, Nigeria

[2]Consultant Public Health Physician, (MBBS, MPH, FWACP), Department of Community Medicine, NAUTH, Nnewi, Nigeria

[3]Consultant Public Health Physician (MBBS, MPH, FMCPH), Department of Community Medicine, University of Abuja, Abuja, Nigeria

[4]Consultant Public Health Physician (MBBS, FMCPH), Department of Community Medicine, NAU/NAUTH, Nnewi, Nigeria

[5]Consultant Public Health Physician (MBBS, FWACP), Department of Community Medicine, NAU/NAUTH, Nnewi, Nigeria

Email: *prosuperhealth50@gmail.com, bright.ifechukwu@gmail.com

Abstract

Background: Abuse of medicines is becoming a serious problem in many parts of the world, with negative consequences ranging from addiction, psychosis, cardiovascular complications, and premature deaths from unintentional overdose. Objectives: The objective of this study is to assess awareness, knowledge, perception and attitudes toward the abuse of prescription medicines (PM) among medicines prescribers and dispensers in Nigeria. Design and Participants: A descriptive cross-sectional study was carried out among pharmacists, other pharmacy staff in retail pharmacies, licensed patent medicines vendors (chemical sellers), and medical doctors in Nnewi, Nigeria. Data were collected through self-completed questionnaire supervised by trained research assistants, between December 2013 and April 2014. Three hundred and seventy-five participants were recruited for this study. Data Analysis: The Statistical Package for the Social Sciences (SPSS) version 17 for windows was used for data analysis. Bivariate and multivariate analyses were carried

---

*Corresponding author.

out to evaluate differences and associations based on selected variables. Results: The perception was high 294 (78.4%) among respondents that PM abuse was a problem in the community. Knowledge of health problems associated with PM abuse was also high at 226 (60.3%). However the attitude of the respondents towards early detection of PM abuse among their patients/clients was discouraging. Education, educational status, work status and gender significantly predict good knowledge and positive attitude about PM abuse. Conclusion: Findings from this study will assist health authorities to formulate appropriate health promotion interventions to control and prevent abuse of prescription medicines. Actions directed at early intervention, capacity building, education, public health initiatives and law enforcements will hopefully curb the menace of PM abuse in Nnewi, Nigeria.

Keywords

Prescription Medicine Abuse, Knowledge, Attitude, Nnewi, Nigeria

1. Introduction

Abuse of medicines is becoming a serious public health problem in many parts of the world. Prescription medicine (PM) abuse is described as using a medication without prescription, taking medication in a higher quantity or in another manner than prescribed, or using it for another purpose than prescribed [1]. This includes prescription medicines such as stimulants (e.g. amphetamines), anxiolytics (e.g. benzodiazepines), opioid analgesics as well as over-the-counter medicines such as cough and cold medicines abused for psychoactive effects.

According to the Centers for Disease Control (CDC), the percent of people taking at least one prescription drug increased by 50 percent between the years of 2007 and 2010 [2]. While the abuse of illicit drugs goes down, more and more people begin to abuse "legal" prescription medicines. This is a fast-growing trend in the United States [3] and developing countries such as Nigeria [4]. Even more alarming is the fact that young people aged 15 to 24 years is the fastest growing demographic of prescription drug abuse.

Prescription drugs are easy to abuse because they are so easy to find and not just getting them from the doctor. The National Institute on Drug Abuse reports that most people who abuse prescription drugs get them from relatives or friends. This can be done as people share their prescriptions with others—or even as abusers steal them from medicine cabinets or purses [3] [5].

Another factor that contributes to prescription medicine abuse is the fact that so many people think that because medications are legal, they are safe. Unfortunately, this is not true, despite the perception. Prescription drugs are only safely used by those to whom they have been prescribed, and only when following directions. In fact, these so-called "legal" drugs are not actually legal when they are not taken according to physician instructions [6].

Individuals abuse prescription medicines for various reasons that may include: in order to get high; as self-medication for anxiety, pain, or sleep problems; or to enhance cognition [7]. It could also be used as secondary drug among those who abuse alcohol and illicit drugs [8]. However, these reasons/purposes may vary by gender, age and other factors. Since medications are usually consumed at high doses, the abuse of opioids, central nervous system depressants, and stimulants can lead to addiction. Other negative consequences of prescription medicine abuse include psychosis, seizures, cardiovascular complications, unintentional overdose and premature deaths from respiratory depression and drug interactions [7].

Pharmacists, other pharmacy staff in retail pharmacies, licensed patent medicines vendors (chemical sellers), and medical doctors are important stakeholders in the prescribing and dispensing of medicines. Substance abusers obtain prescription medicines through over-prescribing by a physician, obtaining multiple prescriptions from different physicians, stealing from homes and pharmacies/patent medicines vendors (chemical) shops, obtaining medicines from family and friends, re-purchasing medicines from patients leaving pharmacies/chemical shops, and through other illegal means [9] [10].

Therefore, apart from physicians who prescribe medicines, pharmacists, other pharmacy staff in retail pharmacies involved in the dispensing of medicines, and licensed proprietary patent medicines vendors (PPMVs) are important stakeholders in substance abuse prevention. It is important that they are aware of this problem and

Awareness, Knowledge, Perception and Attitude towards Prescription Medicines Abuse among...

17

should have sufficient knowledge to identify medication abuse. They also play crucial role in educating individuals with substance abuse problems. For example, a study in the US [11] found that pharmacists who received substance abuse and addiction training in pharmacy schools were more comfortable and confident in providing counseling to patients and referring patients to drug abuse treatment.

Abuse of medicines is a public health problem in many parts of the world [12]. Therefore a comprehensive effort involving relevant stakeholders in the prescription and distribution of medicines is required to prevent misuse of medicines from becoming a serious problem in Nigeria. To the best of our knowledge, no research study involving relevant stakeholders in the prescription and distribution of medicines has been carried out in any single study in Nigeria. The results of this study will provide valuable information, for planning health promotion and for developing preventive measures against abuse and misuse of medicines for non-medicinal purposes and to promote the practice of rational use of medicines.

The objectives of this study include assessing awareness, knowledge, perception and attitudes of prescribers and dispensers of medicines toward the abuse of PMs in Nnewi, Nigeria and determining the respondents' socio-demographic predictors of their knowledge and attitude towards PM abuse.

2. Material and Methods

2.1. Study Area

Nnewi is the second largest town in Anambra State, Nigeria located east of the river Niger and about 22 km southeast of Onitsha and within the tropical rain forest region of Nigeria. Nnewi, as a historical town has many cultural events adorned with festivities and monuments. The town has several private and government-owned health facilities including, health posts, primary health centers and a teaching hospital. Others include licensed private hospitals, clinics, pharmacy shops and proprietary patent medicine vendor (PPMV) stores. These health facilities are manned by health care practitioners including prescribers (mainly doctors) and dispensers (mainly pharmacists, other pharmacy staff, PPMVs etc.).

2.2. Study Design and Sample Selection

A descriptive cross-sectional study was carried out among 375 respondents made up of: 40 pharmacists, 85 pharmacy staff in retail pharmacies, 67 licensed patent medicines vendors (PPMVs) also called chemical sellers, 100 other drug handlers like nurses and laboratory staff, and 83 medical doctors in Nnewi, Nigeria. Pharmacists, and medical doctors were recruited through their professional associations while licensed chemical sellers were recruited using a list obtained from the Pharmacists Council of Nigeria (*i.e.* Government agency responsible for regulation of Pharmacy Practice in Nigeria). The other pharmacy staff were recruited from the pharmacies selected for the study. From each group, participants were selected using simple random sampling technique from a sampling frame of members. The selected participants were identified and approached to complete the questionnaires.

2.3. Data Collection

Data was collected through self-completed questionnaire supervised by trained research assistants. Contact was made with the leaders of the hospitals; pharmacies (sts)', medical doctors' and licensed patent medicines vendors' (PMVs') association to gain their support and to mobilize their members to self-complete the questionnaires, which were distributed at their various places of practice during one of their regular meetings. The research was conducted between December 2013 and April 2014. To encourage honest responses, participants were required to disclose their names and other personal identifiers on the questionnaire.

2.3. Sample Size Calculation

Using Tabachnick and Fidell (2007) sample size estimation for regression analysis as stated by Pallant [13], and assuming 10% attrition rate to further improve the validity of this study, 375 respondents were recruited.

2.4. The Questionnaire

Items on the questionnaire included socio-demographic variables such as age and gender, and questions to assess awareness, knowledge, perception and attitudes towards abuse of medicines.

2.5. Data Analysis

Data was analyzed using the Statistical Package for Social Sciences (SPSS) version 17 for windows. Results were presented as frequencies, percentages and summary statistics such as mean and standard deviation. Bivariate and multivariate analyses were carried out to evaluate differences and associations between selected variables.

3. Result Tables and Figures

Table 1 shows that the predominant age group among the respondents is 20 - 30 years (44.8%), while the 51 - 60 years age group made up only 3.7% of the respondents. The mean age of respondents was 33.2 ± 8.9 years, while the median age was 35 years. There were 83 (22.1%) medical doctors and 40 (10.7%) pharmacists among the respondents. The rest were other drug handlers like PPMVs, pharmacy technicians etc. A large proportion, 147 (39.2%) had attained at least post-secondary education lower than university degree and majority 198 (52.8%) had acquired 2 - 5 years working experience.

Figure 1 depicts that majority 294 (78.4%) of the respondents perceive PM abuse as a problem while 79 (21.1%) were not sure of their perception.

Table 2 shows that 17.6% of the respondents cited frequent unscheduled visits/consultations by some patients to request for refills of prescription medicines" as noticeable evidence of PM abuse among them. Similarly 17.1% cited the fact that some patients regularly claim to have lost their prescription forms and request for replacement" as another evidence. Also 16.5% of the doctor respondents believe that when some patients consume prescription medicines much faster than indicated, it is a sign that they indulge in PM abuse. On the other hand, 25.3% of pharmacists/PPMVs etc believed that when some customers buy prescription medicines more frequently than normal, it is clear evidence that they indulge in PM abuse. About 19.7% of this group also stated that if some customers came to purchase the same type of prescription medicine with multiple prescriptions made by the same or different doctors, then that is an indication that they indulge in PM abuse.

Figure 2 is a depiction of knowledge about health problems associated with PM abuse. A large number of the respondents (226; 60.3%) associated all the listed health problems with PM abuse. One hundred and fifteen (30.7%) linked addiction to PM abuse while 70 (18.7%) associated it with accidental overdose.

Figure 3 depicts about 21.1% of respondents are aware that self-medication for emotional or physical pain is a non-medical reason for which people need prescription medicine; whereas 18.4% said people use PM to induce sleep. About 72.5% are aware that all the non-medical reasons listed are reasons for PM abuse.

Table 3 shows that significantly higher proportion of doctors than other health workers rate their knowledge of PM abuse as adequate, p < 0.005.

Table 4 shows that significantly higher proportion of doctors (85.5%) than non-doctors (48.9%) have received any training on drug and PM abuse (p < 0.01). Similarly, markedly higher proportion of doctors (90.4%)

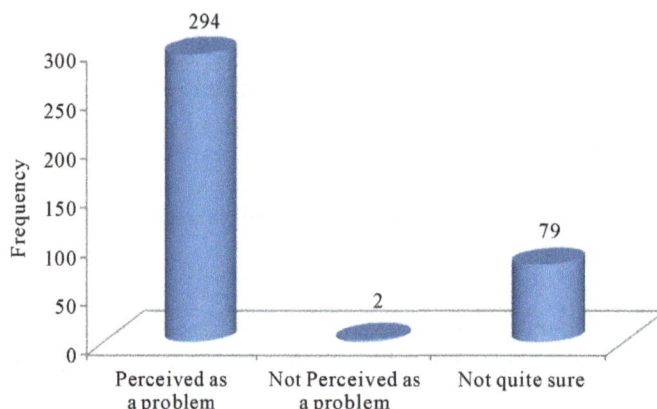

Figure 1. Perception of prescription medicine abuse as a problem in the community.

Table 1. Socio-demographic variables of respondents.

Socio-demographic variables	Frequency	Percent
Age group (Years)		
<20	10	2.7
20 - 30	168	44.8
31 - 40	127	33.9
41 - 50	56	14.9
51 - 60	14	3.7
Total	**375**	**100**
Mean age ± SD	33.2 ± 8.9 Years	
Gender		
Male	176	46.9
Female	199	53.1
Total	**375**	**100**
Occupation		
Pharmacist	40	10.7
Pharmacy technicians	36	9.6
Trained Pharmacy assistants	49	13.0
Doctors	83	22.1
PPMV	67	17.9
Other drug handlers (nurses, laboratory attendants)	100	26.7
Total	**375**	**100**
Educational level		
Secondary education or less	49	13.0
Post-secondary qualification lower than bachelor's degree	147	39.2
Bachelor's degree	145	38.7
Master's degree	18	4.8
PhD degree	16	4.3
Total	**375**	**100**
Year of experience (Years)		
≤1	64	17.1
2 - 5	198	52.8
6 - 10	48	12.8
11 - 20	43	11.5
21 - 30	14	3.7
31 - 35	8	2.1
Total	**375**	**100**
Mean year of experience ± SD	6.3 ± 6.9 years	
Employment status		
Self employed	139	37.1
Employee (of hospital, pharmacy or PPMV)	236	62.9
Total	**375**	**100**

Table 2. Respondents' awareness of early evidence of PM abuse by clients.

Evidence of abuse of PM noticed by doctors	Number (%) of doctors who are aware
Some patients were receiving prescription for the same prescription medicine from other undisclosed doctors	(7.5)
Frequent unscheduled visits/consultations by some patients to request for refills of prescription medicines	(17.6)
Some patients regularly claim to have lost their prescription forms and request for replacement	(17.1)
Some patients consume prescription medicines much faster than indicated	(16.5)
Evidence of abuse of PM noticed by pharmacists/PPMVs	**Number (%) of pharmacists/PPMVs etc who are aware**
Some customers were buying prescription medicines more frequently than normal	(25.3)
Some customers came to purchase the same type of prescription medicine with multiple prescriptions made by the same or different doctors	(19.7)
Some customers presented forged or altered prescription forms	(11.2)
Some customers were buying large quantities of cough medicines or cold medicines at a single purchase	(7.5)
Some customers were buying cough medicines or cold medicines too frequently than normal	(16.5)

Table 3. Rating of knowledge of PM abuse and drug addiction in general.

Knowledge Rating	Number (%) of respondents		X^2	p-value
	Doctors No (%)	Other respondents No (%)		
Very inadequate	6 (7.2)	65 (22.3)		
Inadequate	6 (7.2)	58 (19.9)		
Unsure	6 (7.2)	44 (15.1)	17.6	p < 0.005
Adequate	40 (48.2)	120 (41)		
Very adequate	7 (8.4)	35 (12)		
Total	83	292		

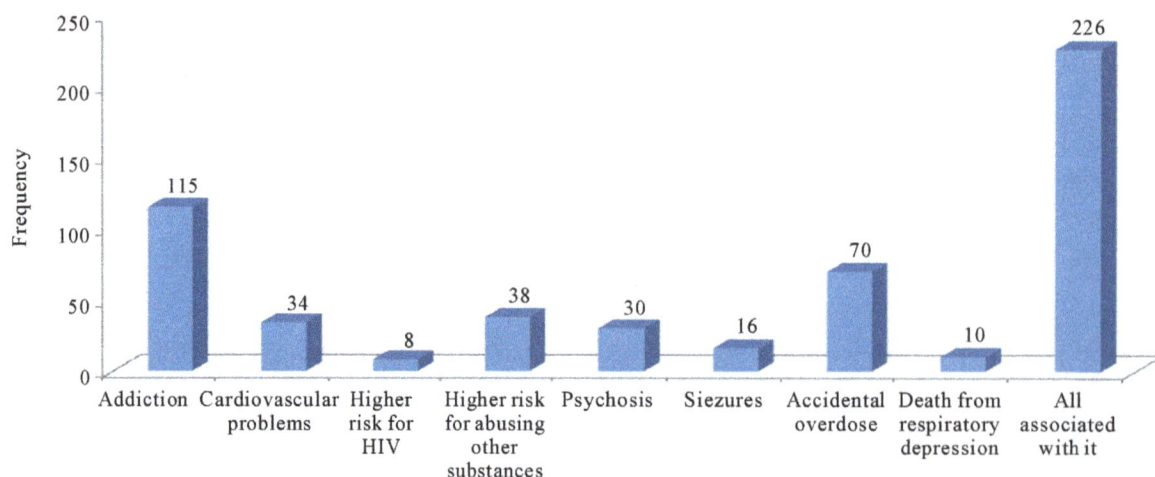

Figure 2. Respondents' knowledge of health problems associated with abuse of PM.

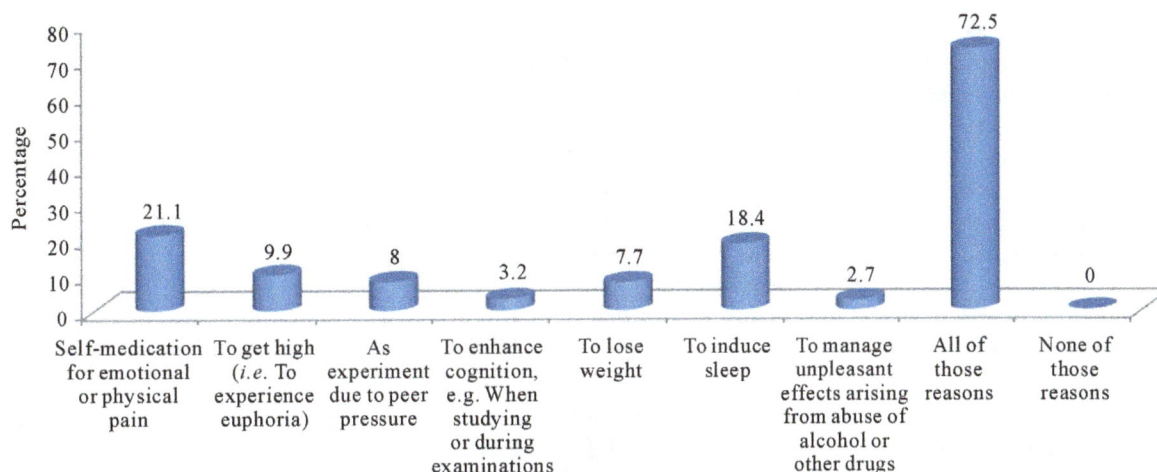

Figure 3. Awareness of non-medical purposes for which people need prescription medicine.

Table 4. Attitude of respondents towards prescription medicine abuse.

Attitude items	Number (%) of respondents		X^2	p-value
	Doctors No (%)	Other respondents No (%)		
Perception of role in prevention of PM abuse				
Very unimportant/Unimportant	11 (13.3)	58 (19.9)		
Unsure	6 (4.8)	8 (2.7)	4.51	p > 0.05
Important/Very important	66 (81.9)	226 (77.4)		
Total	83 (100)	292 (100)		
Received any training on DA including PM abuse				
Yes	71 (85.5)	143 (48.9)		
No	12 (14.5)	149 (51)	30.1	p < 0.01*
Total	83 (100)	292 (100)		
Willing to attend a training session on DA including PM abuse				
Yes	70 (84.3)	258 (88.4)		
No	13 (15.7)	34 (11.6)	0.97	p > 0.5
Not sure	0	0		
Total	83 (100)	292 (100)		
Ever spoken to a client about abuse of PM				
Yes	69 (83.1)	220 (75.3)		
No my clients did not need it	8 (9.6)	34 (11.6)	3.05	p > 0.05
No even though my clients need it	6 (7.2)	38 (13)		
Willingness to provide counseling to clients about PM abuse				
Yes	75 (90.4)	204 (69.9)		
No	8 (9.6)	88 (30.1)	12.8	p < 0.025*
Not sure	0	0		
Willingness to refer PM abusers for treatment in future				
Yes	64 (77.1)	250 (85.6)		
No	13 (15.7)	7 (2.4)	26.5	p < 0.01*
Not sure	6 (7.2)	35 (12)		

than non-doctors (69.9%) are willing to provide counseling services to clients about PM abuse (p < 0.025). Furthermore, significantly higher proportion of non-doctors (85.6%) than doctors (77.1%) expressed willingness to refer PM abusers for treatment in future (p < 0.01).

Figure 4 is a picture of comparative analysis between doctors and other respondents for each of the identified barriers to counseling clients against PM abuse. Significantly higher proportion of doctors (27.7%) than the other respondents (4.5%) identified lack of time as s barrier to counseling clients about PM abuse (p < 0.01). Conversely, markedly higher proportion of non-doctor responders (45.2%) than the doctor responders (12%) said the clients ignore the advice given to them (p < 0.01).

Furthermore, significantly higher proportion of doctors (44.5%) than other responders (25.3%) felt they had no barriers to counseling of their clients against PM abuse (p < 0.02). Also markedly higher proportion (9.9%) of the non-doctor respondents than doctors (2.4%) said they did not possess the necessary skills to counsel clients (p < 0.01).

In **Table 5**, occupation as a doctor is predictive of good knowledge and attitude towards PM abuse: adjusted OR of 1.90 (1.23 - 4.13); p < 0.005 and adjusted OR of 1.39 (1.17 - 4.11); p < 0.01 respectively. The same is applicable to the occupation as pharmacist: adjusted ORs of 2.11 (1.21 - 3.24); p < 0.005 and 1.93 (1.71 - 3.84); p < 0.01, respectively. Moreover, education at the bachelor's degree level upwards is significantly predictive of good knowledge about PM abuse: adjusted ORs of 1.15 (0.59 - 4.14); p < 0.01, 1.06 (0.61 - 3.95); p < 0.01 and 1.53 (0.46 - 3.72); p < 0.04 respectively. Responders who have worked for 2 - 5 years and 6 - 10 years respectively are significantly predictive of knowledge of PM abuse: adjusted ORs of 1.21 (0.75 - 4.53); p < 0.001 and 1.10 (0.91 - 3.87); p < 0.01 respectively. Those who have worked for 2 - 5 years, 6 - 10 years and 31 - 35 years are also predictive of good attitude towards PM abuse: adjusted ORs of 1.93 (1.15 - 3.65); p < 0.01, 1.32 (1.12 - 3.83); p < 0.01 and 1.88 (1.50 - 3.61) respectively. Age, gender and employment status are also significantly predictive of PM abuse among the respondents.

4. Discussion

Prescription medicine abuse has assumed epidemic proportions among patients and clients in Nigeria [1]. Doctors, Pharmacists and other medicine handlers and prescribers have pivotal roles to play in controlling and standardizing the use of prescription medicine among their clients and patients. Therefore their knowledge, perception and attitudes towards the problem are of utmost interest in the search for a permanent solution.

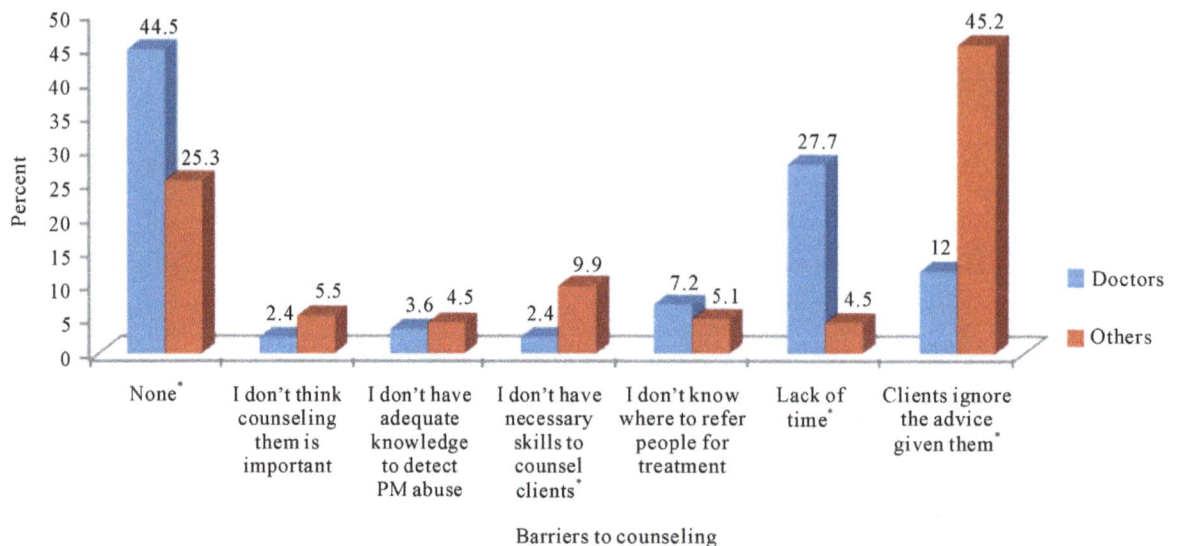

Figure 4. Barriers to counseling of clients about abuse of PM. NB: *significant differences; *"Lack of time" significant difference between doctors and others at p < 0.01 (z = 5.57); *"Clients ignore the advice given them" significant difference between doctors and others at p < 0.01 (z = 5.3); *"No barriers to counseling" significant difference between doctors and others at p < 0.02, (z = 3.37); *"Lack of necessary skills to counsel clients" significant difference between doctors and others at p < 0.01 (z = 5).

Table 5. Socio-demographic predictors of good knowledge and attitude towards PM abuse.

Socio-demographic characteristics that predict good knowledge[†]	Crude OR	Adjusted OR (95% CI)	p-value
Occupation			
Pharmacist	3.40	2.11 (1.21 - 3.24)	0.005
Pharmacy technicians	1.37	0.87 (0.46 - 2.73)	0.17
Trained Pharmacy assistants	1.82	0.98 (0.37 - 2.19)	0.07
Doctors	3.21	1.90 (1.23 - 4.13)	0.005
*PPMV			
Other drug handlers (nurses, laboratory attendants)			
Educational level			
*Secondary education or less	1.29		
Post-secondary qualification lower than bachelor's degree	1.53	0.34 (0.19 - 2.02)	0.13
Bachelor's degree	2.74	1.15 (0.59 - 4.14)	0.01
Master's degree	2.32	1.06 (0.61 - 3.95)	0.01
PhD degree	2.07	1.53 (0.46 - 3.72)	0.04
Year of experience (Years)			
*≤1	1.10		
2 - 5	1.31	0.90 (0.47 - 2.10)	0.10
6 - 10	3.42	1.21 (0.75 - 4.53)	0.005
11 - 20	2.36	1.10 (0.91 - 3.87)	0.01
21 - 30	1.41	1.25 (1.01 - 2.00)	0.16
31 - 35	1.83	1.42 (1.28 - 2.93)	0.07
Socio-demographic characteristics that predict positive Attitude[††]	Crude OR	Adjusted OR (95% CI)	p-value
Age group (Years)			
*<20	1.21		
20 - 40	3.64	1.03 (0.86 - 4.26)	0.01
41 - 60	2.71	1.18 (1.01 - 3.37)	0.01
Gender			
*Male	1.75		
Female	2.81	1.31 (0.91 - 3.76)	0.01
Employment status			
*Self employed	1.12		
Employee (of hospital, pharmacy or PPMV)	2.78	1.25 (0.79 - 3.38)	0.01
Year of experience (Years)			
*<1	1.20		
2 - 5	1.43	1.01 (0.72 - 2.11)	0.15
6 - 10	2.77	1.93 (1.15 - 3.65)	0.01
11 - 20	2.65	1.32 (1.12 - 3.83)	0.01
21 - 30	1.98	1.41 (1.23 - 2.71)	0.05
31 - 35	2.93	1.88 (1.50 - 3.61)	0.01
Occupation			
Pharmacist	2.84	1.93 (1.71 - 3.84)	0.01
Pharmacy technicians	1.67	1.21 (1.13 - 2.50)	0.10
Trained Pharmacy assistants	1.83	1.47 (1.21 - 2.84)	0.07
Doctors	2.71	1.39 (1.17 - 4.11)	0.01
*PPMV	1.16		
Other drug handlers (nurses, laboratory attendants)	1.92	1.48 (1.12 - 2.23)	0.06

[†]Good knowledge is given by knowledge of all the items plotted in **Figure 2** and **Figure 3**; [††]Positive attitude here is given by a combination of 4 or more of the items in **Table 4**.

The large proportion (78.2%) of respondents who perceive PM abuse as a problem in the community is not entirely surprising considering their impressive academic credentials-only 13% possess secondary educational qualification or less, the rest have post-secondary, masters and even doctorate degrees. The high perception of PM abuse was also reported among health workers in another study [6]. The same explanation can be offered for their impressive knowledge of health problems associated with PM abuse. Unfortunately, this has not translated into desired state of alertness, suspicion and positive attitudes necessary to galvanize effective control mechanisms to stem the tide of the PM abuse in our communities. For example the respondents have displayed a generally poor index of suspicion and awareness towards the early signs of PM abuse by their clients. Only 7.5% of doctor respondents could pinpoint the fact that "when patients received prescription for the same prescription medicine from other undisclosed doctors" that is early evidence of PM abuse. Equally among the non-doctor respondents only 7.5% could link to early evidence of PM abuse, the situation whereby their customers "buy large quantities of cough medicines or cold medicines at a single purchase".

It takes a high index of suspicion by all health workers to recognize early signs of PM abuse among their clients. Prescription drug abuse does come with warning signs. Some of these include dramatic changes in behavior like withdrawal from one's social life, dramatic drops in grades at school, or in performance at work, abrupt mood swings on a regular basis, increased annoyance, secrecy, paranoia and irritability [14]. Others include dramatic changes in appearance; sudden weight loss proceeded by loss of appetite. However, if there is a change in grooming and hygiene, that can also be a sign of prescription medicine abuse. Prescription drug addicts eventually stop taking proper care of themselves [14]. One may notice that a friend, relative or child stops bathing as often, or pays little attention to the neatness and cleanliness of clothes and hair [14]. Also if someone has been taking a prescription drug for a long time, without seeming to improve in condition, it could be a sign of prescription drug abuse. Someone addicted to prescription drugs may fake symptoms in order to continue receiving medication. Another indication is if the user keeps switching doctors. This may be a ploy to get extra prescriptions [14]. Another warning sign is an increase in the amount of the prescription drug taken [14].

It is worrisome that the respondents in this study are not very confident about their knowledge of PM abuse and drug abuse in general. Every health worker should be able to recognize the earliest sign of PM abuse bearing in mind though, that the presence of just one sign of prescription drug abuse is unlikely to indicate a problem. Many of the above signs also indicate other problems that may not be related. The key is to look for more than one indication of possible prescription drug abuse [15]. The more the indications of prescription drug abuse that are manifest, the higher the likelihood that there really is a problem. Equally important indicator of PM abuse is the presence of drug related paraphernalia such as more empty bottles in trash cans, always carrying about a bottle of pills [15]. Also, the observant health worker should keep track of own stock of medications. If the stock seems to be depleting at a faster than normal pace, it could mean that someone is stealing them for "recreational" purposes—or even to sell to others. Furthermore, a client who is always looking for money which (could merely indicate that one has fallen on hard times), may also be exhibiting another sign of prescription drug abuse [16]. Addicts need to pay for more drugs. This takes money. If someone is selling his or her treasured possessions, stealing or always asking for money to buy vague things that they "need", it could be an indication of a prescription drug addiction [16].

A comparative analysis of the attitude of the respondents to PM abuse reveals that significantly higher proportion of doctors than non-doctors received training on drug abuse including PM abuse. This has apparently led to a higher proportion of doctors expressing greater willingness to offer counseling services to their clients about PM abuse. This finding underscores the need for regular training of all prescribers and dispensers on PM abuse. Furthermore, the finding that the female gender significantly predicts positive attitude to PM abuse seems to agree with the belief that females are more compassionate and more likely to notice minute details than men [17].

The barriers to counseling of clients against PM abuse needs special mention. It is instructive to note that markedly higher proportion of non-doctor responders than doctors said that the clients ignore the advice given to them concerning PM abuse. Effort should be directed at public enlightenment with the message that non-doctors (dispensers) also possess the necessary counseling skills that should be adhered to. Also the non-doctor health workers should be encouraged to undergo regular training on PM abuse in order to sharpen their counseling skill necessary to command the respect of the clients. This becomes even more pertinent in view of the belief by some non-doctors in this study that they did not possess the necessary skills to counsel clients. On the other hand, a significantly higher proportion of doctors than non-doctors cited "lack of time" as a barrier to counseling. It has become an accepted norm that clinicians hardly have time to spare for counseling order than that for quick clinical appraisal and prescription of drugs [18]. This attitude adversely affects good patient-clinician relationship which has both emotional and informational components [19].

An exploration of the socio-demographic predictors of good knowledge and attitude towards PM abuse reveals that occupations as doctor and pharmacist are predictive of good knowledge and positive attitude towards PM abuse. These are well trained professionals who must have received some formal kinds of didactic instructions on the subject matter in course of their formal training [20]. However, the poor doctor/patient and even worse pharmacist/patient ratios [21] [22] make it imperative that other health workers must also possess desired knowledge and attitude towards PM abuse through regular informal training sessions. This will put them in good stead to also effectively participate in this fight against PM abuse. Similar regular informal training should also be given to health workers who possess below bachelor's degree qualifications as this study has shown that only respondents with bachelors' degree and above have significantly predicted good knowledge and positive attitude towards PM abuse.

Employment status is also significantly predictive of PM abuse among the respondents. Government workers stick to the rules regarding the right knowledge and attitude for them to keep their jobs. On the other hand, the self-employed private practitioner gives account of his work activities to nobody but himself and enjoys the liberty to unfortunately practice his trade according to his whims and caprices. This must be discouraged and in order to stem the tide of PM abuse, government should insist on the same standard of practice for both public and private enterprises.

5. Conclusion

Prescription medicine abuse is increasingly recognized as a serious and growing problem in Nigeria. The perception, awareness and knowledge about PM abuse as a problem in the communities are high among the health worker respondents especially the doctors. However the attitude of the respondents towards early detection of PM abuse among their patients/clients is poor and discouraging. Lack of time especially by doctors, failure of clients to adhere to counsel by health workers, lack of continuing education and lack of necessary skills constitute barriers to counseling against PM abuse. On the other hand, occupation as a doctor or pharmacist, high educational level, working as government employee and female gender are all significantly predictive of good knowledge and positive attitude towards PM abuse.

6. Recommendation

1) Early intervention: Early intervention is meant to provide doctors and other health care professional with the necessary tools to detect PM abuse in its early stages. Additionally, information gathered can further help discover trends and figure out how to better funnel resources into PM abuse prevention.

2) Capacity building: All health workers especially non doctors and the less educated ones in the private sector must be made to mandatorily undergo regular trainings on PM abuse. To increase accessibility to such trainings, they could be organized at the trade union levels and then invite qualified resource persons to conduct the trainings.

3) Education is an important element of prescription medicine abuse prevention. Education and knowledge go beyond spreading the word about the dangers of using prescription drugs for non-medical purposes. Accumulated data on PM abuse should be analyzed to provide trend information to health care professionals and to the public. This can help local prevention programs pinpoint specific problems and decide where the most effective use of resources would be.

4) Public health initiatives: In addition to disseminating information, the government should be interested in taking an active role in creating public health initiatives that can reduce PM abuse. Data gathered can be used by states to develop appropriate laws and set up programs that can help prevent abuse. Public health initiatives can also provide appropriate monitoring through pharmacies and other health care professionals.

5) Law enforcement: Prescription drug monitoring programs should be designed to help law enforcement officials. Databases should be set up to help with information and evidence gathering. Illegal activities associated with prescription drug abuse can be tracked and prosecuted, when appropriate. This can be a deterrent for some when it comes to PM abuse, and it can encourage practitioners to be more conscientious about prescribing drugs to their patients.

Ethical Approval

Ethical approval for the study was obtained from Research Ethics Committee, Nnamdi Azikiwe University Teaching Hospital (NAUTH), Nnewi, Nigeria. Permission was obtained from the pharmacies, the pharmacists', medical doctors' and licensed patent medicines vendors (chemical sellers)' associations. Verbal consent was obtained from study participants and they were informed that participation is voluntary—they were free to withdraw at any stage without any unpleasant consequences. All information was handled with confidentiality.

Dissemination of Findings

Findings have been prepared as manuscripts to be published in relevant scientific journal and will also be presented in a conference. Reports will be delivered to the leaders of the three associations, and appropriate health authority in Nigeria, with recommendations based on the study findings.

Conflict of Interest

The authors hereby declare that they have no conflict of interest in this research.

Funding

Personal income was used to fund this study—there was no external source of funding.

References

[1] NIDA (2013) Drug Facts: Prescription and Over-the-Counter Medications. http://www.drugabuse.gov/publications/drugfacts/prescription-over-counter-medications

[2] Substance Abuse and Mental Health Services Administration (2011) Results from the 2010 National Survey on Drug Use and Health: Summary of National Findings, NSDUH Series H-41, HHS Publication No. (SMA) 11-4658. Substance Abuse and Mental Health Services Administration, Rockville. http://store.samhsa.gov/home

[3] National Survey on Drug Use and Health (2004) Characteristics of Primary Prescription and OTC Treatment Admissions: 2002. Office of Applied Studies, Substance Abuse and Mental Health Services Administration, Washington DC.

[4] Orhii, P. (2012) Prescription of Medicines in Nigeria...Abuse and implications for the Health of Nigerians' A Presentation by Director General (NAFDAC) at the Physicians Week 2012 organized by Nigerian Medical Organization (NMA) Oyo State Branch, 23rd October 2012.

[5] Drug Abuse Warning Network (2006) Emergency Department Visits Involving ADHD Stimulant Medications. Office of Applied Studies, Substance Abuse and Mental Health Services Administration, Washington DC.

[6] Lessenger, J.E. and Feinberg, S.D. (2008) Abuse of Prescription and Over-the-Counter Medications. *Journal of the American Board of Family Medicine*, **21**, 45-54. http://dx.doi.org/10.3122/jabfm.2008.01.070071

[7] NIDA (2011) Research Report Series: Prescription Drugs: Abuse and Addiction. www.erikbohlin.net/Handouts/personality...of_addiction.htm

[8] Onyeka, I.N., Uosukainen, H., Korhonen, M.J., Beynon, C., Bell, J.S., Rönkainen, K., Föhr, J., Tiihonen, J. and Kauhanen, J. (2012) Sociodemographic Characteristics and Drug Abuse Patterns of Treatment-Seeking Illicit Drug Abusers in Finland, 1997-2008: The Huuti Study. *Journal of Addictive Diseases*, **31**, 350-362. http://dx.doi.org/10.1080/10550887.2012.735563

[9] McCabe, S.E. and Boyd, J.C. (2005) Sources of Prescription Drugs for Illicit Use. *Addictive Behaviors*, **30**, 1342-1350. http://dx.doi.org/10.1016/j.addbeh.2005.01.012

[10] Gianutsos, G. (2009) Prescription Drug Abuse: Strategies to Reduce Diversion. http://www.uspharmacist.com/continuing_education/ceviewtest/lessonid/106448

[11] Lafferty, L., Hunter, T.S. and Marsh, W.A. (2006) Knowledge, Attitudes, and Practices of Pharmacists Concerning Prescription Drug Abuse. *Journal of Psychoactive Drugs*, **38**, 229-232. http://dx.doi.org/10.1080/02791072.2006.10399848

[12] Oshikoya, K.A. and Alli, A. (2006) Perception of Drug Abuse amongst Nigerian Undergraduates. *World Journal of Medical Sciences*, **1**, 133-139.

[13] Pallant, J. (2010) SPSS Survival Manual. 4th Edition, McGraw-Hill, Berkshire.

[14] Partnership for a Drug Free America's Website on Signs of Drug Abuse. http://www.theantidrug.com/drug-information

[15] Symptoms and Signs of Drug Abuse. http://drugabuse.com/library/symptoms-and-signs-of-drug-abuse

[16] National Institute on Drug Abuse. The Science of Drug Abuse and Addiction. www.drugabuse.gov/publications/drugs-brains-behavior

[17] Greater Good: The Science of a Meaningful Life. www.addme.com/reports/greatergood.berkeley.edu

[18] Kleinman, A. (2013) From Illness as Culture to Caregiving as Moral Experience. *New England Journal of Medicine*, **368**, 1376-1377. http://dx.doi.org/10.1056/NEJMp1300678

[19] Kelley, J.M., Kraft-Todd, G., Schapira, L., Kossowsky, J. and Riess, H. (2014) The Influence of the Patient-Clinician Relationship on Healthcare Outcomes: A Systematic Review and Meta-Analysis of Randomized Controlled Trials. *PLoS ONE*, **9**, e101191. http://dx.doi.org/10.1371/journal.pone.0094207

[20] University of Southern California School of Pharmacy Committee on Curriculum Development. http://pharmacyschool.usc.edu/

[21] Africapedia; Creating the Best Source of Facts and Trends on Africa. www.africapedia.com/DOCTOR-TO-PATIENT-RATIO-IN-AFRICA

[22] Fasinu, P. (2008) Between Doctors and Pharmacists in Nigeria and the Attendant Health Consequences. NigeriaWorld, Feature Article.

3

A Time to Event Analysis of Adverse Drug Reactions Due to Tenofovir, Zidovudine and Stavudine in a Cohort of Patients Receiving Antiretroviral Treatment at an Outpatient Clinic in Zimbabwe

Tinashe Mudzviti[1,2*], Nyasha T. Mudzongo[1], Samuel Gavi[3], Cleophas Chimbetete[2], Charles C. Maponga[1,4], Gene D. Morse[4]

[1]School of Pharmacy, University of Zimbabwe, Harare, Zimbabwe
[2]Newlands Clinic, Harare, Zimbabwe
[3]Department of Clinical Pharmacology, College of Health Sciences, Harare, Zimbabwe
[4]Center of Excellence in Bioinformatics and Life Sciences and The School of Pharmacy and Pharmaceutical Sciences, University at Buffalo, SUNY, Buffalo, NY, USA
Email: *tmudzviti@yahoo.co.uk

Abstract

Background: Achieving the long terms goals of antiretroviral treatment (ART) requires a careful approach during treatment initiation that takes into account patient's psychosocial state, availability and accessibility of treatment combinations, and adherence support. Adverse drug reactions that occur during the initial phases have a bearing on treatment outcomes and thus need to be monitored and treated. Objective: This study was done to assess length of time (survival time) it took for clinically significant adverse drug reactions to occur in patients taking Nucleoside Reverse Transcriptase Inhibitors (N(t)RTI) available for treatment of Human Immunodeficiency Virus (HIV) infection in Zimbabwe. Methods: A retrospective cohort of patient data collected from January 2009 to December 2012 was extracted from an Electronic Health Record database. Data from patients who were initiated on antiretroviral (ARV) drug regimens containing N(t)RTI drugs were analysed for survival time. A sample of 205 patient files was extracted for the time period for survival analysis using adverse drug reactions due to N(t)RTI drugs. Results: After data extraction, a total of 205 patient records were used in determining the time to event analysis of ADR's in the cohort. The age range for the patients included in the study was 9 - 76 with a mean of 41 years (s.d = 14.8). Patients initiated on stavudine had a lower survival time before a clinically significant

---

*Corresponding author.

ADR compared to tenofovir (−365 days, p-value < 0.0005). Patients on zidovudine also had a less time before a significant reaction compared to those on tenofovir (−230 days; p-value = 0.008). Patients on zidovudine fared better compared to those on stavudine (−134 days; p-value < 0.0005). The mean survival time was highest for tenofovir (618 days), followed by zidovudine (388 days), and then stavudine (254 days).Conclusion: Patients on tenofovir have a longer survival time before a clinically significant adverse reaction. Treatment programmes need to continue commencing patients on tenofovir containing regimens as patients can be maintained for longer periods on this regimen.

Keywords

Survival Analysis, Electronic Medical Records, Adverse Drug Reactions

1. Introduction

The introduction of new antiretroviral (ARV) drug classes continues to improve the available options for patients on treatment making it easier for care providers to tailor treatments to a single patient. These developments have made it easier to achieve the goals of ARV treatment in many patients and thus improving overall survival and quality of life. Addition of new drug combinations and regimens is complemented by the patient's ability to adhere to prescribed treatment in the long term. Adherence has been identified as one of the most important factors in ensuring robust treatment outcomes in patients. Adherence to antiretroviral treatment has also been shown to be dependent on a number of factors like pill burden, existence of psychosocial support structure, the patient's readiness to start treatment, age [1]; and possibly the most important factor of all the type and severity of adverse drug reactions experienced by the patient [2] [3].

Ideally a patient on ARV treatment should be maintained on the first and initial treatment regimen for as long as possible. In many cases patients may change treatment combinations within a year of initiating therapy because of adverse drug reactions that warrant treatment change [4]. Virologic suppression by various nucleoside reverse transcriptase inhibitors (NRTI) containing drug regimens has been shown to be equal including rates of drug switching, however differences occurred in adverse drug reaction profiles of the NRTI drugs [4]. In resource limited countries the choice on NRTI drugs to initiate or maintain patients on is limited with most countries resorting to the use of stavudine (D4T), zidovudine (AZT) or tenofovir (TDF) as part of NRTI backbone.

So far only a few studies set in resource-poor-settings and using routine program data have compared TDF, d4T (30 mg), and AZT-based regimens maybe because data on TDF is limited particularly in sub-Saharan Africa where the drug has been in use for a short duration. In Zambia they compared single drug substitutions and composite mortality and loss-from-care endpoint and findings will be outlined below as with the other two. In Lesotho they assessed single drug substitutions and all-cause mortality. Bygrave and colleagues in South Africa using longer term data and including virologic response, and robust loss-from-care outcomes have compared on the following outcomes: single drug substitutions, HIV RNA suppression, CD4 count increase, loss-from care, and mortality [5].

Tenofovir containing drug regimens in some cases showed better treatment outcomes and a favourable safety profile compared to stavudine and zidovudine [5] [6]. The relative safety of tenofovir as shown in clinical studies and its ability for sustained immune recovery has seen a lot of changes in treatment guidelines, with tenofovir being the N(t)RTI of choice [7]. Tenofovir generally has lower substitution rates compared to zidovudine and stavudine containing regimens [5] [8]-[10]. In spite of the evidence that currently exist that points to differences in efficacy and safety of NRTI's in management of HIV infection, a lot of countries do not have options for HIV patients. Most HIV infected patients in developing countries have either been on stavudine or zidovudine containing regimens before the introduction of tenofovir. New World Health Organization (WHO) recommendations to use tenofovir in favour of zidovudine or stavudine have been slowly implemented across Zimbabwe. Due to the changes in treatment guidelines patients are continuously being upgraded to new regimens. The main objective of this study was to determine the time to clinically significant adverse drug reactions in a cohort of treatment naïve patients on different N(t)RTI containing ARV regimens.

2. Methods

We carried out a retrospective analysis of a cohort of patients who were initiated on ARV treatment at Newlands Clinical in Harare, Zimbabwe. The clinic provides outpatient care and treatment to HIV infected patients from marginalized urban and peri-urban communities. Data were collected from patients who were initiated on ARV treatment from January 2009 to December 2012 and had been switched to another NRTI drug due to a clinically significant adverse drug reaction. The clinic uses an Electronic Medical Record Health System called ePOC (electronic point of care) enabling an integration of HIV and TB therapy. Time to event was considered to be the time a patient started taking treatment up to the time NRTI was substituted due to a clinically significant adverse reaction. Covariates that were collected included age, gender, level of education, employment status, date of HIV diagnosis, date of ARV treatment initiation. Statistical analysis was done using STATA Version 13, a total of 205 patient records were extracted for analysis during the period under review. Ethical approval for the study was provided by the Joint Research and Ethics Committee of the University of Zimbabwe (JREC/306/13).

3. Results

A study sample of 205 patient files is extracted from ePOC. The demographic characteristics of the study participants are shown in **Table 1**.

The age range for the patients included in the study was 9 - 76 with a mean of 41 years (s.d = 14.8). The majority of the participants were female and most participants were on a zidovudine containing regimen. The mean number of days before a clinically significant adverse drug reaction due to an N(t)RTI was lowest for stavudine (254 days), followed by zidovudine (388 days) and tenofovir (618 days).

Table 2 shows that patients on stavudine had a lower survival time before a clinically significant ADR compared to tenofovir (−365 days, p-value < 0.0005). Patients on zidovudine also had a less time before a significant reaction compared to those on tenofovir (−230 days; p-value = 0.008). Patients on zidovudine fared better compared to those on stavudine (−134 days; p-value < 0.0005).

Patients on tenofovir had a longer survival time before a clinically significant adverse drug reaction followed by those on zidovudine; patients on stavudine had the lowest survival time (**Table 3**).

Figure 1. Survival in the three groups of N(t)RTI's (AZT vs. TDF vs. D4T).

4. Discussion

Our study showed that the type of NRTI agent used had an impact on the time to occurrence of an adverse effect.

Table 1. Demographic characteristics of study participants.

Characteristic	Frequency, n(%)
Age	
9 - <20	26 (12.7)
20 - <30	17 (8.3)
30 - <40	44 (21.5)
40 - <50	64 (31.2)
50 - <60	34 (16.6)
≥60	20 (9.8)
Gender	
Male	91 (44.4)
Female	114 (55.6)
N(t)RTI	
Zidovudine	116 (56.6)
Stavudine	69 (33.7)
Tenofovir	20 (9.8)

Table 2. Linear regression-comparison of time before treatment change due to ADR by N(t)RTI.

NRTI	Observed Coefficient	Bootstrap Standard Error (5000 reps)	P-Value	95% Confidence Interval
Tenofovir vs. Stavudine	−365	86.4	<0.0005	−535; −196
Tenofovir vs. Zidovudine	−230	86.2	0.008	−399; −61
Zidovudine vs. Stavudine	−134	33.0	<0.0005	−200; −70

Table 3. Mean survival time for patients initiating on AZT, D4T, and TDF.

N(t)RTI	Restricted Mean (days)	Standard Error	95% Confidence Interval
Tenofovir	618	80.8	460.4 - 777.3
Zidovudine	388	24.3	340.9 - 436.2
Stavudine	254	22.3	210.0 - 297.3

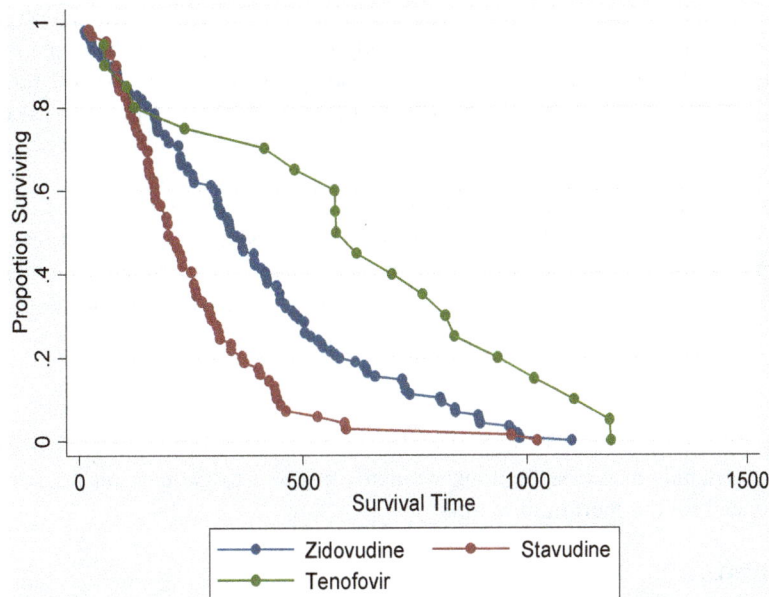

Figure 1. Shows significant difference in survival probability between patients initiated on the three N(t)RTI's; stavudine, zidovudine, and tenofovir. The likelihood-ratio test statistic of homogeneity by N(t)RTI gave a chi-square test statistic $\{chi^2(2) = 15.3, P\text{-value} = 0.0005\}$.

The results showed that a greater proportion of patients maintained tenofovir therapy for longer periods compared to zidovudine and stavudine respectively. The mean number of days before a clinically significant adverse drug reaction due to an N(t)RTI was lowest for stavudine (254 days), followed by zidovudine (388 days) and tenofovir (618 days). Bygrave and colleagues have also reported on outcomes and toxicities among patients on TDF, zidovudine, and d4T-based first-line ART in a routine treatment cohort in Lesotho [5]. Before the 2010 ART recommendations, only a few countries in Africa (Zambia, Namibia, Lesotho, and Botswana) had adopted TDF as part of the first line treatment regimen. Thus the researchers of this study noted a scarcity of reporting of outcomes on TDF compared with other regimens in low-resource settings. All adult patients initiating antiretroviral therapy from January 1, 2008, to December 31, 2008, were included in the analysis and followed until December 31, 2009. They reported that patients on zidovudine were more than twice as likely to experience a toxicity-driven regimen substitution compared with tenofovir (adjusted hazard ratio: 2.32, 95% confidence interval: 1.23 to 4.40); for patients on stavudine, the risk of a toxicity-driven regimen switch was almost 6 times higher than tenofovir (adjusted hazard ratio: 5.43, 95% confidence interval: 3.31 to 8.9. They concluded that a tenofovir-based first-line regimen is supportive of simplified care by reducing the rate of regimen substitutions compared with stavudine-based and zidovudine-based regimens [5].

Njuguna *et al*. in their study described incidence rates of drug substitutions and regimen switches due to virological failure among patients receiving regimens containing D4T, AZT or TDF in a large peri-urban area in Gugulethu, Cape Town, South Africa. They also sought to characterize the reasons and risk factors for ADR-related drug substitutions. This retrospective cohort study included HIV positive, ART naïve adults aged >18 years. Follow-up was censored at first drug change and analysis focused on NRTI changes only. Results indicated that virologic suppression rates at 1 year, regimen switching due to virologic failure and overall losses to the programme were similar across the three groups. TDF had the lowest incidence rate of drug substitutions (2.6 per 100 person-years) compared to 17.9 for D4T and 8.5 per 100 person-years for AZT. ADRs accounted for the majority of drug substitutions of D4T. They concluded that regimen switches and virologic suppression were similar for patients exposed to TDF, D4T and AZT, suggesting that all regimens were equally effective. However, TDF was found to be better tolerated with a substantially lower rate of drug substitutions due to ADRs [11].

In our study, the likelihood ratio test statistic of homogeneity yielded a chi square value of 15.28 and a p value of 0.00048053 which implies that the differences noted are significant; The lowess smoother curve demonstrated that stavudine had the most number of switches within the first 500 days of treatment. In the Kaplan Meir analyses tenofovir had the highest proportion of participants surviving at any given time followed by zidovudine and lastly stavudine. This supports what is already known in literature that a tenofovir based regimen performs better than AZT and D4T. An example of such a study which reported on this outcome is a study by Velen *et al*. [6]. Whilst Velen *et al*., looked at proportions of patients that developed adverse events as a result of an N(t)RTI, our study set to determine the duration that patients were maintained an a regimen until toxicities resulting in a switch emerged.

This study supports the continued expansion and roll out of tenofovir as the preferred first line N(t)RTI in the management of ART naïve patients. Just as well, when a patient eventually fails first-line ART, AZT is the NRTI of choice for patients initiating second line therapy. It is however important to note that in Zimbabwe the national guidelines still list D4T as a possible NRTI option for patients who have not been able to tolerate the other alternatives.

5. Conclusion

There was a statistically significant difference in the time to N(t)RTI switch as a result of adverse drug event. Patients on TDF tolerated this medicine for longer when compared to patients on AZT whilst D4T was the NRTI which was tolerated for the shortest duration.

Acknowledgements

The authors would like to thank Newlands Clinic for the support. This manuscript was supported by Award Number D43TW007991 from the Fogarty International Center. The content is solely the responsibility of the authors and does not necessarily represent the official views of the Fogarty International Center or the National Institutes of Health. For the remaining authors, there are no conflicts of interests to declare. Tinashe Mudzviti is a fellow of the Letten Foundation Research Centre.

References

[1] Langat, N.T., Odero, W. and Gatongi, P. (2012) Antiretroviral Drug Adherence by HIV Infected Children Attending Kericho District Hospital, Kenya. *East African Journal of Public Health*, **9**, 101-104.

[2] Rajesh, R., Sudha, V., Varma, D. and Sonika, S. (2012) Association between Medication Adherence Outcomes and Adverse Drug Reactions to Highly Active Antiretroviral Therapy in Indian Human Immunodeficiency Virus-Positive Patients. *Journal of Young Pharmacists*, **4**, 250-260. http://dx.doi.org/10.4103/0975-1483.104369

[3] Falang, K.D., Akubaka, P. and Jimam, N.S. (2012) Patient Factors Impacting Antiretroviral Drug Adherence in a Nigerian Tertiary Hospital. *Journal of Pharmacology and Pharmacotherapeutics*, **3**, 138-142.

[4] Njuguna, C., Orrell, C., Kaplan, R., Bekker, L.G., Wood, R. and Lawn, S.D. (2013) Rates of Switching Antiretroviral Drugs in a Primary Care Service in South Africa before and after Introduction of Tenofovir. *PLoS ONE*, **8**, e63596. http://dx.doi.org/10.1371/journal.pone.0063596

[5] Bygrave, H., Ford, N., van Cutsem, G., Hilderbrand, K., Jouquet, G., Goemaere, E., *et al*. (2011) Implementing a Te-

nofovir-Based First-Line Regimen in Rural Lesotho: Clinical Outcomes and Toxicities after Two Years. *Journal of Acquired Immune Deficiency Syndromes*, **56**, e75-e78. http://dx.doi.org/10.1097/QAI.0b013e3182097505

[6]   Velen, K., Lewis, J.J., Charalambous, S., Grant, A.D., Churchyard, G.J. and Hoffmann, C.J. (2013) Comparison of Tenofovir, Zidovudine, or Stavudine as Part of First-Line Antiretroviral Therapy in a Resource-Limited-Setting: A Cohort Study. *PLoS ONE*, **8**, e64459. http://dx.doi.org/10.1371/journal.pone.0064459

[7]   Cassetti, I., Madruga, J.V., Suleiman, J.M., Etzel, A., Zhong, L., Cheng, A.K., *et al.* (2007) The Safety and Efficacy of Tenofovir DF in Combination with Lamivudine and Efavirenz through 6 Years in Antiretroviral-Naive HIV-1-Infected Patients. *HIV Clinical Trials*, **8**, 164-172. http://dx.doi.org/10.1371/journal.pone.0064459

[8]   Arribas, J.R., Pozniak, A.L., Gallant, J.E., Dejesus, E., Gazzard, B., Campo, R.E., *et al.* (2008) Tenofovir Disoproxil Fumarate, Emtricitabine, and Efavirenz Compared with Zidovudine/Lamivudine and Efavirenz in Treatment-Naive Patients: 144-Week Analysis. *Journal of Acquired Immune Deficiency Syndromes*, **47**, 74-78. http://dx.doi.org/10.1097/QAI.0b013e31815acab8

[9]   Chi, B.H., Mwango, A., Giganti, M., Mulenga, L.B., Tambatamba-Chapula, B., Reid, S.E., *et al.* (2010) Early Clinical and Programmatic Outcomes with Tenofovir-Based Antiretroviral Therapy in Zambia. *Journal of Acquired Immune Deficiency Syndromes*, **54**, 63-70.

[10] Spaulding, A., Rutherford, G.W. and Siegfried, N. (2010) Tenofovir or Zidovudine in Three-Drug Combination Therapy with One Nucleoside Reverse Transcriptase Inhibitor and One Non-Nucleoside Reverse Transcriptase Inhibitor for Initial Treatment of HIV Infection in Antiretroviral-Naive Individuals. *Cochrane Database of Systematic Reviews* (*CDSR*), **10**, Article ID: CD008740.

[11] Njuguna, C., Orrell, C., Kaplan, R., *et al.* (2013) Rates of Switching Antiretroviral Drugs in a Primary Care Service in South Africa before and after Introduction of Tenofovir. *PLoS ONE*, **8**, e63596. http://dx.doi.org/10.1371/journal.pone.0063596

4

Evaluation Efficacy and Safety of Vortioxetine 20 mg/d versus Placebo for Treatment Major Depressive Disorder: A Systematic Review and Meta-Analysis of Randomized Controlled Trials

Masoud Behzadifar[1,2], Hamidreza Dehghan[1], Korush Saki[3], Meysam Behzadifar[4], Abouzar Keshavarzi[1], Maryam Saran[5], Ali Akbari Sari[6*]

[1]Department of Health, Yazd University of Medical Sciences, Yazd, Iran
[2]Health Management and Economics Research Center, Iran University of Medical Sciences, Tehran, Iran
[3]Department of Medicine, Shahid Beheshti University of Medical Sciences, Tehran, Iran
[4]Department of Medicine, Ilam University of Medical Sciences, Ilam, Iran
[5]Department of Medicine, Tehran University of Medical Sciences, Tehran, Iran
[6]Department of Health Management and Economics, Tehran University of Medical Sciences, Tehran, Iran
Email: *akbarisari@tums.ac.ir

Abstract

Major depressive disorder, a common debilitating illness, is one of the leading causes of disability and disease worldwide. Different drugs for the treatment of patients with major depression can be used. Vortioxetine for the treatment of major depressive disorder was approved by the Food and Drug Administration (FDA) in 2013. This study aimed to evaluation efficacy and safety Vortioxetine 20 mg/d compared placebo in major depressive disorder. To conduct this study, we searched Pub Med, Cochrane library, Scopus, and Central Register of Controlled Trials. This study by including randomized controlled trials (RCTs) that evaluated this study by including randomized controlled trials (RCTs) that evaluated Vortioxetine 20 mg/d in patients with major depressive disorder. Data analysis was conducted by standard mean different ratios (SMD) with 95% confidence intervals (CIs), P values and odds ratios (ORs) for adverse events with 95% confidence intervals (CIs) and P values; heterogeneity testing and sensitivity analysis was also performed in this study. We found that 4 articles met the inclusion criteria and were finally used for this meta-analysis. Results showed statistical significance in the MADRS (Montgomery-Åsberg Depression Rating Scale), SMD = −4.75

---

*Corresponding author.

with 95% CI [−6.84, −2.65] and P value < 0.00001), for Clinical Global Impression Scale-Improvement (CGI-I) SMD was −4.34 with 95% CI [−6.41, −2.27] and P value < 0.00001, and for Sheehan Disability Scale (SDS) SMD was −2.62 with 95% CI [−3.99, −1.25] and P value < 0.00001. The pooled analysis for safety demonstrated for diarrhea OR = 0.92 with 95% CI [0.46, 1.83] , P value = 0.09, for dry mouth OR = 1.74 with 95% CI [1.07, 2.83] , P value = 0.80, for dizziness OR = 1.62 with 95% CI [0.72, 3.66] , P value = 0.05, for fatigue OR = 1.17 with 95% CI [0.34, 4.08], P value = 0.07, for headache OR = 1.28 with 95% CI [0.91, 1.79], P value = 0.60 and for nausea OR = 4.78 with 95% CI [3.43, 6.67], P value = 0.61. Vortioxetine 20 mg/d versus placebo showed a significant difference for nausea and dry mouth, but no significant differences were observed for the four adverse effects. In several studies of the drug Vortioxetine 20 mg/d, the treatment of major depressive illness has been more effective for evaluating the effectiveness of this drug, which must be more clinical studies of sound.

Keywords

Major Depressive Disorder, Vortioxetine 20 mg, Systematic Review, Meta-Analysis

1. Introduction

Major depressive disorder (MDD), a common debilitating illness, is one of the leading causes of disability and disease worldwide [1]. The quality of life of patients suffering from major depression diminishes. This disease causes impairment of physical, mental, and social functions and can be patient [2]. In addition, people with major depressive illness spend a lot to pay for treatment [3]. According to the World Health Organization reports, about 350 million people worldwide suffer from major depressive illness [2]. Given that most antidepressants are available to patients, the evidence shows that about 60 to 70 percent of these people make these drugs an appropriate response to health [4]. Patients with major depression often have such symptoms or signs: depressed mood, low of interest, low pleasure usual activities, changes in eating or sleeping, difficulty concentrating, suicidal thoughts and fatigue. Many treatment options for drug for major depressive disorder, antidepressants can often cause adverse effects. It is estimated that 15% of patients with major depression relapsed disease 35% of them are [5]. Major depression in physical diseases diagnosed has been proven in many studies. Expected depression is to be the second largest contributor to the world's disease burden by 2020 [3] [4]. In patients with major depression reported: COPD, multiple sclerosis, Parkinson's disease, diabetes mellitus, asthma, rheumatic arthritis, migraine, inflammatory bowel disease, cancer, stroke, heart disease, back problems and epilepsy [6]. Different drugs for the treatment of patients with major depression can be used. Vortioxetine for the treatment of major depressive disorder was approved by the Food and Drug Administration (FDA) in 2013. Vortioxetine is a selective serotonin reuptake inhibitor (SSRI) that binds to the presynaptic serotonin reuptake site, increasing the level of serotonin (5-HT) in the neuronal synapse and selectively binding to a variety of other serotonin receptors. It selectively binds to and acts as an antagonist of 5-HT3, 5-HT1D and 5-HT7 receptors, as a partial agonist to 5-HT1B receptors, and as an agonist of 5-HT1A receptors [7]-[10]. The objective of this article is systematic review and meta-analysis evaluation efficacy and safety of Vortioxetine 20 mg/d compared placebo in patients with major depressive disorder in randomized clinical trials.

2. Materials and Methods

2.1. Search Strategy

We searched Pub Med, Cochrane library, Scopus, CRD, Central Register of Controlled Trials to January 2015. Our searches will not be limited by language, publication status or setting. We also searched ClinicalTrials.gov, International depressive disorder Conference and the Anxiety Disorders and Depression Conference. For the reference lists of articles contact authors of included studies to acquire other data that may either be unpublished (**Figure 1**). Data collection, summary and analysis of the identification in this systematic review will be presented as a PRISMA [11]. Two review authors (Masoud. B, Meysam. B) will independently searched. First,

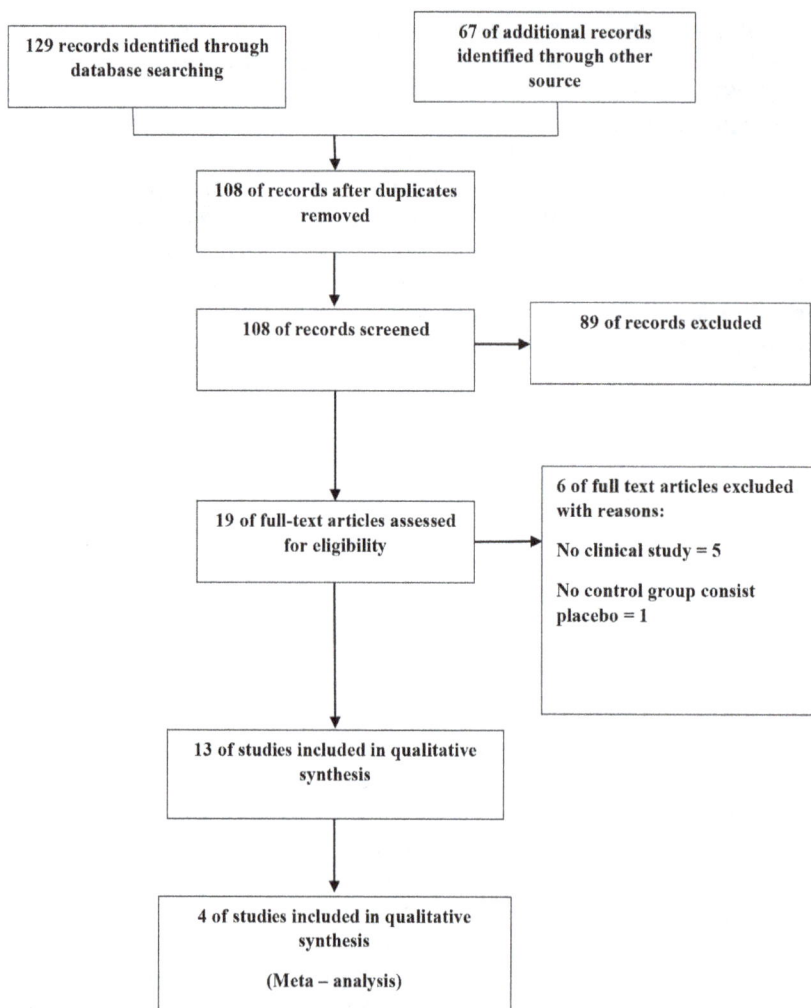

Figure 1. Flowchart of included studies.

screening the titles and abstracts of RCTs, Secondly, (H.D, A.AS) review author will independently full text of all trials. Compared the contents of each review author's list, and Conflicts were resolved by discussion.

2.2. Inclusion Criteria

Clinical trials testing the efficacy of Vortioxetine 20 mg for the short-term treatment (8 wks.) of major depressive disorder were eligible for inclusion. Included studies had to be RCTs comparing Vortioxetine 20 mg with placebo. Patients needed to meet the criteria for major depressive disorder used in the individual trials. Studies were excluded if the main outcome was prevention of relapse or if treatment outcomes based on rating scales of major depressive disorder were not available.

2.3. Data Extraction

We collected data on participant characteristics, treatment details, study procedures, efficacy measures and Adverse Events (AEs). These data included, for example, group (treatment, placebo), size sample, age, sex, duration of treatment, baseline MADRS, doses and study location. Outcome data related to the characteristics of the individual trial and the reported results were extracted for each trial. For instance, the mean changes or reported numbers for Adverse Events were extracted from the individual study when appropriate. The efficacy measures were the mean change from baseline in on Montgomery-Åsberg Depression Rating Scale (MADRS), Clinical Global Impression Scale-Improvement (CGI-I), Sheehan Disability Scale (SDS) study [12]-[14].

2.4. Quality Assessment

We will to assess the quality of studies, used Cochrane Collaboration "Risk of bias" assessment tool [15], including Random sequence generation, Allocation concealment, Blinding of participants and personnel, Blinding of outcome assessment ,incomplete outcome data, Selective reporting and other bias (**Figure 2**).

2.5. Quality of RCTs Included

The study quality was assessed with Jadad scores [16]. The Jadad score is an instrument used to assess the quality of randomized clinical trials (RCTs). It includes three items as follows: randomization, blindness and dropouts. The score standards and the results of our included studies are shown in **Table 1**, respectively. Were rated as providing good methodological quality based on a Jadad score of 1 - 5. So the total scores for all included articles indicated a high study quality.

2.6. Statistical Analysis

In the review, we assessed values, Montgomery-Åsberg Depression Rating Scale (MADRS), Clinical Global Impression Scale-Improvement (CGI-I), Sheehan Disability Scale (SDS) and adverse effects randomized into the Vortioxetine 20 mg/day and placebo groups for each trial were statistically combined using the Mantel-Haenszel random effects model. The effects were expressed as Standard mean different ratios (SMD) with 95% confidence intervals (CIs) and P values. The incidence of adverse effects between the Vortioxetine 20 mg/day and placebo groups was also determined using the Mantel-Haenszel model, and the results were expressed as the Odds Ratio (ORs) with the 95% CI and P values. The heterogeneity across each effect size was evaluated with using the I^2 and Chi-squared tests statistic. This measure evaluates how much of the variance among studies can be attributed to the actual differences among the studies rather than to chance. A magnitude of considerable heterogeneity is usually I^2 = 75% - 100% [16]. A sensitivity analysis was performed to rule out the possibility that any single study strongly influenced the pooled effect. Publication bias was assessed by a funnel plot, Egger's test [17], and Begg's rank correlation test [18]. All the statistical analyses were performed using Review Manager (Rev Man 5.3) software and Stata 12 software.

3. Results and Discussion

3.1. Efficacy

Overall, we found 4 articles met the inclusion criteria and were finally used for this meta-analysis (**Table 2**). This article consist Boulenger JP [19], Mahableshwarkar AR [20], Jacobsen PL [21] and trial no NCT01255787 [22]. A total of five studies with 1337 patients, 609 in the 20 mg/day Vortioxetine group and 728 patients in the placebo group. The standard mean different ratios (SMD) for Montgomery-Åsberg Depression Rating Scale (MADRS) with Vortioxetine 20 mg compared to placebo was −4.75 with 95% CI [−6.84, −2.65] and P value < 0.00001 and heterogeneity for MADRS scale was I^2 = 99%, The Standard mean different ratios (SMD) for Clinical Global Impression Scale-Improvement (CGI-I) was −4.34 with 95% CI [−6.41, −2.27] and P value < 0.00001 and heterogeneity for SMD was I^2 = 99% and Standard mean different ratios (SMD) for Sheehan Disability Scale (SDS) was −2.62 with 95% CI [−3.99, −1.25] and P value < 0.00001 and heterogeneity for SDS was I^2 = 98% (**Figure 3**).

Table 1. Jadad score quality assessment of the included studies.

Name study	Randomization	Blindness	Dropouts	Jaded scores
Boulenger 2014	1	2	1	4
Jacobsen 2013	1	2	1	4
Mahableshwarkar 2013	1	2	1	4
Trial NCT01255787 2104	1	2	1	4

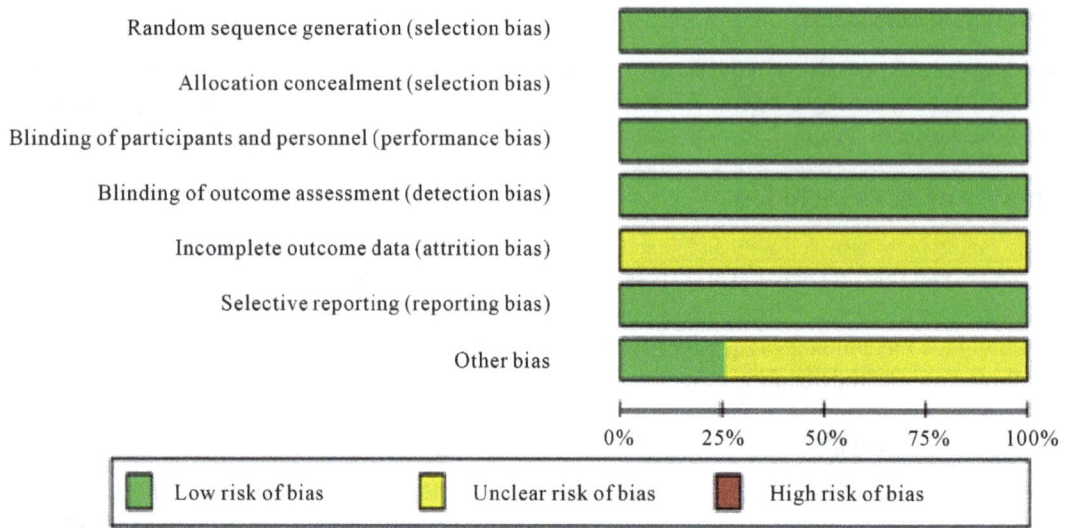

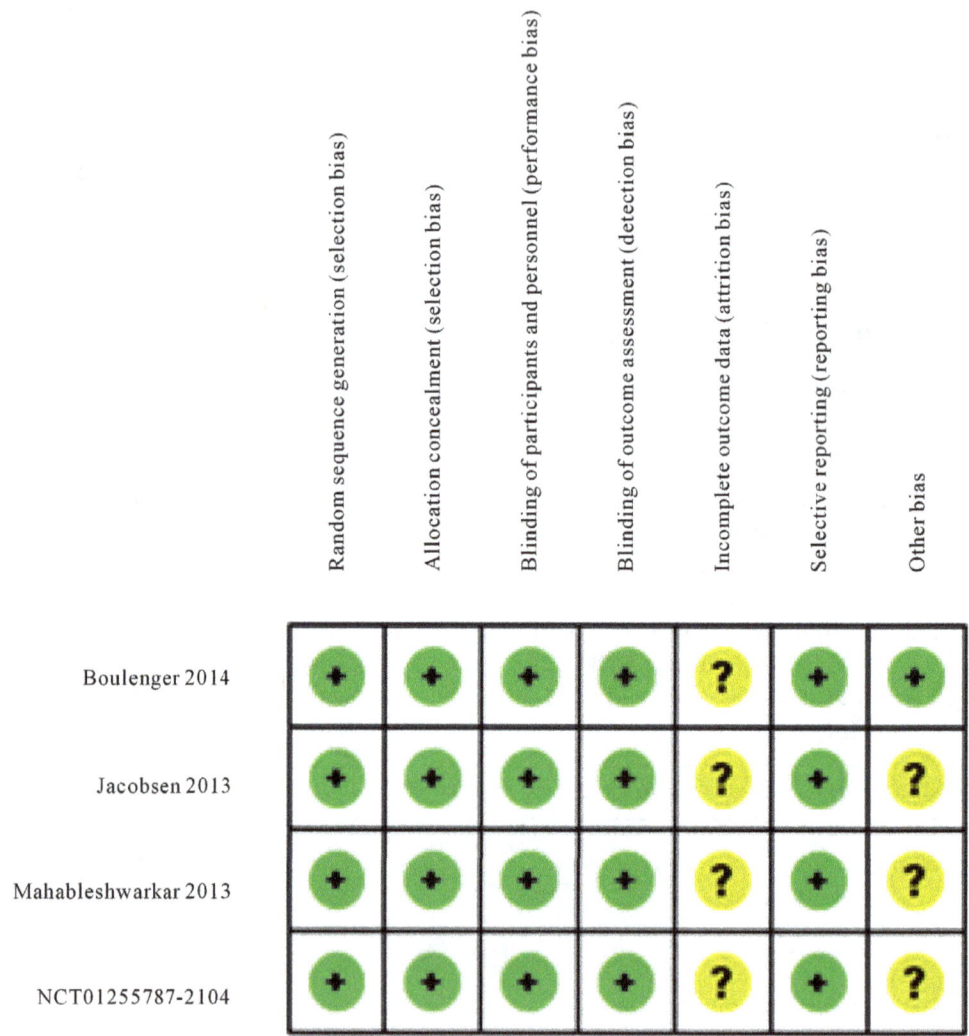

Figure 2. Risk of bias graph in the included studies.

Table 2. Summary of the included studies in the meta-analysis.

Author, year	Group	Cases, n	Age, years	Sex, M:F	Duration of treatment WK	Baseline MADRS score[a]	Doses VTX[b]	Study location	Entry score by MADRS
Boulener *et al.* 2014	Treatment	151	46.2 ± 13.4	60:91	8	31.2 ± 3.4	15, 20 mg	Europe	≥26
	Placebo	158	48.1 ± 13.1	48:110		31.5 ± 3.6			
Mahableshwarkar *et al.* 2013	Treatment	154	42.8 ± 12.40	40:114	8	32.0 ± 4.36	15, 20 mg	Usa	≥26
	Placebo	161	42.4 ± 12.55	45:116		31.6 ± 4.18			
Jacobsen *et al.* 2013	Treatment	150	43.1 ± 13.09	43:107	8	32.4 ± 4.30	10, 20 mg	Usa	≥26
	Placebo	157	42.3 ± 11.61	47:110		32.0 ± 3.99			
Trial NCT01255787 2014	Treatment	154	44.0 ± 11.79	61:93	8	31.7 ± 3.73	5, 10, 20 mg	Europe-Asia	≥26
	Placebo	152	43.6 ± 11.57	61:91		31.6 ± 3.56			

[a]The Montgomery-Åsberg Depression Rating Scale (MADRS) is a depression rating scale consisting of 10 items, each rated 0 to 6. The 10 items represent the core symptoms of depressive illness. The overall score ranges from 0 (symptoms absent) to 60 (severe depression); [b]Vortioxetine.

MADRS:

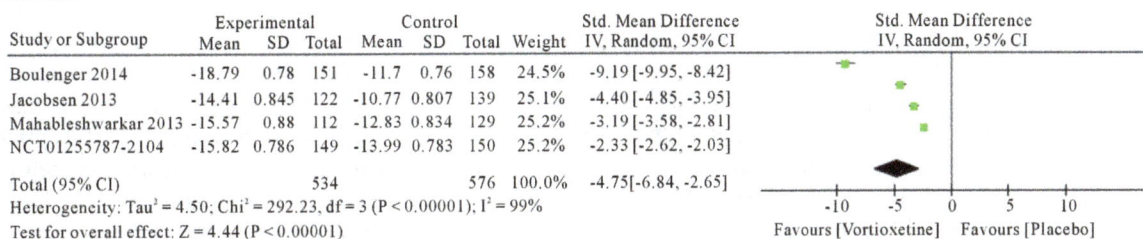

CGI-I:

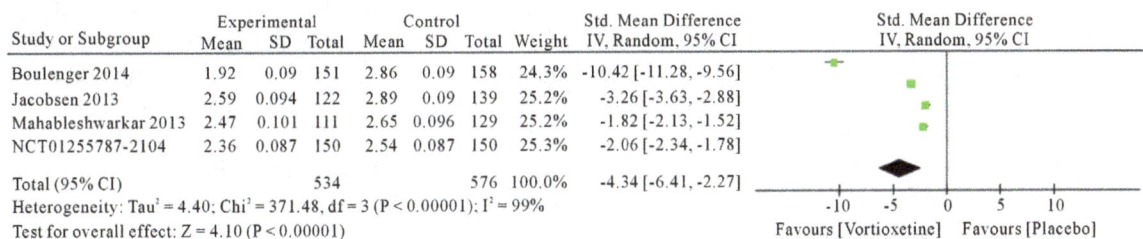

SDS:

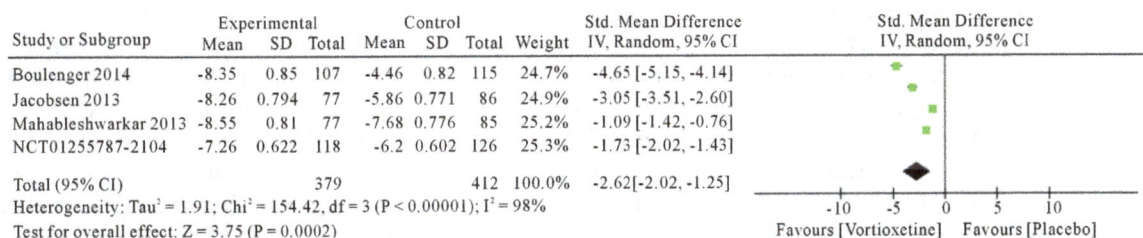

Figure 3. Forest plot of standard different mean ratios (SMD) and 95% confidence intervals (CIs) of change from baseline in the Montgomery-Åsberg Depression Rating Scale (MADRS), Clinical Global Impression Scale-Improvement (CGI-I) and Sheehan Disability Scale (SDS) total score at week 8 in the included studies.

3.2. Safety

Drug safety evaluation for symptoms that have been observed in studies for was meta-analysis. The most common side effects were diarrhea, dry mouth, dizziness, fatigue, headache and nausea.

Results the 20 mg/day Vortioxetine compared to placebo showed for diarrhea OR = 0.92 with 95% CI [0.46,

1.83], P value = 0.09, for dry mouth OR = 1.74 with 95% CI [1.07, 2.83], P value = 0.80, for dizziness OR = 1.62 with 95% CI [0.72, 3.66], P value = 0.05, for fatigue OR = 1.17 with 95% CI [0.34, 4.08], P value = 0.07, for headache OR = 1.28 with 95% CI [0.91, 1.79], P value = 0.60 and for nausea OR = 4.78 with 95% CI [3.43, 6.67], P value = 0.61 (**Figure 4**).

3.3. Sensitivity Analysis

Sensitivity analysis not found that the pooled remission rate was significantly influenced when we excluded the study from .trial no NCT01255787.

3.4. Analysis for Publication Bias

Analysis for publication bias showed, no publication bias was observed for MADRS, CGI-I and SDS (Egger's test: P = 0.006, P = 0.010, P = 0.105 respectively, and Begg's test: P = 0.042, P = 0.174, P = 0.174, respectively). Results showed no publication bias was observed for Adverse Events contain Diarrhea, Dry mouth, Dizziness, Fatigue, Headache and Nausea in the included studies (Egger's test: P = 0.823, P = 0.257, P =0.617, P = 0.149, P = 0.227, P = 0.205, P = 0.197 respectively and Begg's test: P = 1.000, P = 0.174, P = 0.497, P = 0.174, P = 0.174, P = 0.174, respectively).

This study evaluated the efficacy, safety of Vortioxetine 20 mg/d compared with placebo treatment in patients with major depressive disorder. We identified four RCTs examining the efficacy of Vortioxetine 20 mg/d versus placebo for treatment major depressive disorder. The present meta-analysis demonstrated the superior efficacy of Vortioxetine compared with placebo for the treatment of major depressive disorder in terms of mean change MADRS scale (SMD = −4.75). Our results showed that the treatment of the Vortioxetine 20 mg/day group based on both depression rating SDS (SMD = −2.62) and CGI-H (SMD = −4.34) was greater than the placebo group. The decrease in depression symptoms seems too associated with 20 mg/d of Vortioxetine versus placebo. Vortioxetine 20 mg/d were statistically significantly superior to placebo in three scales. Efficacy has been replicated at the 20 m/g doses in adults, demonstrated efficacy in study Boulenger et al., Mahableshwarker et al., Jacobsen et al. and trial NCT01255787. In the studies Alvarez et al. [23], Mahableshwarkar et al. [24], Jain et al. [25], Katona et al. [26], and Henigsberg et al. [27] showed Vortioxetine efficacy. Improve symptoms in patient by major depressive disorder Obtained in these studies. Results of Adverse Events (AEs) showed a significant for dry mouth OR = 1.74 [1.07 - 2.83] and nausea OR = 4.78 [3.43 - 6.67]. But no significant differences were observed for the other four adverse effects. AEs discontinuation rates were generally low. It suggested that the negative results in previous double-blind, random-controlled studies may have been due to an inadequate sample size, which can be overcome by the meta-analytic method. These findings indicate that compared to placebo, 20 mg/d mg/day Vortioxetine significantly improved depressive symptoms in patients with major depressive disorder. In the randomized clinical analyzed, the common adverse effects of Vortioxetine include diarrhea, dizziness, dry mouth, nausea, headache and fatigue.

The limitations of this meta-analysis include the following: the inclusion of patients only during the acute phase, which did not enable us to analyze the long-term efficacy and safety of Vortioxetine in treating major depressive disorder. The included studies did not include data on the onset time of Vortioxetine's efficacy, and thus, we did not compare the onset time between 20 mg/d Vortioxetine and placebo. All included trials were supported by the Takeda company, Ltd. All included studies did not include the efficacy and adverse effects based on sex; thus, we could not evaluate gender differences. Due to the limited number of the published articles, we did not analyze the efficacy and safety of different doses of Vortioxetine in the treatment of major depressive disorder. The small number of included studies and the relatively small sample size, which may influence the reliability of the results. However, depression is frequently associated with coronary heart diseases [28], diabetes mellitus [29], stroke [30], pregnancy, and the postpartum period [31]. Thus, the use of Vortioxetine should also benefit the physical state of these patients. Due to the small number of trials in our meta-analysis, our results warrant additional studies to verify these findings. In the future, additional large-scale and well-designed Studies are needed to determine the optimal dose, the most appropriate treatment group, and the efficacy and safety of Vortioxetine combined with other antidepressants in treating depression [32].

4. Conclusion

We found that Vortioxetine may be another treatment option for major depressive disorder. However, our results

Diarrhea:

Study or Subgroup	Experimental Events	Total	Control Events	Total	Weight	Odds Ratio M-H, Random, 95% CI
Boulenger 2014	11	151	6	158	23.0%	1.99 [0.72, 5.52]
Jacobsen 2013	11	150	14	157	27.9%	0.81 [0.35, 1.84]
Mahableshwarkar 2013	12	154	10	161	26.7%	1.28 [0.53, 3.05]
NCT01255787-2104	5	154	14	152	22.4%	0.33 [0.12, 0.94]
Total (95% CI)		609		628	100.0%	0.92 [0.46, 1.83]
Total events	39		44			

Heterogeneity: Tau^2 = 0.26; Chi^2 = 6.51, df = 3 (P = 0.09); I^2 = 54%
Test for overall effect: Z = 0.24 (P = 0.81)

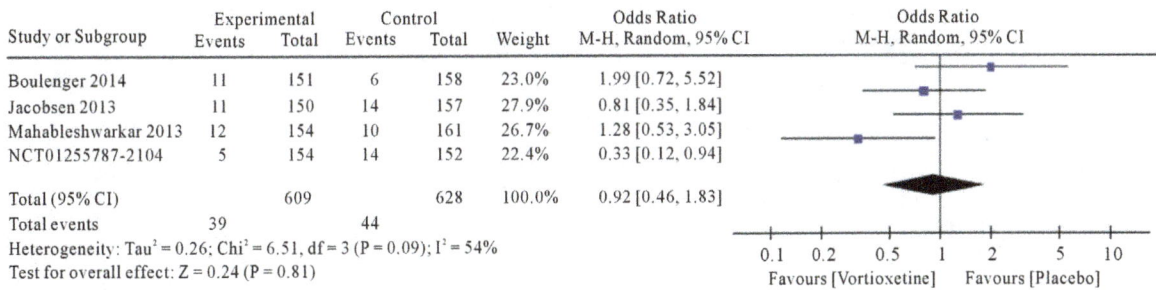

Dry mouth:

Study or Subgroup	Experimental Events	Total	Control Events	Total	Weight	Odds Ratio M-H, Random, 95% CI
Boulenger 2014	9	151	5	158	19.0%	1.94 [0.63, 5.93]
Jacobsen 2013	7	150	5	157	17.3%	1.49 [0.46, 4.80]
Mahableshwarkar 2013	22	154	16	161	50.3%	1.51 [0.76, 3.00]
NCT01255787-2104	9	154	3	152	13.4%	3.08 [0.82, 11.62]
Total (95% CI)		609		628	100.0%	1.74 [1.07, 2.83]
Total events	47		29			

Heterogeneity: Tau^2 = 0.00; Chi^2 = 0.98, df = 3 (P = 0.80); I^2 = 0%
Test for overall effect: Z = 2.23 (P = 0.03)

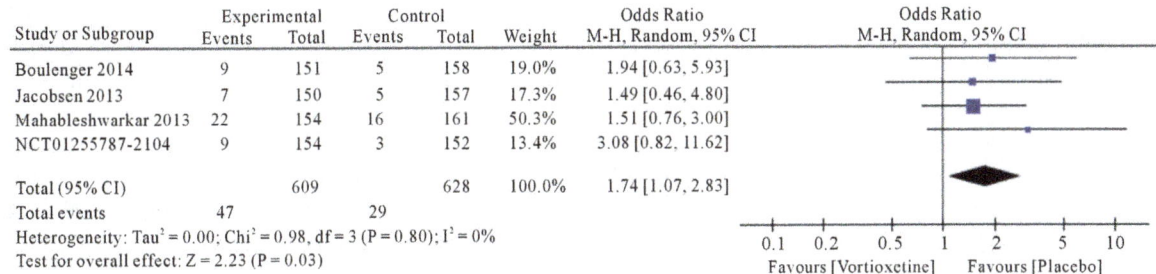

Dizziness:

Study or Subgroup	Experimental Events	Total	Control Events	Total	Weight	Odds Ratio M-H, Random, 95% CI
Boulenger 2014	7	151	10	158	25.4%	0.72 [0.27, 1.94]
Jacobsen 2013	9	150	9	157	26.1%	1.05 [0.41, 2.72]
Mahableshwarkar 2013	20	154	5	161	25.1%	4.66 [1.70, 12.74]
NCT01255787-2104	10	154	5	152	23.4%	2.04 [0.68, 6.12]
Total (95% CI)		609		628	100.0%	1.62 [0.72, 3.66]
Total events	46		29			

Heterogeneity: Tau^2 = 0.43; Chi^2 = 7.81, df = 3 (P = 0.05); I^2 = 62%
Test for overall effect: Z = 1.16 (P = 0.25)

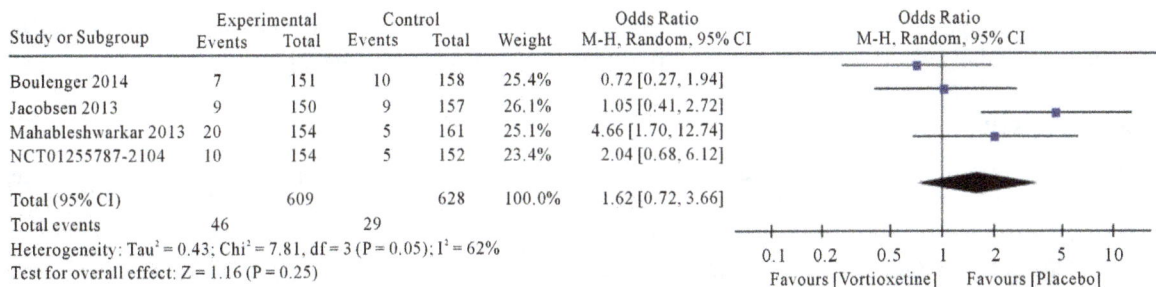

Fatigue:

Study or Subgroup	Experimental Events	Total	Control Events	Total	Weight	Odds Ratio M-H, Random, 95% CI
Boulenger 2014	5	151	4	158	29.8%	1.32 [0.35, 5.01]
Jacobsen 2013	0	150	9	157	13.4%	0.05 [0.00, 0.90]
Mahableshwarkar 2013	8	154	4	161	31.6%	2.15 [0.63, 7.29]
NCT01255787-2104	5	154	2	152	25.2%	2.52 [0.48, 13.18]
Total (95% CI)		609		628	100.0%	1.17 [0.34, 4.08]
Total events	18		19			

Heterogeneity: Tau^2 = 0.90; Chi^2 = 7.09, df = 3 (P = 0.07); I^2 = 58%
Test for overall effect: Z = 0.25 (P = 0.80)

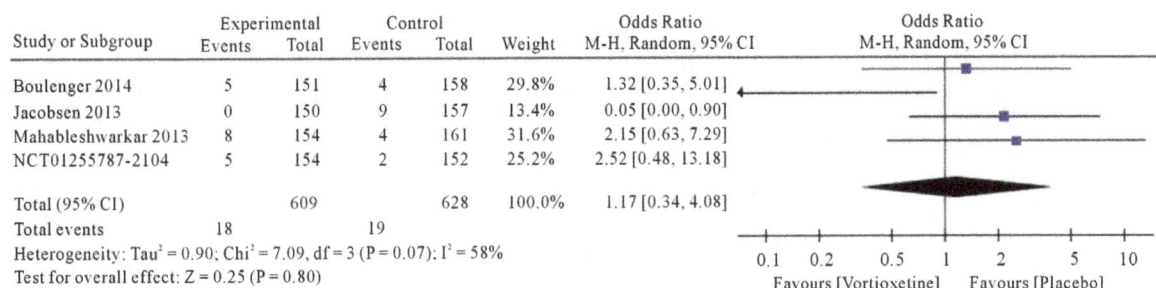

Headache:

Study or Subgroup	Experimental Events	Total	Control Events	Total	Weight	Odds Ratio M-H, Random, 95% CI
Boulenger 2014	19	151	12	158	19.8%	1.75 [0.82, 3.74]
Jacobsen 2013	24	150	17	157	25.7%	1.57 [0.81, 3.05]
Mahableshwarkar 2013	20	154	21	161	26.5%	1.00 [0.52, 1.92]
NCT01255787-2104	23	154	21	150	27.9%	1.08 [0.57, 2.04]
Total (95% CI)		609		626	100.0%	1.28 [0.91, 1.79]
Total events	86		71			

Heterogeneity: Tau^2 = 0.00; Chi^2 = 1.85, df = 3 (P = 0.60); I^2 = 0%
Test for overall effect: Z = 1.43 (P = 0.15)

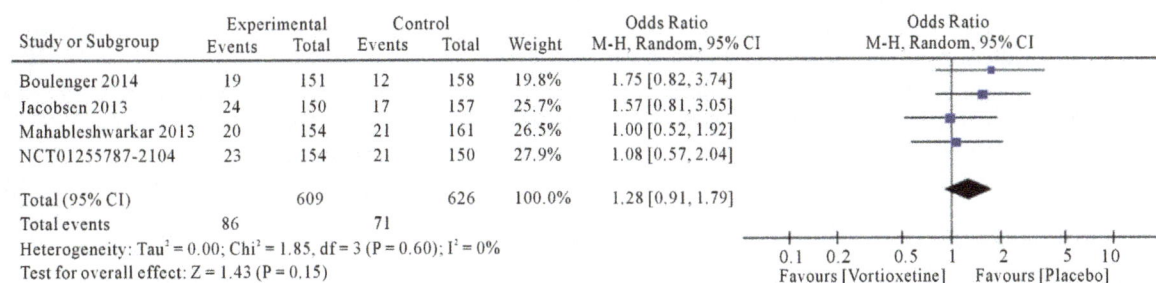

Nausea:

Study or Subgroup	Experimental Events	Total	Control Events	Total	Weight	Odds Ratio M-H, Random, 95% CI
Boulenger 2014	48	151	16	158	28.8%	4.14 [2.22, 7.69]
Jacobsen 2013	44	150	8	157	17.6%	7.73 [3.50, 17.09]
Mahableshwarkar 2013	57	154	18	161	31.9%	4.67 [2.59, 8.42]
NCT01255787-2104	37	154	11	152	21.6%	4.05 [1.98, 8.30]
Total (95% CI)		609		628	100.0%	4.78 [3.43, 6.67]
Total events	186		53			

Heterogeneity: Tau^2 = 0.00; Chi^2 = 1.83, df = 3 (P = 0.61); I^2 = 0%
Test for overall effect: Z = 9.21 (P < 0.00001)

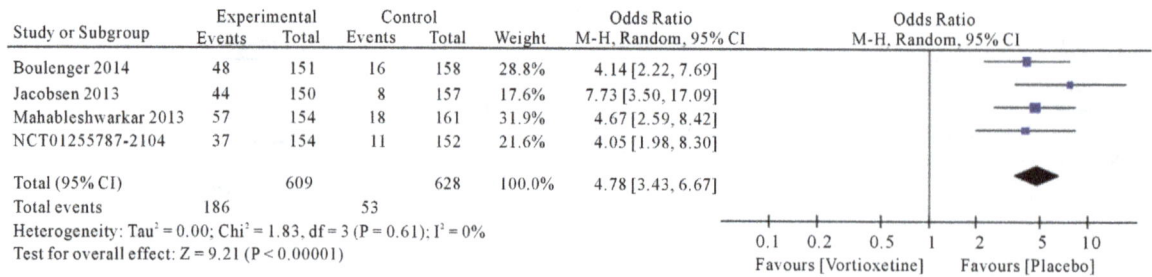

Figure 4. Forest plot of Odds ratio (OR) and 95% confidence intervals (CIs) of Diarrhea, Dry mouth, Dizziness, Fatigue, Headache and Nausea AEs in the included studies.

should be interpreted and translated into clinical practice with caution, small effect sizes of the clinical trials included in present the meta-analysis. Adequately powered, well-designed, and direct-comparison clinical trials should also more clearly address the comparative efficacy of Vortioxetine and different antidepressants. The current meta-analysis of published RCTs has shed light on the benefits of 20 mg/d Vortioxetine for the treatment of major depression disorder. As a novel antidepressant, there is increasingly greater interest in Vortioxetine. In several studies of the drug Vortioxetine 20 mg/d, the treatment of major depressive illness has been more effective for evaluating the effectiveness of this drug, which must be more clinical studies of sound.

Acknowledgements

This study was part of the MSc (Health Technology Assessment (HTA)) thesis of first author (Masoud Behzadifar). The authors would like to thank all participants who made this study possible.

References

[1] Ferrari, A.J., Charlson, F.J., Norman, R.E., *et al.* (2013) Burden of Depressive Disorders by Country, Sex, Age, and Year: Findings from the Global Burden of Disease Study 2010. *PLoS Medicine*, **10**, e1001547.

[2] World Health Organization Mental Health Depression. http://www.who.int/mediacentre/factsheets/fs369/en/

[3] Murray, C.J. and Lopez, A.D. (1997) Alternative Projections of Mortality and Disability by Cause 1990-2020: Global Burden of Disease Study. *The Lancet*, **349**, 1498-1504. http://dx.doi.org/10.1016/S0140-6736(96)07492-2

[4] Souery, D., Papakostas, G.I. and Trivedi, M.H. (2006) Treatment Resistant Depression. *Journal of Clinical Psychiatry*, **67**, 16-22.

[5] Liu, M.T., Maroney, M.E. and Hermes-DeSantis, E.R. (2015) Levomilnacipran and Vortioxetine: Review of New Pharmacotherapies for Major Depressive Disorder. *World Journal of Pharmacology*, **4**, 17-30. http://dx.doi.org/10.5497/wjp.v4.i1.17

[6] Halperin, D. and Reber, G. (2007) Influence of Antidepressants on Hemostasis. *Dialogues in Clinical NeuroSciences*, **9**, 47-59.

[7] National Institute of Mental Health What Is Depression? http://www.nimh.nih.gov/health/topics/depression/index.shtml

[8] Centers for Disease Control and Prevention Depression. http://www.cdc.gov/mentalhealth/basics/mental-illness/depression.htm

[9] American Psychiatric Association (2013) DSM-5 Task Force. Diagnostic and Statistical Manual of Mental Disorders. 5th Edition, American Psychiatric Association, Washington DC.

[10] Wesolowska, A., Tatarczynska, E., Nikiforuk, A. and Chojnacka-Wojcik, E. (2007) Enhancement of the Anti Immobility Action of Anti-Depressants by a Selective 5-HT$_7$ Receptor Antagonist in the Forced Swimming Test in Mice. *European Journal of Pharmacology*, **555**, 43-47. http://dx.doi.org/10.1016/j.ejphar.2006.10.001

[11] Liberati, A., Altman, D.G., Tetzlaff, J., Mulrow, C., Gøtzsche, P.C., Ioannidis, J.P.A., *et al.* (2009) The PRISMA Statement for Reporting Systematic Reviews and Meta-Analyses of Studies That Evaluate Health Care Interventions: Explanation and Elaboration. *PLoS Medicine*, **6**, e1000100. http://dx.doi.org/10.1371/journal.pmed.1000100

[12] Montgomery, S.A. and Asberg, M. (1979) A New Depression Scale Designed to Be Sensitive to Change. *The British*

Journal of Psychiatry, **134**, 382-389. http://dx.doi.org/10.1192/bjp.134.4.382

[13] Forkmann, T., Scherer, A., Boecker, M., Pawelzik, M., Jostes, R. and Gauggel, S. (2011) The Clinical Global Impression Scale and the Influence of Patient or Staff Perspective on Outcome. *BMC Psychiatry*, **11**, 83. http://dx.doi.org/10.1186/1471-244X-11-83

[14] Leon, A.C., Olfson, M., Portera, L., Farber, L. and Sheehan, D.V. (1997) Assessing Psychiatric Impairment in Primary Care with the Sheehan Disability Scale. *The International Journal of Psychiatry in Medicine*, **27**, 93-105. http://dx.doi.org/10.2190/T8EM-C8YH-373N-1UWD

[15] Higgins, J.P., Altman, D.G., Gøtzsche, P.C., Jüni, P., Moher, D., Oxman, A.D., Savovic, J., Schulz, K.F., Weeks, L. and Sterne, J.A. (2011) The Cochrane Collaboration's Tool for Assessing Risk of Bias in Randomized Trials. *BMJ*, **343**, Article ID: d5928.

[16] Jadad, A.R., Moore, R.A., Carroll, D., Jenkinson, C., Reynolds, D.J., Gavaghan, D.J. and Mc Quay, H.J. (1996) Assessing the Quality of Reports of Randomized Clinical Trials: Is Blinding Necessary? *Controlled Clinical Trials*, **17**, 1-12. http://dx.doi.org/10.1016/0197-2456(95)00134-4

[17] Egger, M., Davey Smith, G., Schneider, M. and Minder, C. (1997) Bias in Meta-Analysis Detected by a Simple, Graphical Test. *BMJ*, **315**, 629-634. http://dx.doi.org/10.1136/bmj.315.7109.629

[18] Begg, C.B. and Mazumdar, M. (1994) Operating Characteristics of a Rank Correlation Test for Publication Bias. *Biometrics*, **50**, 1088-1101. http://dx.doi.org/10.2307/2533446

[19] Boulanger, J.P., Loft, H. and Olsen, C.K. (2014) Efficacy and Safety of Vortioxetine (Lu AA21004), 15 and 20 mg/day: A Randomized, Double-Blind, Placebo-Controlled, Duloxetine-Referenced Study in the Acute Treatment of Adult Patients with Major Depressive Disorder. *International Clinical Psychopharmacology*, **29**, 138-149. http://dx.doi.org/10.1097/YIC.0000000000000018

[20] Mahableshwarkar, A.R., Jacobsen, P.L., Serenko, M., *et al.* (2013) A Duloxetine-Referenced, Fixed-Dose Study Comparing Efficacy and Safety of 2 Vortioxetine Doses in the Acute Treatment of Adult MDD Patients (NCT01153009) (Poster). *American Psychiatric Association 166th Annual Meeting*, San Francisco, 18-22 May 2013.

[21] Jacobsen, P.L., Mahableshwarkar, A.R., Serenko, M., *et al.* (2013) A Randomized, Double-Blind, Placebo-Controlled Study of the Efficacy and Safety of Vortioxetine 10 mg and 20 mg in Adults with Major Depressive Disorder (NCT01163266) (Poster). *American Psychiatric Association 166th Annual Meeting*, San Francisco, 18-22 May 2013.

[22] Efficacy and Safety Study of Vortioxetine (Lu AA21004) for Treatment of Major Depressive Disorder. NCT01255787. http://clinicaltrials.gov/show/NCT01255787

[23] Alvarez, E., Perez, V., Dragheim, M., Loft, H. and Artigas, F. (2012) A Double-Blind, Randomized, Placebo-Controlled, Active Reference Study of Lu AA21004 in Patients with Major Depressive Disorder. *International Journal of Neuropsychopharmacology*, **15**, 589-600. http://dx.doi.org/10.1017/S1461145711001027

[24] Mahableshwarkar, A.R., Jacobsen, P.L. and Chen, Y. (2013) A Randomized, Double-Blind Trial of 2.5 mg and 5 mg Vortioxetine (Lu AA21004) versus Placebo for 8 Weeks in Adults with Major Depressive Disorder. *Current Medical Research & Opinion*, **29**, 217-226. http://dx.doi.org/10.1185/03007995.2012.761600

[25] Jain, R., Mahableshwarkar, A.R., Jacobsen, P.L., Chen, Y. and Thase, M.E. (2013) A Randomized, Double-Blind, Placebo-Controlled 6-wk Trial of the Efficacy and Tolerability of 5 mg Vortioxetine in Adults with Major Depressive Disorder. *International Journal of Neuropsychopharmacology*, **16**, 313-321. http://dx.doi.org/10.1017/S1461145712000727

[26] Katona, C., Hansen, T. and Olsen, C.K. (2012) A Randomized, Double-Blind, Placebo-Controlled, Duloxetine-Referenced, Fixed-Dose Study Comparing the Efficacy and Safety of Lu AA21004 in Elderly Patients with Major Depressive Disorder. *International Clinical Psychopharmacology*, **27**, 215-223. http://dx.doi.org/10.1097/YIC.0b013e3283542457

[27] Henigsberg, N., Mahableshwarkar, A.R., Jacobsen, P., Chen, Y. and Thase, M.E. (2012) A Randomized, Double-Blind, Placebo-Controlled 8-Week Trial of the Efficacy and Tolerability of Multiple Doses of Lu AA21004 in Adults with Major Depressive Disorder. *The Journal of Clinical Psychiatry*, **73**, 953-959. http://dx.doi.org/10.4088/JCP.11m07470

[28] Penninx, B.W., Beekman, A.T., Honig, A., Deeg, D.J., Schoevers, R.A., van Eijk, J.T. and van Tilburg, W. (2001) Depression and Cardiac Mortality: Results from a Community-Based Longitudinal Study. *Archives of General Psychiatry*, **58**, 221-227. http://dx.doi.org/10.1001/archpsyc.58.3.221

[29] Schlienger, J.L. (2013) Type 2 Diabetes Complications. *La Presse Médicale*, **42**, 839-848. http://dx.doi.org/10.1016/j.lpm.2013.02.313

[30] Robinson, R.G. and Spalletta, G. (2010) Post Stroke Depression: A Review. *Canadian Journal of Psychiatry*, **55**, 341-349.

[31] Di Florio, A., Forty, L., Gordon-Smith, K., Heron, J., Jones, L., Craddock, N. and Jones, I. (2013) Perinatal Episodes

across the Mood Disorder Spectrum. *JAMA Psychiatry*, **70**, 168-175.
http://dx.doi.org/10.1001/jamapsychiatry.2013.279

[32] Fu, J. and Chen, Y. (2015) The Efficacy and Safety of 5 mg/d Vortioxetine Compared to Placebo for Major Depressive
      Disorder: A Meta-Analysis. *Psychopharmacology*, **232**, 7-16. http://dx.doi.org/10.1007/s00213-014-3633-z

5

In Vitro and *in Vivo* (Mouse) Evaluation of Drug-Drug Interactions of Repaglinide with Anti-HIV Drugs

Vijay Saradhi Mettu[1], P. Yadagiri Swami[2*], P. Abigna[2], A. Ravinder Nath[1], Geeta Sharma[3]

[1]Department of Pharmacy, University College of Technology, Osmania University, Hyderabad, India
[2]Department of Chemistry, University College of Science, Osmania University, Hyderabad, India
[3]Forma Therapeutics Singapore, Singapore City, Singapore
Email: mettusaradhi@gmail.com, *parikibandla@gmail.com

Abstract

Repaglinide is type 2 short acting anti-diabetic drug which is primarily metabolized by CYP2C8 and CYP3A4 and is also a substrate of influx transporter OATP1B1. HIV drugs are potent inhibitors of CYP3A4 and OATP transporters. Several drug-drug interactions (DDIs) were noticed when protease inhibitors (PIs) coadministered with drugs metabolized by CYP3A4. The PIs are also potent mechanism based inhibitors, out which ritonavir is most potent. In the current study we evaluated *in vitro* (mouse and human liver microsomes) and *in vivo* DDIs of repaglinide with anti-HIV drugs. Out of the following tested drugs (Amprenavir, Indinavir, Nelfinavir, Ritonavir, Saquinavir, Delavirdine, Maraviroc, Efavirenz, Nevirapine and Ketoconazole) Amprenavir (APV), Ritonavir (RTV) and Ketoconazole (KTZ) showed inhibition of OH-repaglinide formation in human and mouse liver microsomes. The positive reversible inhibitions were further tested for irreversible inhibitions where we didn't observe any irreversible inhibitions. *In vitro* inhibitions were further evaluated in the *in vivo* pharmacokinetics (mouse) where repaglinide pharmacokinetics was altered by RTV and KTZ. The DDIs in both studies were very strong; the dose of repaglinide is reduced to 20 fold. In conclusion, there could be possible DDIs when RTV dosed with repaglinide; we have also demonstrated that mouse could be useful preclinical tool when used in conjunction with *in vitro* screening models for DDIs.

Keywords

Repaglinide, Drug-Drug Interaction, Repaglinide Km, Repaglinide Bioanalytical Method

---

*Corresponding author.

1. Introduction

People living with diabetes would reach 366 Vs 171 million by 2030, out of which 90 to 95% are type 2 diabetic patients. Apart from chronic diabetic related problems such as nephropathy, neuropathy and accelerated atherosclerosis, the following groups of people with diabetics and HIV can be identified: 1) patients with preexisting diabetics contact HIV; 2) patients who are diagnosed to have diabetics at the onset of HIV; 3) HIV patients diagnosed with gestational diabetics; 4) patients who develop diabetics after HIV therapy [1].

Patients with HIV and diabetics would be on polytherapy and these subjects would be more prone to DDIs. HIV drugs notably PIs are potent inhibitors of drug metabolizing enzymes and drug transporters. Majority of PIs showed irreversible inhibition of CYP3A4 which is major metabolizing enzyme in human contributing to metabolism of about 50% of marked drugs [2]. In a previous study in our lab we had seen that except indinavir all tested PIs demonstrated irreversible inhibition of CYP3A4 (Ritonavir, Indinavir, Nelfinavir, Saquinavir and Amprenavir) and these results were in agreement with published results [3]. Many of the anti-HIV drugs like RTV are also OATP inhibitors [4].

Pharmacokinetic drug interactions were observed in repaglinide with drugs which are inhibitors of CYP3A4, CYP2C8 and transporter OATP1B1. The DDIs were severe in case of CYP2C8 and OATP1B1. However the inhibitions were severe in case of CYP inhibitions than that in transporters inhibitions. More than double repaglinide AUC (144%) was noticed when coadministered with cyclosporine, a potent OATP1B1 inhibitor. Severe DDIs were observed when gemfibrozil was coadministered with repaglinide; an eight fold increase in repaglinide AUC was seen. This drug interaction was further enhanced with introduction of itraconazole. OATP inhibition seems to be involved only at higher doses. In a separate study subtherapeutic doses (<300 mg) of gemfibrozil in healthy volunteers caused mechanism based inhibition by formation of metabolite (gemfibrozil 1-O-β-glucuronide) with higher levels of repaglinide [5].

Furthermore, AUC of repaglinide was higher with subjects with higher activity of CYP2C8*1/*3 genotype than with lower activity of CYP2C8*1/*1 genotype. According to EMEA's (committee for Proprietary Medicinal Products) using this combination was declared as contraindication [5]. On the other hand selective inhibitor of CYP2C8 by trimethoprim increases the AUC of repaglinide by 61% in healthy subjects [5].

Rifampicin a antitubercular drugs which is prototype inducer of CYP3A4 and OATP inhibitor, interfered the pharmacokinetics of repaglinide. The exposure of repaglinide is influenced by rifampicin treatment for example repaglinide AUC was decreased by 31% when repaglinide is treated one hour after the last dose of rifampicin. In a separate study, AUC of repaglinide was decreased to 57% when ingested 12.5 hours after last dose rifampicin [6]. Yet in another study AUC of repaglinide is affected by 50% and 80% when repaglinide administrated concomitantly and 24 hours after the last treatment of rifampicin respectively [6]. From this study we can hypothesize that ripaglinide disposition would be effected by OATP transporter, which makes repaglinide available for metabolism and CYP3A4 which plays a role in metabolism. Influencing CYP3A4 and OATP would alter the PK of the repaglinide. HIV drugs which are known CYP3A4 inhibitors and OATP inhibitors would alter pharmacokinetics of repaglinide. http://www.hiv-druginteractions.org published by liver pool university indicated some possible DDIs of anti-HIV drugs when repaglinide was coadministrated. They indicated that close monitoring or dose adjustment was required when repaglinide dosed with atazanavir, darunavir, fosamprenavir, indinavir, lopinavir, nelfinavir, ritonavir, saquinavir and tipranavir.

In the current study we evaluated the effect of repaglinide metabolism in HLM and MLM, furthermore tested the mechanism based inhibition in HLM and MLM. RTV and KTZ were also tested for DDIs in mouse model. KTZ was used as positive control for CYP3A4 inhibition in *in vitro* and *in vivo*.

2. Materials and Methods

Drugs and Chemicals. Midazolam, ketoconazole, ritonavir, amprenavir, indinavir, nefinavir, Maraviroc, Delavirdine and Nevirapine purchased from Kemprotec (United Kingdom). MLM XenoTech, LLC (Kansas City). Verapamil, repaglinide, polyethylene glycol 400, NADPH from Sigma-Aldrich (St Lous, MO, USA) nateglinide, efavirenz gift from Dr. Reddy's and Hetero Drugs (Hyderabad, India) respectively. All the chemicals used were HPLC grade.

Animals. *In vivo* mouse studies were performed according to the Guidelines for the Care and Use of Laboratory Animals that was approved by the Committee of Ethics of Animal Experimentation of J.S.S college of Pharmacy, Ooty. 8 to 12 weeks old Female Balb/c mice used in the same facility. Animals were housed in a temperature- and humidity-controlled room with a 12-h light/dark cycle. Animals were fed with standard animal diet (Harlan mice diet); food and water was provided ad libitum. Mice were fasted overnight before oral dose and fed after 2 hours of dosing, for multiple dosing mice were fasted on the last dose.

Enzyme Kinetics (HLM & MLM). To determine the Km and Vmax values (the apparent enzyme kinetic constants), repaglinide was incubated in duplicates with an incubation mixture containing HLM or MLM with 0.2 mg/ml protein (repaglinide concentration 0.334, 1, 3, 9, 27, 81, 243 μM) and MgCl$_2$ (3.3 mM) in 100 mM potassium phosphate buffer pH 7.4, after 5 mins equilibration in water bath at 37°C the reaction was started with NADPH (NADPH (1.3 mM), 0.2 ml total volume). The reaction was terminated with acetonitrile containing internal standard (nateglinide 500 ng/ml). The samples were stored at -80°C and analyzed later. All the incubations were accepted only if midazolam metabolism was $\geq$90%.

IC$_{50}$ & Time Dependent IC$_{50}$. Incubation conditions were similar to the enzyme kinetic experiment, unless otherwise specified. Repaglinide concentration was tested at the Km value for both HLM and MLM, inhibitor concentrations for APV were (50, 16.665, 5.555, 1.851, 0.615, 0.205 μM), RTV and KTZ (10, 3.334, 1.111, 0.370, 0.123, 0.041, 0.013, 0.004 μM). The reaction was terminated after 30 minutes of incubation and incubation accepted as in the Km experiment non dilution method was used for time dependent IC$_{50}$ (repaglinide at Km concentration), inactivators were incubated along with NADPH for 30 mins, after which substrate was added and incubated for 5 mins [7] [8]. This was answered in enzyme kinetics. After the incubation samples were stored at -80°C and analyzed later, the incubation pass criteria was as specified earlier.

In vivo **studies.** Oral dosing formulation for repaglinide and inhibitors were formulated in 10% Ethanol: 60% PEG400: 30%: 5% dextrose in water (D5W). With these cocktail vehicles all the drugs were in solution state. The weighed drugs were transferred to mortar and pestle, vehicles were added in following order, ethanol, PEG 400 and D5W. After adding ethanol compound was triturated followed by PEG 400 and D5W. All the formulations were made fresh before dosing. Repaglinide was dosed 1 hour after inhibitor dosing, sampling time was started after repaglinide dosing. Blood samples were centrifuged to separate plasma and analyzed using HPLC-mass spectrometry. Composite sampling is taken from retro orbital. After dosing of repaglinide the following time points were taken 0, 0.5, 1, 2, 4, 8 and 24 hours. The collected samples were stored at -80°C until analysis.

Analytical Methods. All sample analysis was carried out using high performance liquid chromatography (HPLC)—tandem mass spectrometry methods. The HPLC elute was introduced via electrospray ionization. Mass spectral analysis was performed using multiple reaction monitoring with the following transitions (positive ionization mode) m/z amprenavir 506.4 $\rightarrow$ 155.7, indianvir 614.5 $\rightarrow$ 421.3, nelfinavir 568.1 $\rightarrow$ 330.1, saquinavir 671.9 $\rightarrow$ 570.5, ritonavir 721.9 $\rightarrow$ 296.3, ketoconazole 531.1 $\rightarrow$ 82, efavirenz 316.2 $\rightarrow$ 244.2, repaglinide 453 $\rightarrow$ 230.4 and nateglinide 318.3 $\rightarrow$ 125.

The mass spectrometry 3200 QTRAP (ABI Sciex, Applied Biosystems) connected with HPLC Agilent 1100 MSD system (Agilent Technologies, Palo Alto, CA) and auto sampler CTC PAL (Leap Technologies, Carrboro, NC). Chromatography was performed by using Phenomenex Luna C-18 column (particle size 3 μm, 50 $\times$ 2 mm) preceded by Phenomenex C-18 guard column (Phenomenex, Torrance, CA), column temperature was set to 40°C, injection volume 10 μL. Mobile phase consisting of 10mM ammonium formate in 0.1% formic acid with acetonitrile with a flow rate 500 μL for *in vitro* and *in vivo* samples. The run time and gradient (ACETONITRILE %) as follows 0 min to 0.5 min 70%, 0.5 min to 2.5 min 30%, 2.5 min to 2.6 min 2%, 2.6 min to 3.2 min 100% and 3.2 min to 4 min 100%.

Sample Preparation. *In vitro* samples were precipitated with acetonitrile containing IS (nateglinide) at 500 ng/ml, centrifuged and injected into the LC-MS/MS. The plasma samples were extracted using liquid-liquid extraction method. In brief to 20 μl plasma sample 1 ml of methyl tertiary butyl ether is added and shaken for 10 min, freezed and supernatant is dried and reconstituted with 200 μl water methanol 1:1. 10 μl of sample is injected into LC-MS/MS.

3. Data Analysis

In vitro Data Analysis

Enzyme kinetics for repaglinide and midazolam were estimated by standard equation using GraphPad Prism software equation:

$$V = \frac{V_{max}[S]}{Km+[S]}$$

IC$_{50}$ and MBI IC$_{50}$ were determined by nonlinear regression analysis with GraphPad Prism software (version 5, GraphPad Software Inc., SanDiego).

To determine the enzyme inactivation kinetics constant for Human and mouse liver microsomes, the natural logarithm of remaining OH-midazolam and OH-repaglinide is plotted against the pre-incubation time incubated with inhibitors.

Pharmacokinetic Analysis. *In vivo* data analysis was carried out with noncompartmental analysis by using WinNonlin Professional (version 4.0.1; Pharsight, Mountain View, CA). In brief, the Cmax and Tmax were recorded by visual observation of the data. The area under the plasma concentration-time curve (AUC $_{tot}$) was calculated using linear and log trapezoidal summations.

Statistical Analysis. The statistical significance ($p < 0.05$) between treated (repaglinide dosed with perpetrators) and control (repaglinide alone) groups were established by Dunnett's multiple comparison test.

4. Results and Discussions

The tested HIV drugs are well known CYP3A4 inhibitors and most of them are irreversible inhibitors, notably the PIs for example, AMP, Nelfinavir, RTV, Saquinavir and Delavirdine [3]. To test possible hits we screened inhibitors at 50 µM and incubated with one µM of repaglinide, incubation conditions were described as in method described in Km and Vmax section. Out of *in vitro* screens in HLM and MLM we identified AMP, KTZ, Efavirenz and RTV demonstrated inhibition of metabolism of repaglinide. To further test these hits Km and Vmax values were generated in HLM and MLM (**Figure 1(a)** & **Figure 1(b)**). Furthermore the repaglinide is incubated at Km with different concentration of inhibitors, we have observed inhibitions at top 3 concentrations of inhibitors for KTZ, AMP and RTV because of which we could not generate exact IC-$_{50}$ values. RTV and AMP are known mechanism based inhibitors (MBI); these two compounds were further evaluated for MBI's along with KTZ which is included as negative control. In MBI (time dependent inhibitions) we have not noticed differences in inhibitions when compared with reversible inhibitions.

The *in vitro* hits tested in *in vivo* using mouse as an animal model. The DDIs at 0.1 mg/kg of repaglinide and RTV and KTZ (doses 45 and 40 mg/kg respectively, dose was normalized to human plasma concentrations) (**Figure 2(a)** & **Figure 2(b)**) were so strong that mice were either moribund or dead. The dose of repaglinide was reduced to 5 fold (0.02 mg/kg) and dosed, same kind of toxicity is observed. Noticing strong DDIs the dose of repaglinide is reduced to 20 fold (0.005 mg/kg), where we did not observe any adverse effects (the cage behavior was normal). This dose was used to for repaglinide to evaluated pharmacokinetics DDIs with KTZ and RTV. Repaglinide dosed with KTZ in mouse, the Cmax of repaglinide increased from undetectable levels (less than 2 ng/ml) to 11.63 ng/ml, which could be due to CYP3A4 inhibition. Similarly in the clinic KTZ and clarithromycin which are strong CYP3A4 inhibitors increased the Cmax of repaglinide significantly with less effect on AUC, indicating that CYP2C8 would take over the metabolism when CYP3A4 is inhibited [5]. In a separate study when CYP3A4 induced and OATP inhibited by rifampicin the DDI were stronger than inhibition CYP3A4 alone. This is further strengthened by potent inhibition of gemfibrozil which is CYP2C8 irreversible inhibitor and also inhibitor of OATP transporter. Gemfibrozil DDI indicates that the repaglinide Pharmacokinetics will be altered greatly with interfering with CYP2C8 and influx transporter OATP, than CYP3A4 alone. This also indicates that the OATP plays major role in disposition of repaglinide. This implies that inhibition of CYP enzyme

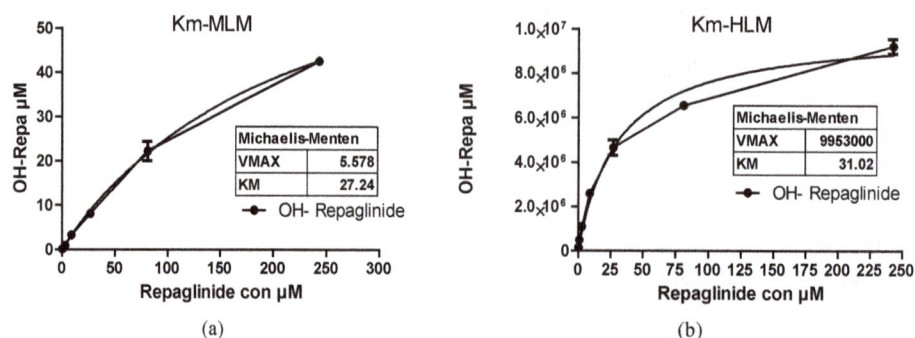

Figure 1. (a) Repaglinide Km estimation in MLM; (b) Repaglinide Km estimation in HLM, the concentration ranging from 0.334 µM to 243 µM for both MLM and HLM.

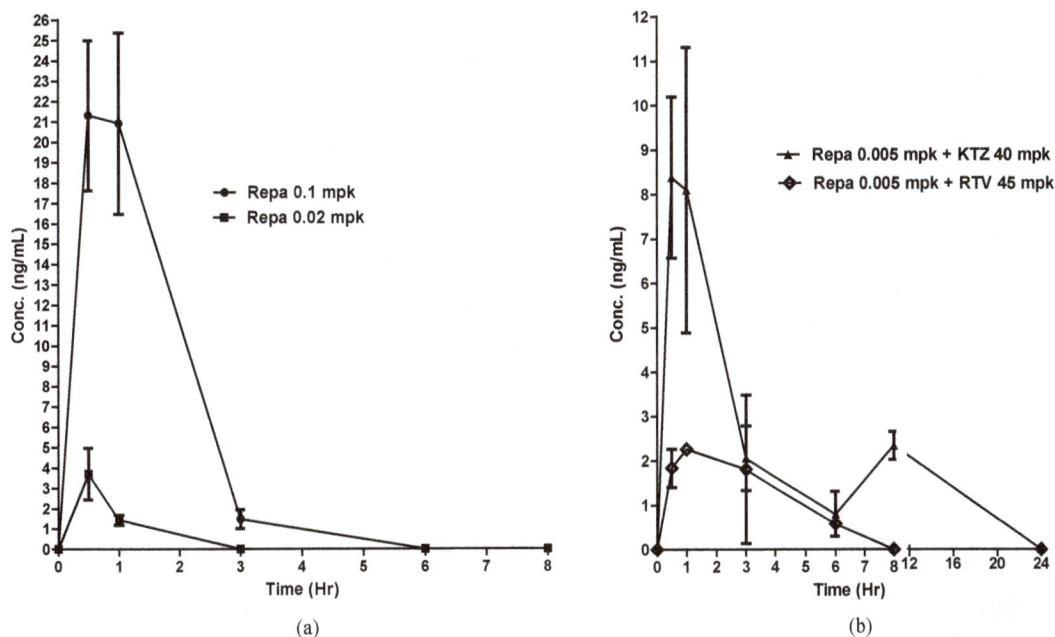

Figure 2. (a) Pharmacokinetic profile of repaglinide in mice (n = 3) at 0.1 mg/kg and 0.02 mg/kg. Repaglinide dosed at 0.005 mg/kg was not detected when dosed alone; (b) Repaglinide 0.005 mg/kg dosed after a single dose RTV and KTZ one hour prior dosing of repaglinide. Doses of RTV and KTZ were 45 and 40 mg/kg respectively (n = 3). KTZ significantly increased the Cmax and AUC of repaglinide with (P < 0.001 & P < 0.05) respectively.

(3A4 and 2C8, either of them or both) along with OATP would have higher change in pharmacokinetics of repaglinide [9]. In the current study the Cmax (P < 0.001) and AUCall (p < 0.05) was significantly increased by KTZ when compared to repaglinide dosed alone.

Similarly, RTV (45 mg/kg) is a prototype irreversible CYP3A4 inhibitor and OATP inhibitor, increased repaglinide (0.005 mg/kg) concentration when dosed with RTV, the Cmax increased from below detection levels to 2.88 ng/ml and also able to calculate AUC (5.91 hr*ng/ml). Although the significance not shown at lower dose of repaglinide (0.005 mg/kg), we have to be aware that when tested at 0.1 and 0.02 mg/kg mice were moribund or dead (the significance not obtained due to higher standard deviation). In comparison with KTZ and clarithromycin (which showed clinical DDIs with repaglinide) which are CYP3A4 reversible and irreversible inhibitors respectively, RTV and AMP, both are potent irreversible inhibitor than clarithromycin and additionally RTV is also potent and non specific inhibitor the OATP and AMP is moderate inhibitor of OATP1B1 [4] [10] [11], the possibility of RTV or AMP DDIs with repaglinide are high.

5. Conclusion

In conclusion the current result demonstrated high possibility of DDIs when RTV or AMP dosed with repaglinide due to strong DDIs in liver microsomes furthermore RTV showed DDIs in *in vivo* mouse model. Based on the current results future clinical trials can be planned with lower dose of repaglinide with RTV and AMP with close monitoring of patients.

References

[1]   Kalra, S., Kalra, B., Agrawal, N. and Unnikrishnan, A.G. (2011) Understanding Diabetes in Patients with HIV/AIDS. *Diabetology and Metabolic Syndrome*, **1**, 2.

[2]   Shimada, T., Yamazaki, H., Mimura, M., *et al.* (1994) Interindividual Variations in Human Liver Cytochrome P450 Enzymes Involved in the Oxidation of Drugs, Carcinogens and Toxic Chemicals. *Journal of Pharmacology and Experimental Therapeutics*, **270**, 414-423.

[3]   Ernest 2nd, C.S., Hall, S.D. and Jones, D.R. (2005) Mechanism-Based Inactivation of CYP3A by HIV Protease Inhibitors. *Journal of Pharmacology and Experimental Therapeutics*, **312**, 583-591.
       http://dx.doi.org/10.1124/jpet.104.075416

[4]   Karlgren, M., Vildhede, A., Norinder, U., Wisniewski, J.R., Kimoto, E., Lai, Y., Haglund, U. and Artursson, P. (2012) Classification of Inhibitors of Hepatic Organic Anion Transporting Polypeptides (OATPs): Influence of Protein Expression on Drug-Drug Interactions. *Journal of Medicinal Chemistry*, **55**, 4740-4763. http://dx.doi.org/10.1021/jm300212s

[5]   Holstein, A., Beil, W. and Kovacs, P. (2012) CYP2C Metabolism of Oral Antidiabetic Drugs-Impact on Pharmacokinetics, Drug Interactions and Pharmacogenetic Aspects. *Expert Opinion on Drug Metabolism & Toxicology*, **12**, 1549-1563. http://dx.doi.org/10.1517/17425255.2012.722619

[6]   Varma, M.V., Lin, J., Bi, Y.A., Rotter, C.J., Fahmi, O.A., Lam, J.L., El-Kattan, A.F., Goosen, T.C. and Lai, Y. (2013) Quantitative Prediction of Repaglinide-Rifampicin Complex Drug Interactions Using Dynamic and Static Mechanistic Models: Delineating Differential CYP3A4 Induction and OATP1B1 Inhibition Potential of Rifampicin. *Drug Metabolism and Disposition*, **41**, 966-974. http://dx.doi.org/10.1124/dmd.112.050583

[7]   Paris, B.L., Ogilvie, B.W., Scheinkoenig, J.A., Ndikum-Moffor, F., Gibson, R. and Parkinson, A. (2009) A. *In Vitro* Inhibition and Induction of Human Liver Cytochrome p450 Enzymes by Milnacipran. *Drug Metabolism and Disposition*, **37**, 2045-2054. http://dx.doi.org/10.1124/dmd.109.028274

[8]   Parkinson, A., Kazmi, F., Buckley, D.B., Yerino, P., Paris, B.L., Holsapple, J., Toren, P., Otradovec, S.M. and Ogilvie, B.W. (2011) An Evaluation of the Dilution Method for Identifying Metabolism-Dependent Inhibitors of Cytochrome P450 Enzymes. *Drug Metabolism and Disposition*, **39**, 1370-1387. http://dx.doi.org/10.1124/dmd.111.038596

[9]   Scott, L.J. (2012) Repaglinide: A Review of Its Use in Type 2 Diabetes Mellitus. *Drugs*, **2**, 249-272. Review. Erratum in: Drugs. 2012, **72**, 744-755. http://dx.doi.org/10.2165/11207600-000000000-00000

[10] Kajosaari, L.I., Laitila, J., Neuvonen, P.J. and Backman, J.T. (2005) Metabolism of Repaglinide by CYP2C8 and CYP3A4 *in Vitro*: Effect of Fibrates and Rifampicin. *Basic & Clinical Pharmacology & Toxicology*, **97**, 249-256. http://dx.doi.org/10.1111/j.1742-7843.2005.pto_157.x

[11] Vijay Saradhi, M., Yadagiri Swami, P. and Ravinder Nath, A. (2013) *In Vitro* and *in Vivo* (Mouse) Evaluation of Drug Drug Interactions of Glibenclamide with HIV Protease Inhibitors. *International Conference on Pharmacology and Drug Discovery*, NUS, Singapore.

6

Comparison of Two Pour-On Formulations of Ivermectin against Gastrointestinal Worms, Fleas and Lice in Naturally Infected Stray Dogs

Froylán Ibarra-Velarde[1], Yolanda Vera-Montenegro[1], Joaquín Ambía Medina[2],
Karla Sánchez-Peralta[1], Pedro Ochoa Galván[3]

[1]Departamento de Parasitología, Facultad de Medicina Veterinaria y Zootecnia, Universidad Nacional Autónoma de México, México, D.F., México
[2]Laboratorio Salud Animal, México, D.F., México
[3]Departamento de Génetica, Facultad de Medicina Veterinaria y Zootecnia, Universidad Nacional Autónoma de México, México, D.F., México
Email: ibarraf@unam.mx

Abstract

The aim of the present study was to evaluate the efficacy of two commercial pour-on ivermectin formulations against intestinal parasites (IP), fleas and lice in naturally infested stray dogs. Eighteen crossbreed dogs with eggs of IP as well as adult fleas and lice were included in the trial. On day 0, the dogs were randomly divided into 3 groups of 6 animals each: a group receiving a single pour-on treatment with 0.5% ivermectin (500 mcg/kg), a group treated similarly with 0.2% ivermectin (200 mg/kg), and a control group. Fecal and skin analyses were carried out on days 0, 7, 14, 21 and 28 to determine the reduction of eggs and the number of fleas and lice. Weight gain was also measured on day 28. On day 30, the dogs were humanely sacrificed in order to count adult IP. Efficacy was measured as the percentage of the reduction of eggs per gram fecal mass (EPGF), of adult IP, fleas and lice relative to the control group. For the eggs of IP, ivermectin at 0.5% showed an efficacy of 100% against ascarids and 79% against *Ancylostoma caninum*. ivermectin at 0.2% removed 90.2% of the ascarids and 50.4% of *A. caninum*. For adult IP, the efficacy of 0.5% ivermectin against *Toxocara canis* and *A. caninum* was 100%, and for 0.2% ivermectin it was 62.4% and 76.4% for *T. canis* and *A. caninum*, respectively. Both compounds were 100% effective against lice and 96% and 71.1% efficacious against fleas, respectively. However, neither treatment was effective against *Dypilidium caninum*. Weight gain in treated dogs was statistically different from that of the controls (p < 0.05). We concluded that 0.5% pour-on ivermectin showed better efficacy than 0.2% pour-on ivermectin in the reduction of eggs and adult intestinal parasites and fleas; it was similarly efficacious against lice.

Keywords

Ivermectin, Intestinal Worms, Fleas and Lice, Stray Dogs

1. Introduction

Infections with intestinal parasites (IP), fleas and lice in dogs and cats are very common all over the world [1]. They are the major factors responsible for public health losses and some times for public health risks and causing zoonotic diseases in human and animals [2]-[4]. For instance, the cat flea *Ctenocephalides felis* is the cause of severe discomfort and irritation in humans, dogs and cats. It is also responsible for the production of allergic dermatitis [5]. This flea can also serve as the vector of typhus-like rickettsia and is the intermediate host for filarids and cestodes. In addition, fleas, being hematophagous insects, can produce iron deficiency anemia in heavy infestations, particularly in young animals. They have been reported to produce anemia in dogs, cats, goats, cattle and sheep [6]-[8]. Murine typhus, caused by the organism *Rickettsia typhi*, is a mild febrile disease characterized by the development of headaches, chills, and skin rashes in humans with an infrequent involvement oin the kidneys and the central nervous system [9]. With the increase in feline plague cases in the western US, there are some concerns over the importance of *C. felis* as a possible vector. *Ctenocephalides felis* serves as an intermediate host of the subcutaneous filarid nematode of dogs *Dipetalonema reconditum* [10].

On the other hand, macrocyclic lactones, such as avermectin and milbemycins, show a high anti-parasitic activity against nematodes, fleas and lice in dogs and many other animals. It is available in injectable, oral, or topical formulations for use in animals [11]-[13]. It is frequently used in combination with other drugs [14]-[17]. Nowadays, considering its wide spectrum of activity, it is one of the drugs most employed to control some helminths and artropods.

However, even though investigations with ivermectins on internal and external parasites in ruminants and horses are widely documented [18]-[22], the research on the efficacy of pour-on ivermectin formulations in dogs is somewhat scarce [3]-[23]. In Mexico, where disease-carrying IP, fleas and lice in dogs are abundant, no controlled test on the impact of pour-on ivermectin has been carried out, either on the weight differences of treated animals or on the specific identification of the parasites present before and after treatment of the dogs.

The aim of the present study is to compare the efficacy of two pour-on ivermectin formulations against IP, fleas and lice as well as the weight differences and specific identification of parasites in naturally infested stray dogs from Mexico.

2. Materials and Methods

Study design. In the present study, eighteen 5 to 12 month-old stray dogs (crossbreed) of both sexes and weights between 4 and 15 kg were selected on the basis of the high numbers of egg per gram of the faeces (EPGF) of intestinal parasites or adult fleas and lice.

Drugs. 1) Vermisan Pour-on® (Laboratorios Salud Animal, S.A de C.V) containing ivermectin at 0.5% for pour-on application.

2) Dermodex® (CPMax S.A de C.V.) containing ivermectin at 0.2% for pour-on application.

Conduction of the study. On day 0, the dogs were divided into 3 groups (G) of 6 animals each. They were individually caged to avoid inter group re-infestation. Group 1 (G1) received a single treatment with ivermectin at 0.5% applied percutaneously (pour-on) at 500 mg/kg^{-1} (1 ml/10kg body weight).

G2 received a single treatment with ivermectin at 0.2% topically (pour-on) applied at 200 mg^{-1}/Kg (1 ml/10 kg body weight), according to label instructions.

G3 served as a non-treated control.

Coprological analyses. Simple fecal analyses using the McMaster method was carried out on days 0 (day of treatment), 7, 14, 21 and 28 to determine the percentage of Egg Per Gram of Feces (EPGF).

The administration of any other anthelmintic drug was prohibited for the duration of the study.

Adverse events occurring before and after treatments were recorded for each individual animal. The study was strictly limited to the person preparing and administering the doses and other witnesses present for the preparationand administration of the doses were not permitted to be involved in any observation made as end points for the study e.g. fecal egg counts (FEC).

On day 30 after treatment, the dogs were humanely sacrificed using an overdose of sodium penthobarbital injected into the femoral vein. Once the dogs showed no vital signs, the necropsy was performed on each animal to obtain the intestine and to collect and identify the adult worms.All procedures were carried out with the approval of the Internal Comitee for Use and Care of Animals for Experimentation. In addition, the number of fleas and lice after treatment was also individually recorded to determine the percentage of ectoparasite reduction in all experimental groups. All identification procedures for parasites were carried out according to [10].

Drug efficacy and statistical analysis. Efficacy was measured as the percentage reduction in the EPGF, adult worms, as well as in the number of fleas and lice from the treated groups relative to the untreated control. To do this the following formula was used: [24] [25].

$$\% \, R = T1 - \frac{T2}{T1} \times 100 \text{ where:}$$

% R = The percentage of reduction of EPG, adult worms, fleas and lice.

T1 = The geometric mean of the control group.

T2 = The geometric mean of the treated group.

Differences on the weight gain. This parameter was also measured and aimed at determining if 30 days after a single treatment the dogs showed a statistical difference on the weight gain when compared with that of the non treated control group.

Statistical analysis. The information obtained was submitted to the Kruskall-Wallis test and the Wilcoxon sign test, using the Sientific Analysis System (S.A.S) paquet, 2004.

3. Results

Our parasitological procedures showed that most of the dogs were infested with *Ancylostoma caninum*, *Toxocara canis* and *Dypilidium caninum*.

Coprological analyses. At the beginning of the experiment (day 0), the average number of EPGF in the control group was 4900 and 12,900 for *Toxocara* and *Ancylostoma*, respectively.

The fecal analyses showed the presence of ascarids and *Ancylostoma* eggs, but not the presence of *Dypilidium* eggs (**Table 1**).

Drug efficacy at reducing parasite eggs. The efficacy conferred by ivermectin at 0.5% throughthe percentage of reduction of EPG against ascarids was 100%, 75.5%, 98.7% and 100%, and for Ancylostoma 100%, 87.5%, 83.3% and 79%, for days 7, 14, 21 and 28, respectively. When the efficacy of both drugs was statistically compared, significant differences were found viz. $p < 0.007$, $p < 0.049$, $p < 0.07$ and $p < 0.14$, for days 7, 14, 21 and 28, respectively (**Table 1**).

As it can be observed in **Table 1**, the efficacy exerted at the 7th. day post treatment is high (100%) and it proportionally decreases as the following faecal analyses were carried out.

In the case of ivermectin at 0.2%, the data obtained showed a lower efficacy since the percentages of ascarid reduction of EPG were 46.6%, 100%, 91.6% and 90.2% and for *Ancylostoma* 50.7%, 47.1%, 42.3% and 50.4%, respectively.

It can be said then that the efficacy exerted for both compounds in terms of EPG reduction can be considered similar against ascarids but lower against *Ancylostoma* in the case of Ivermecyin at 0.2%. (**Figure 1**).

Drug efficacy against adult intestinal parasites. Specimens such as *Dypilidium caninum*, *Taenia taeniaeiformis*, *Toxocara canis*, *Toxascaris leonina* and *Ancylostoma caninum* were collected at necropsy (**Figure 2**).

The percentage of efficacy for ivermectin at 0.5% was 100% for *T. canis* and *A. caninum*. For ivermectin at 0.2% the efficacy obtained against adult worms was 62.4% for *T. canis* and 76.4%, for *A. caninum* (**Figure 3**).

Statistical differences were determined with both formulations against *T. canis* ($p < 0.055$) and *A. caninum* ($p < 0.0073$).

No evaluations against *T. taeniaeiformis* and *T. leonina* were carried out since very few specimens of these parasites were recorded (**Figure 3** and **Table 2**).

Also no statistical analyses were performed with the data on *Dypilidium* since it was evident that no efficacy at all was exerted from both compounds against this cestode.

Efficacy against fleas and lice. The percentage reduction forivermectin at 0.5% on fleas was 67.9%, 78.8%, 91.5% and 96% and for ivermectin at 0.2% 57.7%, 66.7%, 59.2% and 71.1%, respectively. The statistical analysis showed significant differences betwen groups ($p < 0.107$), ($p < 0.0076$), ($p < 0.0024$) and ($p < 0.001$)

Table 1. Coprological analysis of Eggs Per Gram of Feces (EPGF) before and after pour-on treatment with ivermectin of dogs naturally infected with intestinal parasites.

Groups (n = 6)	Sex	Weight	Dose	Day of treatment				Days after treatment					
				0		7		14		21		28	
			(ml)	Tox*	Anc**	Tox	Anc	Tox	Anc	Tox	Anc	Tox	Anc
	M	10	1	50	600	0	0	0	0	0	0	0	0
1	M	6	0.6	150	300	0	0	0	0	0	0	0	0
Ivermectin 0.5%	M	4	0.4	650	1350	0	0	150	0	50	0	0	100
	F	8	0.8	100	250	0	0	0	0	0	0	0	0
	F	4	0.4	350	800	0	0	200	0	0	0	0	0
	F	6	0.6	150	200	0	0	200	150	0	300	0	250
Total of EPGF/group				1450	3500	0	0	550	150	50	300	0	350
	F	5	0.5	250	10,250	50	0	0	0	0	0	0	0
2	F	8	0.8	100	150	150	1500	100	1750	50	1150	50	800
Ivermectin 0.2%	M	4	0.4	150	650	0	100	0	0	0	0	0	0
	M	6	0.6	300	1750	0	900	0	650	0	2150	0	1650
	F	15	1.5	100	4450	150	29,100	0	8050	0	17,350	0	14,900
	M	6	0.6	100	3500	100	1000	0	700	0	150	0	100
Total of EPGF/group				1000	20,750	450	32,600	100	11,150	50	20,800	50	17,450
	F	4	---	750	750	0	0	100	4350	0	1750	0	2400
3	M	7	---	100	550	50	0	200	50	150	500	0	9400
Untreated	M	11	---	100	800	250	50	850	100	50	3400	0	7100
Control	F	3	---	3500	9700	2400	350	50	3000	0	8100	0	1450
	M	9	---	350	350	2400	50	5050	50	5050	0	0	1750
	F	11	---	100	750	50	0	100	50	250	500	50	3600
Total of EPGF/group				4900	12,900	5150	450	6350	7600	5500	14,250	50	25,700

1 ml = 20 drops = 200 mcg/kg de pv. *= *Toxocara canis*; **= *Ancylostoma caninum*.

for days 7, 14, 21 and 28, respectively, clearly indicating that the efficacy produced by ivermectin at 0.5% on fleas was higher (**Figure 4**).

In the case of lice, both compounds showed 100% efficacy. Here it is important to mention that the number of lice was lower than the number of fleas; this might be one of the reasons why there were no statistical differences between groups.

4. Discussion

Ivermectin (IVM), a member of the macrocyclic lactone antiparasitic drugs, exhibits a broad spectrum in activity against gastrointestinal (GI) and lung nematodes as well as against ectoparasites of clinical relevance in domestic animals [17]. Since the IVM patent protection has expired, several "similar" (generic) products have entered the veterinary market worldwide; according to official data more than 60 different IVM formulations are currently registered for use in veterinary medicine [17]. However, pour-on presentations for the treatment of

Table 2. Specific identification and percentage of endo and ectoparasites from specimens collected from the untreated control group.

		Endoparasites		
		Specie	No. of specimens	Percentage (%)
Helminths	Cestodes	*Dypilidium caninum*	151	37.9
		Taenia taeniaeformis	1	0.2
	Nematodes	*Toxocara canis*	8	2
		Toxascaris leonina	1	0.2
		Ancylostoma caninum	237	59.5
		Total	398	
		Ectoparasites		
Arthropods	Fleas	*Ctenocephalides canis*	94	62.5
		Ctenocephalides felis	27	18.7
		Pulex irritans	8	5.5
	Lice	*Lignognathus setosus*	11	7.6
		Trichodectes canis	4	2.7
		Total	144	

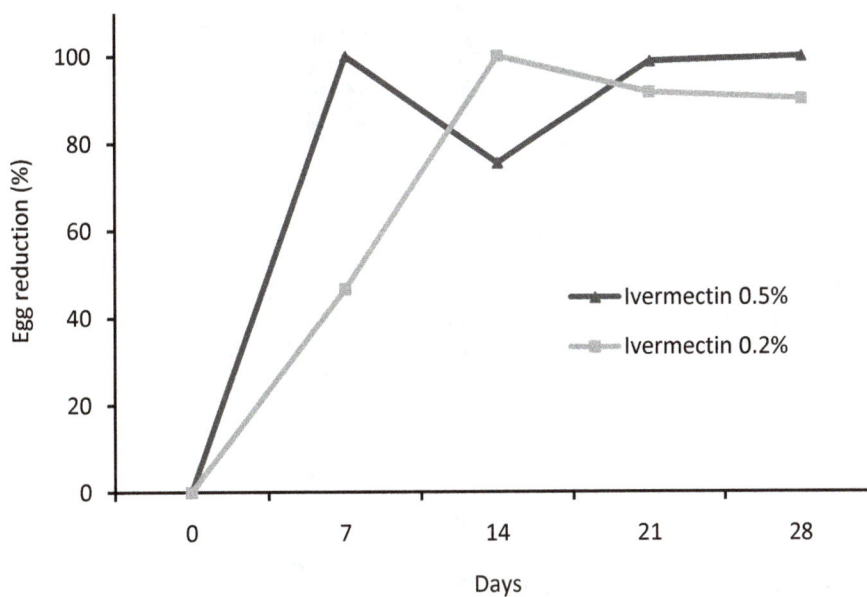

Figure 1. Anthelmintic efficacy of two pour on formulations of ivermectin in the egg reduction of *Toxocara* spp. in stray dogs.

dogs are launched at lower levels and formulations of IVM with a different excipient may exerta different efficacy percentage.

Interpretation of the results, taking into account study limitations and assesment of the current state of knowledge in the context of study results and other evidence were also considered.

As was observed, it seems that the 0.5% formulation of ivermectin is neccesary to remove a higher percentage of Ascarids and Ancylostoma spp., as well as flea infestations, but both formulations are equally effective against lice. However, the IVM administration in dogs may show a toxic effect if it passes the hematoencephalic barrier and reaches the central nervous sytem, a possibility that may increase depending of the dose used. However, it is well known that only certain races of dogs (Collie, Old English sheep dog, Doberman, German Shepherd

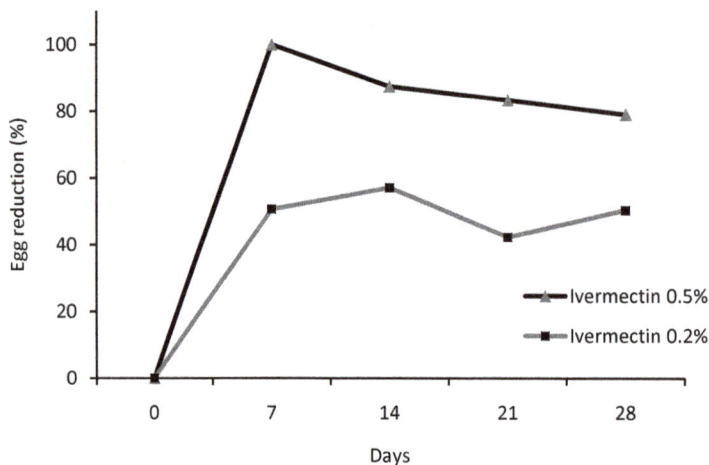

Figure 2. Anthelmintic efficacy of two different formulations of ivermectin in the egg reduction of *Ancylostoma caninum* in stray dogs.

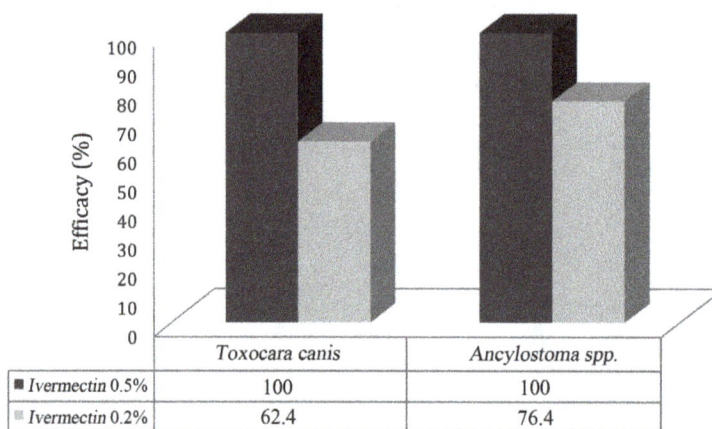

	Toxocara canis	Ancylostoma spp.
Ivermectin 0.5%	100	100
Ivermectin 0.2%	62.4	76.4

Figure 3. Efficacy percentage of two commercial compounds against adult intestinal parasites after single pour-on treatment in naturally infected dogs. No evaluations against *Taenia taeniaeiformis* and *Toxascaris leonina* were carried out since very few specimens of these parasites were recorded.

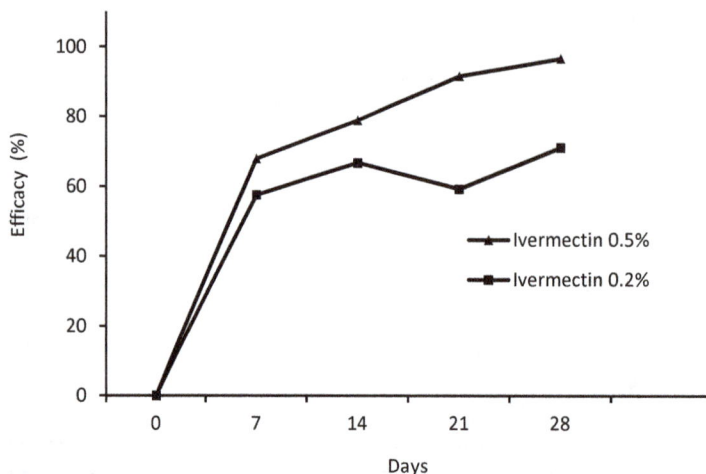

Figure 4. Comparison of the efficacy of two pour-on ivermectin formulations on the flea reduction in stray dogs.

or their breeds), are susceptible to this toxic effect. Here it is important to mention that no adverse effects were observed after the treatment of the experimental dogs with both drugs, and the physical condition of treated animals was clearly improved at the end of the experiment.

Sueur *et al.* [26] mentioned that pour-on aplications requires that the treated animal not be bathed for the 24 hours after the treatment in order to make sure to the active ingredient can penetrate the skin.

Even though the experimental groups had an equal number of male and female dogs, it was not possible to carry out a statistical analysis since the number of parasites was too high or too small and this could produce a confusing effect which does not really show if males are affected with parasites more frequently or in greater proportion than females.

With the regard to weight it is well known than puppies between 2 to 5 kg. show higher parasite EPG burden of ascarids and as the animals grow in age and weight the presence of Ancylostoma EPG is more frequently observed. In the present study this relationship was clearly noted.

5. Conclusions

Ivermectin at 0.5% showed better percentages of efficacy than the 0.2% formulation either in egg reduction or in the elimination and intestinal parasites as well as in the case of fleas. Both compounds showed 100% efficacy against lice.

Further studies should be conducted to determine if there is any toxicity in the use of pour-on presentations of these ivermectins on dogs since the available data up to now is limited.

Acknowledgements

The study is supported by Laboratorios Salud Animal, S.A de C.V, Mexico to the Internal Comitee for Animal Care and Use of Animals for Experimentation-Mexico, for approval to carry out the study.

References

[1]   Beck, W., Boch, K., Mackensen, H., Wiegand, B. and Pfister, K. (2006) Qualitative and Quantitative Observations on the Flea Population Dynamics of Dogs and Cats in Several Areas of Germany. *Veterinary Parasitology*, **137**, 130-136. http://dx.doi.org/10.1016/j.vetpar.2005.12.021

[2]   Kozen, E., Sevimli, F.K., Birdane, F.M. and Adanir, R. (2008) Efficacy of Eprinomectin against *Toxocara canis* in Dogs. *Parasitology Research*, **102**, 397-400. http://dx.doi.org/10.1007/s00436-007-0776-4

[3]   Snyder, D.E., Wyseman, S., Cruthers, L.R. and Slone, R.L. (2011) Ivermectin and Milbemycin Oxime in Experimental Adult Hearthworm (*Dirofilaria immitis*) Infection in Dogs. *Journal of Veterinary Internal Medicine*, **25**, 61-64. http://dx.doi.org/10.1111/j.1939-1676.2010.0657.x

[4]   Ahmad, N., Qaqbool, A., Saeed, K., Ashraf, K. and Qamar, M.F. (2011) Toxocariasis, Its Zoonotic Importance and Chemotherapy in Dogs. *The Journal of Animal & Plant Sciences*, **21**, 142-145.

[5]   Beck, W. and Panchev, N. (2010) Zoonosis Parasitarias. 1ra. Edition, SERVET, Zaragoza.

[6]   Yeruham, I., Rosen, S. and Hadani, A. (1989) Mortality in Calves, Lambs and Kids Caused Severe Infestation with Cat Flea *Ctenocephalides felis felis* (Bouché, 1835) in Israel. *Veterinary Parasitology*, **30**, 351-356. http://dx.doi.org/10.1016/0304-4017(89)90105-2

[7]   Dryden, M.W. (1933) Biology of Fleas of Dogs and Cats. *Pract. Vet.*, **15**, 569-579.

[8]   Gunn, A. and Pitt, S.J. (2012) Parasitology an Integrated Approach. Willey-Blackwell, Oxford.

[9]   Azad, A.F. (1990) Epidemiology of Murine Thyphus. *Annual Review of Plant Biology*, **35**, 553-569. http://dx.doi.org/10.1146/annurev.en.35.010190.003005

[10] Taylor, M.A., Coop, R.L. and Wall, R.L. (2007) Veterinary Parasitology. 3rd Edition, Blackwell Publishing, Oxford, 717.

[11] Obiukwu, M.O. and Onyali, I.O. (2006) Comparative Efficacy of Ancylol, Ivomec, Mebendazole, and Piperazine against *Ancylostoma caninum* in Experimentally Infected Pups. *Animal Research International*, **3**, 540-544.

[12] Ashraf, K., Rafique, S., Hashmi, H.A., Maqbool, A. and Chaudhary, Z.I. (2008) Ancylostomosis and Its Therapeutic Control in Dogs. *Journal of Veterinary and Animal Sciences*, **1**, 40-44.

[13] Khayatnoury, M.H., Garedaghi, Y., Arbati, A.R. and Khalili, H. (2011) The Effect of Ivermectin Pour-On Administration against Natural *Heterakis gallinarum* Infestation and Its Prevalence in Native Poultry. *American Journal of Ani-*

mal and Veterinary Sciences, **6**, 55-58. http://dx.doi.org/10.3844/ajavsp.2011.55.58

[14] Borges, F.A., Silva, H.C., Buzzulini, C., Soares, V.E., Santos, E., Oliveira, G.P. and Costa, A.J. (2008) Endectocide Activity of a New-Long Action Formulation Containing 2.25% Ivermectin + 1.25% Abamectin in Cattle. *Veterinary Parasitology*, **155**, 299-307. http://dx.doi.org/10.1016/j.vetpar.2008.04.019

[15] Hellmann, K., Heine, J., Braun, G., Pandesova, R. and Svoboduva, V. (2011) Evaluation of the Therapeutic and Preventive Efficacy of 2.5% Moxidectin / 10% Imidacloprid (Advocate®, Bayer Animal Health) in Dogs Naturally Infected or at Risk of Natural Infection by *Dirofilaria repens*. *Parasitology Research*, **109**, 77-86. http://dx.doi.org/10.1007/s00436-011-2404-6

[16] Snyder, D.E. and Wyseman, S. (2012) Dose Confirmation and None-Interference Evaluations of the Oral Efficacy of a Combination of Milbemycin Oxime and Spinosad against the Dose Limiting Parasites, Adult Cat Flea (*Ctenocephalides felis*) and Hookworm (*Ancylostoma caninum*) in Dogs. *Veterinary Parasitology*, **184**, 284-290. http://dx.doi.org/10.1016/j.vetpar.2011.11.067

[17] Suarez, G., Alvarez, L., Castells, D., Correa, O., Fagiolino, P. and Lanusse, C. (2013) Relative Bioavailability and Comparative Clinical Efficacy of Different Ivermectin Oral Formulations in Lambs. *BMC Veterinary Research*, **9**, 27-34. http://dx.doi.org/10.1186/1746-6148-9-27

[18] Fagbemi, B.O. (1982) Effect of *Ctenocephalides felis* Infestation on the Performance of West African Dwarf Sheep and Goats. *Veterinary Quarterly*, **4**, 92-95. http://dx.doi.org/10.1080/01652176.1982.9693846

[19] Bresciani, K.D.S., Freitas, D., Buzzulini, C., Chechi, C., Costa, J.P. and Oliveira, G.H.N. (2004) Effect of a 3.5% Ivermectin + Abamectin Association with Weight Gain of Nelore Calves Kept on Pasture. *XXIII World Buiatrics Congress*, Quebec, 11-16 July 2004, 26-27. Center for Research in Animal Health, Intervet.

[20] Rodríguez, D.C., Steckelberg, A., Lopes, W.D.Z., Santana, I.F., Martins, J.R. and Borges, F.A. (2005) Actividade anti-Helmíntica da associação Ivermectina 2.25% + abamectina 1.25% comparativamente a diferentes endectocidas em bovinos e efeito no desenvolvimento ponderal. *A Hora Veterinaria*, **25**, 27-30.

[21] Costa, A.J. and Docentel, A.J. (2004) Atividade endectocida de una inovacao quimioteràpica (Ivermectina + abamectina): Resultados de 12 avalição experimentais. *Revista Brasileira de Parasitologia Veterinária*, **13**, 171-177.

[22] Garg, R., Kumar, K.A., Yadav, C.L. and Banerjal, P.S. (2007) Duration of Anthelmintic Effect of Three Formulations of Ivermectin (Oral, Injectable and Pour-On) against Multiple Anthelmintic-Resistant *Haemonchus contortus* in Sheep. *Veterinary Research Communications*, **31**, 749-755. http://dx.doi.org/10.1007/s11259-007-0054-z

[23] Mandal, S.C. (2006) Veterinary Parasitology at a Glance. International Book Distributing Company, Lucknow, 203 p.

[24] Jacobs, D.E., Arakawa, A., Courtney, C.H., Gemmell, M.A., McCall, J.W., Myers, G.H. and Vanparijs, O. (1994) World Association for the Advancement of Veterinary Parasitology (W.A.A.V.P.) Guidelines Forevaluating the Efficacy of Anthelmintics for Dogs and Cats. *Veterinary Parasitology*, **52**, 179-202. http://dx.doi.org/10.1016/0304-4017(94)90110-4

[25] Marchiondo, A.A., Holdsworth, P.A., Green, P., Blagburn, B.L. and Jacobs, D.E. (2007) World Association for the Advancement of Veterinary Parasitology (W.A.A.V.P.) Guidelines for Evaluating the Efficacy of Parasiticides for the Treatment, Prevention and Control of Flea and Tick Infestation on Dogs and Cats. *Veterinary Parasitology*, **145**, 332-344. http://dx.doi.org/10.1016/j.vetpar.2006.10.028

[26] Sueur,C.L., Bour, S. and Schaper, R. (2010) Efficacy of a Combination of Imidacloprid 10%/Moxidectin 2.5% Spot on (Advocat® for Dogs) in the Prevention of Canine Spirocercosis (*Spirocerca lupi*). *Parasitology Research*, **107**, 1463-1469. http://dx.doi.org/10.1007/s00436-010-2022-8

7

Beta Blockers Use in Cardiac Failure: Does the Current Prescribing Practice at a Large Urban Hospital in Zimbabwe Exhibit Evidence Based Care and Offer Optimal Therapy for Cardiac Failure Patients?

Patrick Rutendo Matowa

Pharmaceutical Technology Department, Harare Institute of Technology, Harare, Zimbabwe
Email: patmat01@yahoo.co.uk

Abstract

Background: Cardiac failure treatment largely focused on symptomatic relief at the expense of the address of the underlying disease process of cardiac remodelling. This old wisdom of practice has been turned around by clinical research findings that have shown that there are agents that reverse cardiac remodelling and offer long-term benefits to cardiac failure patients. This has led to the recommendation of evidence-based practice in chronic heart failure management using reverse modelling agents such as beta blockers. Objectives: To ascertain the prescribing patterns of beta blockers in cardiac failure patients by doctors in a public hospital setting and determine the prevalence of cardiac failure hospitalisation and the age groups involved. Study design: A retrospective medical records review observational study. Methodology: A sample size of 385 cardiac failure cases was used. Data on cardiac failure patients who were once hospitalised at the hospital of study were abstracted from the patients' medical records files using data collection forms. Results: There were 36 (9.4%) patients who were prescribed beta blockers, 7 patients had their beta blocker substituted for another. Atenolol was prescribed to 30 (7.8%) patients, propranolol to 7 (1.8%) and carvedilol to 6 (1.6%) patients. Metoprolol and bisoprolol were not prescribed at all. There were more females (57.9%) than males (42.1%) and the mean age was 41.9 (standard deviation 24.0) years. The prevalence of cardiac failure hospitalisation was 1.54%. Conclusion: The rate of beta blocker prescribing was low. There is need for emphasis on evidence-based treatment options in the management of cardiac failure in Zimbabwe.

Keywords

Cardiac Failure, Beta Blockers, Prescribing Patterns

1. Introduction

Beta blockers are indicated in the following types of heart failure; systolic heart failure, diastolic heart failure and atrial fibrillation. Heart failure therapy has traditionally concentrated largely on symptomatic relief rather than addressing the underlying disease processes. The disease processes are engulfed in cardiac remodelling. Cardiac remodelling encompasses many changes associated with progressive heart failure. Therapeutic interventions aimed at solely correcting a low cardiac output or reduced blood flow; those offering symptomatic relief or improved cardiac emptying, do not necessarily slow heart failure progression or reduce mortality [1]-[4]. Prevention of the progression of heart failure by reversing the remodelling process should be the target for therapy, in addition to improving symptoms and reducing morbidity and mortality [1] [5]. Systems and factors that influence remodelling where therapy can be targeted towards, include the renin angiotensin system, sympathetic nervous system, endothelin, cytokines (Tumor Necrosis Factor, TNF, and interleukins) and nitrous oxide and oxidative stress. Large randomized studies have assessed measures of remodelling that include ejection fraction, left ventricular end-diastolic volume and left ventricular systolic volume, which are important in heart failure progression [1].

Traditionally, beta blockers were avoided in heart failure management. The rationale being that, the sympathetic nervous system over-activity provided an important compensatory protection for the failing heart. Thus blocking this level of compensation using a beta blocker would risk precipitating or worsening heart failure [6] [7].

Subsequent studies and clinical trials have challenged this old school of thought and practice [6] and have demonstrated that beta blockers reduce mortality and morbidity [8] [9]. Although the risks remain, there is a need to strike a balance between those short term risks and long term benefits of using beta blockers. At first, patients may feel worse from the blockade of the sympathetic nervous system activity, thus the need for starting with low doses and gradually increasing to the optimum dose [6]. Multiple clinical trials have proved the benefits of beta blockade in cardiac failure [6]. In all these studies, the beta blockers were administered in conjunction with an angiotensin converting enzyme inhibitor and a diuretic(s). Beta blockade consistently improved left ventricular function and provided additional clinical benefits over and above those achieved on standard therapy alone (*i.e.* Angiotensin converting enzyme inhibitor, ACEI, + diuretic) [6] [10]. Beta blockers reduce morbidity and mortality tremendously, mainly due to reversal of cardiac remodelling which subsequently would improve ejection fraction, left ventricular function and geometry [1] [6] [11]. The trials have shown overwhelming benefits of beta blockers in heart failure, such that the Cardiac Insufficiency Bisoprolol Study II, CIBIS-11, and the Metoprolol CR/XL Randomised Intervention Trial in congestive Heart Failure, MERIT-HF, studies were ended prematurely due to pronounced benefit in the treatment groups. Benefits from beta blockers include improved survival (30% - 35%), reduced need for hospitalisation and reduced symptoms of heart failure [6].

The main aim of beta blockade in chronic heart failure is not short term relief of symptoms but improvement in LV function and long-term outcomes. The long term benefits of beta blockers in heart failure include improved survival, improved control of heart failure, reduced need for hospitalisation, improved quality of life and improved left ventricular ejection fraction [6]. The short term risks of beta blockers in heart failure are worsening heart failure, bradyarrhythmias, prolonged intra-ventricular conduction, hypotension and worsening renal function [6]. These short term risks must be balanced against the long term benefits of using beta blockers in heart failure. Their mechanisms in improving survival in heart failure include antiarrhythmic action, anti-ischaemic action, attenuation of catecholamine toxicity and reduced cardiac remodelling [6].

The use of beta blockers in heart failure has been shown to significantly reduce mortality and hospital admissions by approximately a third. Since heart failure carries a high risk of death and disability, these important benefits of beta blockers should be utilised as a priority by clinicians in the management of heart failure [12].

1.1. Research Problem

Due to rapid urbanisation, dietary changes, lifestyle modifications, risk-prone behaviour and cultural attitudes predominantly in young people in Africa; prevalence of heart failure is on the rise substantially in sub-Saharan Africa [13]. Heart failure is emerging as a dominant form of cardiovascular disease and has massive social and economic relevance due to its high prevalence, mortality, morbidity and negative impact on young economically active individuals. The cases of heart failure in Africans are largely (about 90%) due to hypertension, cardiomyopathy, heumatic diseases, chronic lung diseases and pericardial disease; and remaining largely non-ischaemic [13].

In the abundance of all this overwhelming evidence of the rise in heart failure cases coupled with the discoveries of more effective beta blockers, the Zimbabwean health care system still finds itself stuck with the less effective beta blockers at the expense of the proven ones from many clinical studies. The Zimbabwe national treatment guidelines, Essential Drug List of Zimbabwe (EDLIZ), has no updated recommendations on the use of beta blockers in heart failure in line with new international guidelines which advocate for the use of the more efficacious beta blockers such as carvedilol and metoprolol rather than the outdated and less effective atenolol and propranolol. In as much as the concept of the EDLIZ is appreciated, it is the manner and period it is reviewed that, sometimes, leaves the health care provision disabled. This is so when lifesaving medicines like the newer beta blockers, are overlooked during the review of the treatment guidelines in the gist of them "being expensive or unaffordable". Therefore, lack of evidence based clinical guidelines for the management of heart failure using beta blockers in Zimbabwe is of major concern.

Moreover, current evidence suggests that some primary care physicians underperform in their management of heart failure patients [7] [14]. While most doctors prescribe medication appropriately, some doctors display patterns that are inconsistent with evidence-based medicine [14]. Identifying those patterns can offer intervention opportunities that might otherwise remain unnoticed. Heart failure is a chronic condition that poses a major growing concern, negative impact and threat to the public and country's economy; especially during this era of Human Immunodeficiency Virus (HIV) pandemic. HIV is an important cause of heart failure in most African countries. HIV cardiac related pathology, mainly dilated cardiomyopathy (CM) and TB pericarditis, is on the rise and poses a serious threat to the health care systems in Africa [15].

1.2. Significance of the Study

In order to engage in meaningful economic activities, people have to be in a good and sound state of health. Thus, improving the effectiveness of care and optimising patient outcomes through utilisation of evidence based practice becomes increasingly important.

The study will help identify the prescribing patterns of beta blockers in the public health sector and subsequently indicate the areas the country's health care is faring well and where amendments or updates are necessary, in terms of beta blocker therapy in chronic heart failure patients. This study would help in the formulation of clinical guidelines on how to manage heart failure patients using beta blockers, improving the knowledge of clinicians on the use of beta blockers in heart failure cases and optimisation of beta blockers in heart failure.

2. Aims of Study

The purpose of this study is to establish the prescribing patterns of beta blockers in chronic heart failure patients in one of Harare's major public hospitals; in order to get a picture of whether heart failure patients are receiving optimal evidence based therapy in line with clinical studies supporting the use of certain beta blockers in heart failure. This would help in policy implementations such as the formulation of clinical guidelines for the management of heart failure using beta blockers and also continual education of clinicians on the importance and use of beta blockers in heart failure.

Objectives of Study

1) To assess the prescribing patterns of beta blockers in heart failure patients by doctors in a large urban public hospital, in Harare, and compare against evidence from clinical trials.

2) To identify disease conditions that are common in heart failure.

3) To ascertain the prevalence of heart failure hospitalisations and the age groups involved, at the hospital.

4) To determine the most prescribed beta blockers in heart failure cases at the hospital.

3. Methods

3.1. Study Design

An observational retrospective medical records review study

3.2. Study Tool and Data Collection

Data collection forms were constructed and used by the investigator to abstract information from heart failure patients' medical files.

3.3. Study Setting and Population

One of Harare's major public referral hospitals was used for the study. A total of 385 heart failure cases, as calculated using Cochrane's sample size formula, were identified and studied.

3.4. Inclusion and Exclusion Criteria

The study included all heart failure cases which fell within the sample size, retrospectively from December 2011, and excluded all non-heart failure cases. Age was not taken into account

3.5. Sample Size Calculation

The sample size was calculated using Cochrane sample size formula for a single proportion.

$$n = (z/\Delta)^2 \times p(1-p) \tag{I}$$

where, n is sample size;

z is 1.96 (from statistical tables at 95% confidence interval);

Δ is level of precision ($\pm$ 5);

p is the estimated proportion of an attribute that is present in the population or degree of variability (50 in this case).

This yielded a sample size of 385.

3.6. Sampling Procedure

All heart failure cases of the year 2011 (317 cases) and some from the year 2010 (68 cases) were picked up for study without any form of order or systematic random selection method employed, until the sample size of 385 cases was attained.

3.7. Data Collection Procedure

The hospital medical records department was used as the source for the heart failure cases. Data collection forms were used to capture the relevant information from the selected medical files. Data collected included gender, age, date of admission and discharge, diagnosis, related disease conditions, medical history, whether the patient was on a beta blocker prior to admission, any beta blocker prescribed upon admission, beta blocker dosing schedule, other heart failure medication taken by the patient, cardiovascular examination (ECG, ECHO), any other medical tests done and reason for discharge.

3.8. Ethical Considerations

Authorisation from Joint Research Ethical Committee, JREC, to carry out the study, and also from the Medical Records department, to have access to patient medical records, was sought for and granted.

All patient identification information was not recorded onto the study data collection forms.

3.9. Data Analysis and Model Procedure

Data was statistically analysed using Epi Info package for 1) the frequencies of a particular gender, beta blockers prescribed, associated diseases, death and discharge 3) for the association between disease exposure and beta blocker prescription

Statistical Package used was R software package version 2.15.1 (2013). The modelling environment applied in the statistical analysis aimed to establish if association exists between: 1) disease an individual is exposed to and the physician beta blockers prescribing pattern (prescribe/do not prescribe); and 2) the treatment (standard + beta blockers (BB) or standard + other drugs) and the occurrence of death. An ACEI (enalapril/captopril) and a loop diuretic (furosemide) were used as the standard treatment in the study. The outcome of interest in both cases was binary, making a logistic regression a suitable approach in predicting the outcome.

The model procedure follows a stepwise regression analysis approach. With the stepwise approach we begin by bivariate analysis, to test for association between single exposure variable and outcome of interest.

The prevalence of heart failure hospitalisation was calculated from the total hospitalisations of the year 2011; data was obtained from the medical records department.

4. Results

The results show that there were less males (42.1%) than females (57.9%) hospitalised with heart failure, as shown in **Table 1** below.

The average age of the patients admitted with heart failure was found to be 41.9 years (standard deviation 24.0 and median 41.5), the mean hospitalisation time was found to be 8.3 days (standard deviation 6.8 and median 6.5) and the most affected age group was found to be 30 - 49 years (31.4 of the total cases) as indicated in **Table 2**. There was also a worrisome significant number of young children (0 - 9 years) affected by the disease, 10.6%, as shown in **Table 1**, which is attributed to the advent of HIV/AIDS as most of them were born HIV positive.

Table 1. Gender and age distribution among the cases.

Variable	Frequency	Percentage
Gender	Total (N = 385)	%
Males	162	42.1
Females	223	57.9
AGE (years)	N =	%
0 - 9	41	10.6
10 - 19	38	10.0
20 - 29	44	11.4
30 - 39	60	15.6
40 - 49	61	15.8
50 - 59	39	10.1
60 - 69	35	9.1
70 - 79	45	11.7
80 - 89	19	4.9
90 - 99	3	0.8

Table 2. The mean age and mean hospitalisation times.

Variable	Obs	Total	Mean	SD	min	25%	Median	75%	max
Age (years)	385	116118	41.9	24.0	0.2	24.5	41.5	62.5	92
Hosp. time (days)	385	3186	8.3	6.8	1.0	4.0	6.5	10.5	50

[*]Obs is the number of observed records, "total" represents the age of all the patients put together and the sum-mation of hospitalisation time in days; and SD is the standard deviation.

Table 3 highlights the following: Hypertension was diagnosed in almost half of the patients, with 189 patients (49.1%) being confirmed to be hypertensive. There were 59 cases (15.3%) diagnosed of diabetes, 40 (10.4%) were found to be in renal failure, 35 patients (9.1%) had hypercholesteremia, pneumonia accounting for 35 cases (9.1%) as well and 20 patients (5.2%) were confirmed to have Left Ventricular Dysfunction, LVD. There were 37 cases of anaemia, 12 (3.1%) of which were diagnosed as Zidovudine, AZT, induced. Cardiomyopathy, CM, was also present in a number of patients, with 78 cases being recorded, 25 (6.5%) of which were confirmed as HIV induced and 22 (5.7%) confirmed as post-partum. There were also 4 (1.6%) cases of thyrotoxicosis, 11 (2.9%) cases of infective endocarditis, 10 (2.6%) cases of Atrial Fibrillation, AF, 13 (3.4%) cases with rheumatic heart disease, 34 (8.8%) with Asthma/Chronic Obstructive Pulmonary Disease (COPD) and 15 (3.9%) patients diagnosed of pericarditis.

As indicated in **Table 4**, almost all the patients admitted at the hospital and diagnosed of heart failure where prescribed a diuretic, furosemide, 379 (98.4%). A small number of patients, 36 (9.4%), were prescribed beta blockers. A large number of patients, 309 (80.3%), were prescribed an ACEI. There were 192 (49.9%) cases were prescribed spironolactone and 122 (31.7%) digoxin. Quite a number of patients, 202 (52.5%) were also prescribed antibiotics whilst 64 (16.6%) patients were prescribed analgesics.

Of the 385 patients that were studied, 96 (24.9%) died whilst there were 287 (74.5%) normal hospital discharges due to the patients stabilising and responding well to treatment and one patient absconded whilst another one was discharged on care giver's request, as shown in **Table 5**. Of those who died, eight (8) were on beta blockers.

Table 3. Disease conditions associated with heart failure/concomitant diagnosis.

Variable	Frequency (N =)	Percentage (%)
Hypertension	189	49.1
Diabetes	59	15.3
Hypercholesteremia	35	9.1
Pneumonia	35	9.1
Rheumatic heart disease	13	3.4
Infective endocarditis	11	2.9
Asthma/COPD	34	8.8
LVD	20	5.2
AF	10	2.6
Congenital heart disease	20	5.2
Alcoholism	4	1.0
Anaemia	25	6.5
AZT-induced anaemia	12	3.1
Cardiomyopathy	31	8.1
HIV-induced CM	25	6.5
Post-partum CM	22	5.7
Thyrotoxicosis	6	1.6
Pericarditis	15	3.9
Renal Failure	40	10.4

Table 4. Medication/categories of medicines taken by the study patients.

Type/class of drug	Number of patients (N =)	Percentage (%)
Furosemide	379	98.4
Digoxin	122	31.7
ACEI	309	80.3
Spironolactone	192	49.9
Analgesics	64	16.6
Antibiotics	202	52.5
Beta blockers	36	9.4

Table 5. Cardiovascular (CVS) examination and patient discharge from hospital.

CVS exam	N =	%
ECHO	317	82.3
ECG	315	81.8
Reason for hospital discharge	N =	%
Stable, home on treatment	287	74.5
Absconded	1	0.3
Care giver's request	1	0.3
Died	96	24.9

New Serology Screen

Of all the 385 Congestive Heart Failure, CHF, admissions, 89 (23.1%) patients were confirmed to be HIV negative, 86 (22.3%) patients were confirmed as HIV positive whereas the HIV status of 210 (54.5%) patients was not confirmed, as shown in **Table 6**.

Table 7 and **Graph 1** show that there was a small number of beta blocker prescriptions observed. Atenolol was the most prescribed followed by propranolol and lastly carvedilol. Metoprolol and bisoprolol were not prescribed to any patient

The results shown in **Table 8** indicate that before hospitalisation, 22 (5.7%) patients were already taking beta blockers and after hospitalisation there were 36 (9.4%) cardiac failure patients taking beta blockers. This implies that there were 14 (3.6%) patients who were introduced to beta blocker therapy for the first time while in hospital. In patients who took beta blockers, 8 (22.2%) died and 28 (77.8%) were stabilised and discharged home. Of the patients who died whilst taking beta blockers, four were on propranolol, three were taking atenolol and one was on carvedilol.

The prevalence of cardiac failure hospitalisation for the year 2011 was 1.54% as shown in **Table 9**.

The variables that were found to be statistically related to the prescription outcome include age ($p < 0.0001$), hypertension ($p < 0.01$), diabetes ($p < 0.0001$) and renal failure ($p < 0.05$).

No treatment variables were found to be statistically related to the occurrence of death.

Age showed a positive effect on the prescribing pattern of beta blockers, (older aged are more likely to be occupied), also diabetes showed a positive effect with beta blocker prescriptions (diabetics much more likely to be prescribed beta blockers), as indicated in **Table 10**.

This is the minimal adequate model.

Table 6. HIV status.

HIV+	Frequency	Percentage
No	89	22.1
Yes	86	22.3
Not-confirmed	210	54.6
Total	385	100.0

Table 7. Beta blockers prescribed in the heart failure cases.

Beta blocker	Cases (n =) (total n = 43)	Percentage (%)
Atenolol	30	7.8
Propranolol	7	1.8
Carvedilol	6	1.6
Metoprolol	0	0
Bisoprolol	0	0

Table 8. Beta blocker prescriptions before and after hospitalisation.

Beta blocker prescription	Frequency	Percentage
Prior to admission	22	5.7
After admission	36	9.4
New BB patients	14	3.6

Table 9. Prevalence of heart failure hospitalisation for the year 2011.

Number of CHF hospitalisations	317
Total number of hospitalisation	20,522
Prevalence	1.54%

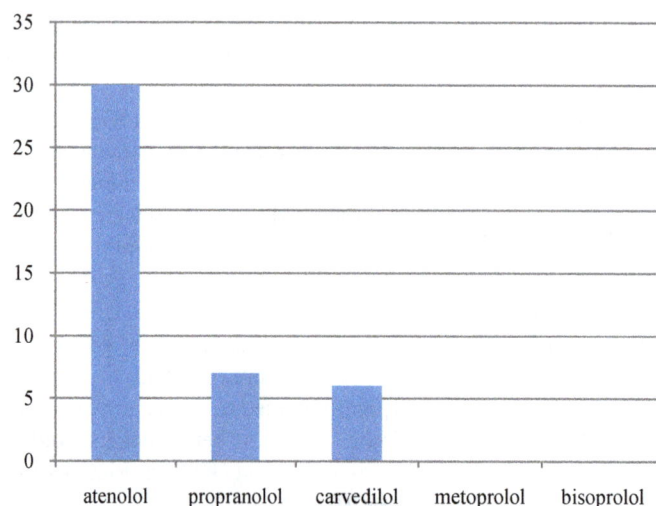

Graph 1. Beta blockers prescribed in the cardiac failure cases.

Table 10. Relationship between variables (odds ratios).

Variable	Odds Ratio (OR)	p-Value
Beta blocker and increased age	1.02	0.0107
Beta blocker and diabetes	2.22	0.0281
Atenolol & hypercholesterolemia	5.56	0.000136
Atenolol and hypertension	5.01	0.004759
Propranolol and age	1.04	0.0332

$$\text{Logit}[\text{odds}] = -2.77 + 0.02\text{AGE} + 0.80\text{DIABETES}$$

The odds of prescribing beta blockers are 1.02 times for a year older individual. The odds of prescribing beta blockers are 2.22 times among the diabetics than the non-diabetic. The observations revealed an association between atenolol and hypertension and hypercholesterolemia, with ORs of 5.01 (p = 0.004759) and 5.56 (p = 0.000136) respectively. Also, propranolol was demonstrated to be associated to age (OR = 1.04, p = 0.0332). Diabetes was also associated with a beta blocker prescription.

5. Discussion

The results show that there were few beta blocker prescriptions by doctors in cardiac failure patients. This could have been due to the fact that most patients present to the hospital with CHF when the disease is at an advanced stage and clinicians tend to shun beta blockers because of the belief that beta blockers worsen heart failure especially in the frail and elderly patients [16] [17]. This reluctance to prescribe beta blockers in CHF by clinicians has been a matter of concern as it may deny patients of life-saving treatment, especially as they reverse modelling. Of the small number of beta blocker prescription observed, atenolol was the most prescribed followed by propranolol and lastly carvedilol. Metoprolol and bisoprolol were not prescribed to any patient. This trend could be because of the local national guidelines which recommend atenolol and propranolol as the beta blockers to use in CHF. Consequently, there haven't been much strides or effort by the practitioners in trying to introduce patients to the more efficacious beta blockers such as carvedilol, metoprolol and bisoprolol [18], as seen by the very few prescriptions of carvedilol and none on metoprolol and bisoprolol. The other factor of the low prescriptions could be related to the availability of the drugs in the hospital which can influence prescriptions of the readily available agents. These results do not compare well with international guidelines that recommend use of clinically proven beta blockers, carvedilol, metoprolol and bisoprolol, in CHF patients. Nevertheless, a significant number of patients who got prescribed beta blockers received protection from the disease and managed to recover and got discharged. Introduction of more efficacious beta blocker agents in the national treatment guidelines (EDLIZ) and prescribing to more chronic heart failure patients could further improve clinical care and significantly reduce mortality, hospitalisation time and symptoms; and improve the patients' quality of life.

There seem to be a gender shift in those affected by CHF. More men than women used to be reported as suffering from CHF but the results showed that more women (57.9%) were affected by the condition than men (42.1%) at the study hospital. This could be due to complications during pregnancies, which can precipitate heart failure, because of early marriages and the HIV infection, more women taking up stressful jobs initially reserved for men and lifestyle changes that have resulted in more women engaging in health-hazard practices such as smoking and beer-drinking.

The study showed that the main contributors to the diagnosed cardiac failure were hypertension 49.1% (189), diabetes 15.3% (59), hypercholesterolemia 9.1% (35), pneumonia 9.1% (35), renal disease 10.4% (10), asthma/ COPD 8.8% (34), rheumatic heart disease 3.4% (13), LVD 5.2% (20), congenital heart disease 5.2% (20), anaemia 9.6 (37), cardiomyopathy 20.3% (78) and pericarditis 3.9% (15). These results are comparable to other studies concluded in sub-Saharan African. In the Heart of Soweto study, carried out in South Africa, the mean age of those with heart failure was 55 years and 57% were women [19]. The gender proportion of those with heart failure in South Africa's Soweto suburb is a mirror image of the Zimbabwe's situation at this major referral hospital. In the Soweto study, the most common diagnosis was hypertension (33%), cardiomyopathy (28%), right heart failure (27%) and rheumatic heart disease [19]. In a study carried out at St Elizabeth Catholic general hospital in Cameroon, the average age for the heart failure cases was 42.5 years. The cardiac failure cases were attributed to valvulopathies (35%), cardiomyopathies (32%), hypertension (15%), pericarditis (7%), COPD (8%) and congenital heart disease (3%) [20]. The Cameroon results are also comparable to this hospital study results. The notable similarities being the mean age, congenital heart disease, COPD and cardiomyopathies. The only major difference is that whilst in Zimbabwe's setting hypertension is the major contributor to heart failure with 49.1%, in Cameroon it only contributes 15%. This could be a genetic difference and/or lifestyle difference.

The results also confirm that hypertension, cardiomyopathy, rheumatic heart disease, chronic lung disease and pericardial disease account for over 90% 0f the heart failure cases in sub-Saharan Africa.

The prevalence of chronic heart failure hospitalisation at this studyhospital was found to be 1.54%. The actual prevalence of heart failure cases is likely to be higher than the hospitalisation prevalence due to a number of factors such as more patients seeking medical help from primary health centres, some patients not affording to seek any medical help and some patients seeking alternative help (traditional or spiritual). According to some studies done, the prevalence of chronic heart failure is on the rise. This has been attributed to consequences of urbanisation, diet, lifestyle modification and risk-prone behaviour [13].

HIV seems to be contributing to the rise in heart failure cases. From the results, there were 12 cases (3.1%) of AZT induced anaemia which subsequently led to heart failure. HIV-induced cardiomyopathy was a bit higher than the anaemia caused by AZT, having 6.5% (25) cases. This can be summed up as having HIV contributing at least 9.6% of the heart failure cases. There were 36 (9.4%) patients who were prescribed beta blockers, 14 patients taking a beta blocker for the first time. This was low as compared to other countries, especially the western world where they have embraced the importance of beta blockers in chronic heart failure [17]. Of the prescribed beta blockers, atenolol was the highly prescribed with a frequency of 30 (7.8%) followed by propranolol with 7 patients (1.8%) and carvedilol prescribed to 6 patients (1.6%). No patient was prescribed metoprolol or bisoprolol. This is in contrast with international guidelines where beta blockers are part of the first line drugs in heart failure management [21] with carvedilol, bisoprolol and metoprolol amongst the recommended beta blocker drugs whilst atenolol and propranolol are not indicated for heart failure treatment [10]. This is an indication that the hospital prescribing patterns are not in tandem with evidence-based practice in heart failure management using beta blockers.

However, the results went on to show that furosemide and an ACEI (captopril/enalapril) were highly prescribed. This combination is used as the standard treatment at the hospital. In testing for an association between the standard treatment plus a beta blocker and death as the outcome; and standard treatment plus other drugs (digoxin or spironolactone or both) and death, it was discovered that there was no association between treatment combination and occurrence of death. This implies that, from the study, no treatment variables were found to be statistically related to the occurrence of death. There was also no statistical association between diseases presented and prescription of metoprolol, bisoprolol and carverdilol. Associations were however found between beta blocker prescription and age, OR = 1.02 (p = 0.0107), beta blocker prescription and diabetes, OR = 2.22 (p = 0.0281), propranolol and age, OR = 1.04 (p = 0.0332), atenolol and hypercholesteremia, OR = 5.56 (p = 0.000136), atenolol and hypertension, OR = 5.01 (p = 0.004759). From the odds ratio results, older people were more likely to be prescribed a beta blocker—the odds of prescribing a beta blocker were 1.02 times for a year older heart failure patient. The odds of prescribing a beta blocker were 2.22 times more for a diabetic heart failure patient than a non-diabetic heart failure patient. This has been elucidated in a study to find out if diabetes mellitus patients who are also heart failure patients benefit as well as the non-diabetic heart failure patients. It was found that the diabetes mellitus patients had a better prognostic benefit from beta blocker therapy than the non-diabetic heart failure patients [22]. Propranolol was found to be prescribed 1.04 times more per year increase in age, making it more likely to be prescribed in the elderly. Prescriptions of atenolol were demonstrated to increase with hypertensive and hypercholesteremic heart failure patients. In hypertension it is because atenolol has been proven to be effective in lowering blood pressure with less adverse effects than propranolol.

Echocardiography and ECG services were used regularly in the diagnosis of chronic heart failure as shown by the high number of patients with those examinations done for their diagnosis; ECHO (317) and ECG (315). In most cases, a patient would be subjected to both examinations. ECHO is regarded as the most accurate diagnostic tool for heart failure [23] and with its regular use at thehospital; patients are getting accurate diagnosis, provided the results are interpreted correctly.

The national treatment guidelines (EDLIZ) recommend the use of propranolol or atenolol under a specialist care when the standard treatment regimen plus other agents such as spironolactone and or digoxin have failed. This has helped in improving patients' outcomes but could be further improved. The guidelines are not up to date with the new evidence-based beta blockers such as bisoprolol, carvedilol and metoprolol recommended by international treatment guidelines like National Institute of Health Care Excellence (NICE). These relatively new beta blockers have been shown in various studies (for example CIBIS-II and MERIT-HF) to offer better prognosis in chronic heart failure patients. Thus, the inclusion of these newly recommended evidence-based agents in the EDLIZ could offer optimal therapy for the patients put on beta blockers and greatly improve their disease condition.

6. Limitations

The study was done in a public hospital setting only. Efforts to include a private hospital were unsuccessful as the authorities could not grant permission for the study to be carried out using their medical records. Time permitting; more hospitals across the country could have been included in the study to have a better picture of the health practice in the whole country. Also, a prospective study involving the outpatients department together with the retrospective one could have been the best study design, but the time limit of the study could not afford the prospective arm to be included as it required more time for completion.

7. Conclusion

There were more women than men diagnosed with cardiac failure at the hospital and the average age of CHF was forty two years. The prescribing rate of beta blockers was observed to be very low. Atenolol was the most prescribed beta blocker, followed by propranolol and lastly carvedilol. Metoprolol and bisoprolol were virtually not prescribed. The prevalence of chronic heart failure hospitalisation was 1.54%. Hypertension, cardiomyopathy, renal failure, pneumonia, asthma/COPD, rheumatic heart disease, LVD, pericarditis and anaemia were the major contributors to cardiac failure. There is lack of evidence based prescribing of beta blockers in cardiac failure in the Zimbabwe's public health care system. The health care system is lagging behind in terms of implementing international guidelines on the use of beta blockers in chronic heart failure.

8. Recommendations

To have a better assessment of the prescribing patterns, more studies in other hospitals across the country have to be carried out. Treatment guidelines on the use of beta blockers in chronic heart failure should be constructed, in line with international guidelines, in order to create an evidence-based practice system. The involvement of all the critical stake holders that includes academia, research groups and the pharmaceutical industry, in the formulation of local guidelines is important so that results of all or most of the completed clinical studies and updated international guidelines are forwarded and discussed for possible consideration into the local guidelines. Of importance as well is the setting up of a special national health committee or consultancy that has the mandate of engaging the ministry of health, the pharmaceutical industry and health practitioners on the updates on evidence-based practice in line with recent clinical evidence or updates and also assessing how best the country's health care system could adopt or move with the changing times so as to afford the best possible treatment options to patients.

Acknowledgements

My heartfelt appreciation goes to the highly contributing Chairman of Clinical Pharmacology at the University of Zimbabwe, Prof CFB Nhachi, for his support and guidance. I greatly appreciate the advice extended to this work by Ms Celia Matyanga, who responded promptly and enthusiastically to my requests for frank comments, despite her congested schedule. I am indebted to all of them, who did their best to bring improvements through their contributions and suggestions. I am also thankful to my family, wife and kids, who directly or indirectly have been helpful in one way or the other. I thank my Dearest Parents for affording me the opportunity to explore life and extend my reach.

And to my late brother, Sylvester, you are always my greatest motivator, may your soul rest in peace.

To my wife and kids, I love you.

May God bless you.

References

[1]   Jay, N. (2000) Cardiac Remodelling—Concepts and Clinical Implications: A Consensus Paper from an International Forum on Cardiac Remodelling. *JAAC*, **45**, 582-596.

[2]   Packer, M., Carver, J.R., Rhodeheffer, R.J., *et al.* (1991) Effect of Oral Milrinone on Mortality in Severe Chronic Heart Failure. *The New England Journal of Medicine*, **325**, 1468-1475. http://dx.doi.org/10.1056/NEJM199111213252103

[3]   Digitalis Investigation Group (1997) The Effects of Digoxin on Mortality and Morbidity in Patients with Heart Failure. *The New England Journal of Medicine*, **336**, 525-533. http://dx.doi.org/10.1056/NEJM199702203360801

[4]   Massie, B.M., Fisher, S.G., Deedwania, P.C., Singh, B.N., Fletcher, R.D. and Singh, S.N., for the CHF-STAT Investigators (1996) Effect of Amiodarone on Clinical Status and Left Ventricular Function in Patients with Congestive Heart Failure. *Circulation*, **93**, 2128-2134. http://dx.doi.org/10.1161/01.CIR.93.12.2128

[5]   Pieske, B. (2004) Reverse Remodelling in Heart Failure—Fact or Fiction? *European Heart Journal Supplements*, **6**, D66-D78. http://dx.doi.org/10.1016/j.ehjsup.2004.05.019

[6]   Fletcher, P. (2000) Cardiovascular Medicines, John Hunter Hospital, Newcastle: Beta Blockers in Heart Failure. *Australian Prescriber*, **23**, No 6.

[7]   Hobbs, F.D.R. (2000) Management of Heart Failure: Evidence versus Practice. Does Current Prescribing Provide Optimal Treatment for Heart Failure Patients? *British Journal of General Practice*, **50**, 735-742.

[8]   Brophy, J.M., Joseph, L. and Rouleau, J.L. (2001) Beta Blockers in Congestive Heart Failure: A Bayesian Meta-Analysis. *Annals of Internal Medicine*, **134**, 550-560. http://dx.doi.org/10.7326/0003-4819-134-7-200104030-00008

[9]   Dobre, D., De Jongste, M.J., Lucas, C., Cleuren, G., van Veldhuisen, D.J., Ranchor, A.V. and Haaijer-Ruskamp, F. (2007) Effectiveness of Beta Blocker Therapy in Daily Practice Patients with Advanced Chronic Heart Failure: Is There an Effect-Modification by Age? *British Journal of Clinical Pharmacology*, **63**, 356-364. http://dx.doi.org/10.1111/j.1365-2125.2006.02769.x

[10]   McMurray, J.J., *et al.* (2012) ESC Guidelines for the Diagnosis and Treatment of Acute and Chronic Heart Failure. *European Heart Journal*, **33**, 1787-1847.

[11]   Eichhorn, E.J. and Bristow, M.R. (1996) Medical Therapy Can Improve the Biological Properties of the Chronically Failing Heart: A New Era in the Treatment of Heart Failure. *Circulation*, **94**, 2285-2296.

[12]   Shibata, M.C., Flather, M.D. and Wang, D.L. (2001) Systematic Review of the Impact of Beta Blockers on Mortality and Hospital Admissions in Heart Failure. *European Journal of Heart Failure*, **3**, 351-357. http://dx.doi.org/10.1016/S1388-9842(01)00144-1

[13]   Ntusi, N.B. and Mayosi, B.M. (2009) Epidemiology of Heart Failure in Sub-Saharan Africa. *Expert Review of Cardiovascular Therapy*, **7**, 169-180.

[14]   Hobbs, F.D., Jones, M.I., Allan, T.F., Wilson, S. and Tobias, R. (2000) European Survey of Primary Care Physician Perceptions on Heart Failure Diagnosis and Management. *European Heart Journal*, **21**, 1877-1887. http://dx.doi.org/10.1053/euhj.2000.2170

[15]   Magula, N.P. and Mayosi, B.M. (2003) Cardiac Involvement in HIV-Infected People Living in Africa: A Review. *Cardiovascular Journal of Southern Africa*, **14**, 231-237.

[16]   Berry, C., Murdoch, D.R. and McMurray, J.J.V. (2001) Economics of Chronic Heart Failure. *European Journal of Heart Failure*, **3**, 283-291. http://dx.doi.org/10.1016/S1388-9842(01)00123-4

[17]   Yilmaz, M.B., Refiker, M., Guray, Y., Guray, U., Altay, H., Dermirkan, B., Caldir, V. and Korkmaz, S. (2007) Prescribing Patterns in Patients with Systolic Heart Failure at Hospital Discharge: Why Beta Blockers Are Under-Prescribed or Prescribed at Low Dose in Real Life. *International Journal of Clinical Practice*, **61**, 225-230. http://dx.doi.org/10.1111/j.1742-1241.2006.01157.x

[18]   Krum, H. (1999) Beta Blockers in Heart Failure. The "New Wave" of Clinical Trials. *Drugs*, **58**, 203-210. http://dx.doi.org/10.2165/00003495-199958020-00001

[19]   Stewart, S., Wilkinson, D., Hansen, C., Vaghela, V., Mvungi, R., McMurray, J. and Sliwa, K. (2008) Predominance of Heart Failure in the Heart of Soweto Study Cohort. Emerging Challenges for Urban African Communities. *Journal of American Heart Association*, **118**, 2360-2367. http://dx.doi.org/10.1161/circulationaha.108.786244

[20]   Yancy, C.W., Fowler, M.B., Colucci, W.S., Gilbert, E.M., Bristow, M.R., Cohn, J.N., Lukas, M.A., Young, S.T. and Parker, M. (2001) Race and Response to Adrenergic Blockade with Carvedilol in Patients with Chronic Heart Failure. *New England Journal of Medicine*, **334**, 1358-1365. http://dx.doi.org/10.1056/NEJM200105033441803

[21]   NICE5 Guidelines, CG5. Chronic Heart Failure; Management of Chronic Heart Failure in Adults in Primary and Secondary Care, July 2003. www.nice.org.uk/guidance/cg5

[22]   Haas, S.J., Vos, T., Gilbert, R.E. and Krum, H. (2003) Are Beta Blockers as Efficacious in Patients with Diabetes Mel-

litus as in Patients without Diabetes Mellitus Who Have Chronic Heart Failure? A Meta-Analysis of Large-Scale Clinical Trials. *American Heart Journal*, **146**, 848-853. http://dx.doi.org/10.1016/S0002-8703(03)00403-4

[23] Fuat, A., Hungin, A.P.S. and Murphy, J.J. (2003) Barriers to Accurate Diagnosis and Effective Management of Heart Failure in Primary Care: Qualitative Study. *BMJ*, **326**, 196. http://dx.doi.org/10.1136/bmj.326.7382.196

8

Health Related Quality of Life among Osteoarthritis Patients: A Comparison of Traditional Non-Steroidal Anti-Inflammatory Drugs and Selective COX-2 Inhibitors in the United Arab Emirates Using the SF-36

Mohammed Hassanein*, Mohammed Shamssain, Nageeb Hassan

Clinical Pharmacy Department, College of Pharmacy and Health Science, Ajman University of Science and Technology, Ajman, United Arab Emirates
Email: *mohammedhassanein@outlook.com

Abstract

Objectives: Osteoarthritis (OA) has a dramatic impact on patients' health related quality of life (HRQoL). Chronic use of analgesics and anti-inflammatory medications for pain management may improve symptoms but on long term may affect HRQoL negatively. The objective of the present study was to compare the impact of two different classes of analgesics, traditional non-steroidal anti-inflammatory drugs (NSAIDs) and selective cyclo-oxygenase-2 (COX-2) inhibitors on HRQoL among osteoarthritis patients using the SF-36 questionnaire. Methods: Clinic based cross-sectional study conducted at Al-Qassimi Hospital, Sharjah, United Arab Emirates (UAE), over a period of six months. Ethical Approval was obtained from the ethics committee at Al-Qassimi Clinical Research Center. Total of 200 osteoarthritis patients fulfilling the inclusion and exclusion criteria were involved in the study. Patients' demographics were collected from their medical records. The Medical Outcome Study Short-Form 36 (SF-36) questionnaire was used to measure patients' HRQoL. SF-36 data were scored using health outcomes scoring software 4.5. Results: Mean age of the subjects was 62.19 ± 9.81 years with females constituting 151 (75.5%) of the patients. In general, females scored lower in most of the HRQoL domains compared to males and there was significant difference between the two groups in the mental health ($p = 0.005$) & mental component ($p = 0.042$) domains. Compared to selective COX-2 inhibitors, patients on NSAIDs scored higher on all domains of SF-36 except physical functioning. There was significant difference in mental health

---

*Corresponding author.

domain for patients treated with NSAIDs ($p = 0.02$). Celecoxib was only better than NSAIDs in osteoarthritis patients with more than one musculoskeletal disorders in the domain of bodily pain ($p = 0.009$). Conclusion: NSAIDs-treated patients did not differ significantly from celecoxib-treated patients in all domains of the SF-36 except for the mental health domain.

Keywords

Osteoarthritis, Health Related Quality of Life, Short Form-36, Traditional Nonsteroidal Anti-Inflammatory Drugs, Selective COX-2 Inhibitors

1. Introduction

Osteoarthritis (OA) is a chronic disease that has a substantial effect on patients' health related quality of life (HRQoL) as well as an extremely high economic burden usually attributed to the treatment side effects [1]. Activities of daily living are negatively affected in OA patients [2]. Its symptoms are debilitating, and accounting for significant disability characterized as the impaired performance of social and physical life tasks [3] [4]. Their impact on patients' functional levels is well known and constitutes difficulties patients have to deal with, which will require long term pharmacological treatment and physical therapies [5].

The deleterious effects and impacts of osteoarthritis are well studied and mainly focusing on its consequences on health status; this is also true for the efficacy of treatments which was also assessed in context of health status and focused only on the objective measures of health status. However, few studies examined the impact of OA and its treatments on patients' HRQoL and the patients' subjective perspective. HRQoL outcomes provide an effective means for clinicians to make clinically sensible decisions by providing further insight into the benefits and drawbacks of treatment options [6] [7].

Pain and stiffness dominate other symptoms usually in early OA, therefore, treatment should focus on the reduction of pain and improvement of functional capacities as well as improvement of patients' HRQoL [8] [9]. Chronic use of analgesics and anti-inflammatory drugs can cause dramatic changes on patients' HRQoL & long term plan is definitely important when safety and patients' HRQoL are considered. Previous studies have shown that both NSAIDs and selective COX-2 inhibitors improved patients' HRQoL when compared to the baseline [2] [3] [10] [11]; however very few studies conducted direct comparison between the two medication classes [12]. It is well recognized now that a key outcome measure for any intervention for OA is measuring the changes in HRQoL as for many other conditions [13].

According to the Emirates Arthritis Foundation (EAF), the estimated prevalence of arthritis in the UAE is 20%, with only 6000 patients having been officially diagnosed [14]. The present study aims to compare the impact of two different classes of analgesics: traditional non-steroidal anti-inflammatory drugs (NSAIDs) and selective cyclo-oxygenase-2 (COX-2) inhibitors on HRQoL among osteoarthritis patients using the Medical Outcome Study SF-36 questionnaire as a measurement tool.

2. Materials and Methods

This was an observational cross-sectional study involving patients with symptomatic osteoarthritis recruited form Al-Qassimi Hospital in the United Arab Emirates. The present study was conducted between October 2013 and March 2014. Ethical Approval was obtained from the Ethics Committee of Al-Qassimi Clinical Research Center located at Al-Qassimi Hospital.

2.1. Study Population

Two hundred patients, 151 females and 49 males who fulfilled the inclusion and exclusion criteria were included in the study. To be eligible for inclusion, patients had to have documented diagnosis of osteoarthritis of any localization for at least 3 months, age $\geq$ 45 years, taking either oral traditional NSAIDs or selective COX-2 inhibitors. Patients on topical NSAIDs, intra-articular hyaluronic injections or taking over the counter chondroitin or glucosamine supplementations were allowed to be involved in the study. Patients newly diagnosed; diagnosis dated back to less than 3 months, patients with concomitant oesteoarticular disorders, or with motor function impairment not due to osteoarthritis (e.g. Rheumatoid Arthritis), patients underwent knee replacement surgery, or on oral glucocorticoids were excluded from the study.

2.2. Data Collection

HRQoL was measured using the Medical Outcome Study Short Form-36 (SF-36) (4 weeks recall). The procedures for data collection were similar among the two groups. Each patient was identified by a code number for the purpose of maintaining patients' confidentiality and data retrieving. All subjects received an informed consent form asking them to participate in the study. Patients' socio-demographic data included gender, age, weight, height & calculated Body Mass Index (BMI). Data regarding localization of OA, presence of any comorbidities or comorbid musculoskeletal disorders, concurrent OA medications, total daily doses of all the medications taken for osteoarthritis & concurrent medications for other conditions were extracted from patients' files only after the questionnaire has been completed by the patient.

Comorbidities were classified into five categories; cardiovascular disorders including (hypertension, dyslipidaemia, ischemic heart diseases & anaemia), endocrine and metabolic disorders including (diabetes mellitus both types, thyroid disorders), respiratory (asthma & COPD), neuropsychiatric (stroke, epilepsy, Parkinson & depression) and renal diseases. Obesity was regarded as one of the comorbidities and was defined by BMI.

2.3. Measurement Tool

The SF-36 [2] [3] [15] is a well-known self-administered and generic health status measure which encompasses 8 domains related to daily life activities and consist of 36 items. Each domain scores from 0 (lowest level of functioning) to 100 (highest level of functioning). Arabic version has been validated for the UAE Population. Both Arabic and English versions were available and readily distributed according to the patient's preferences. During the visit patients were invited to complete the whole questionnaire alone, only if required patients were assisted by a trained health professional or the principle investigator. All respondents were asked to answer the questionnaire based on what they understood.

2.4. Statistical Analysis

The data were analyzed using Statistical Package for Social Science (SPSS version 20). Descriptive analyses were used for socio-demographic data and clinical values. p value ≥ 0.05 was considered significant. Continuous variables were reported using means & standard deviations (SD). Categorical variables were reported by percentage and proportions. SF-36 data was scored using the health outcomes scoring software 4.5. Chi-square test was used to examine the homogeneity of treatment groups for categorical variables. Independent sample t-test was used to assess the difference between traditional NSAIDs and selective COX-2 inhibitors in terms of HRQoL domains.

3. Results

Between October 2013 and March 2014, 200 osteoarthritis patients were eligible to be included in the study and agreed to complete the questionnaire. Written informed consent form was obtained from each patient. The English version of the SF-36 questionnaire was only used marginally by three patients (1.5%). Reasons for non-participation were either patients were not interested or they did not have the time to complete the questionnaire.

Among the enrolled patients, 151 (75.5%) were females and 49 (24.5%) were males. The age range was between 45 & 88 years. Mean age was 62.19 ± 9.81. BMI was calculated using the reported weights and heights. Data on weights and heights was only available for 100 patients collectively. The other 100 patients were treated by SPSS as missing values. The definitions of the certain groups "normal", "overweight" and "obese" were based on the definition of the World Health Organization (WHO). Mean BMI was 32.68 ± 8.82 with females showed slightly higher values compared to males (**Table 1**).

NSAIDs were prescribed for 46.5% of the patients. Celecoxib was the only selective COX-2 inhibitors prescribed (53.5%). With respect to the individual NSAIDs prescribed, meloxicam 7.5 mg was the most common traditional NSAIDs prescribed among the study patients (n = 81) (40.5%), followed by piroxicam 20 mg (2.5%)

Table 1. Physical measurements of subjects. (Mean ± SD).

Parameter	Females (n = 151)	Males (n = 49)	All
Age (Years)	60.77 ± 9.312	66.53 ± 10.1	62.19 ± 9.817 (n = 200)
Height (Cm)	156.8 ± 7.94	167.8 ± 10.0	159.5 ± 9.73 (n = 100)
Weight (Kg)	81.77 ± 23.4	89.58 ± 31.69	83.75 ± 25.77 (n = 100)
BMI	33.0 ± 8.66	31.53 ± 9.38	32.68 ± 8.82 (n = 100)

& diclofenac 50 mg (2.5%) with naproxen 200 mg & ibuprofen 400 mg were marginally prescribed (0.5%) for each, respectively (**Table 2**). Chi-square test did not reveal any significant difference between males and females in terms of the type of medications prescribed, but females were shown to be prescribed more analgesics both traditional NSAIDs & selective COX-2 Inhibitors (celecoxib) more frequently compared to males.

In general, mental health domains and mental health component (mental health, role emotional, social functioning & vitality) were better and less affected than physical health domains (physical functioning, role physical and bodily pain) for both genders. Females scored lower in all domains of SF-36 compared to males except for social functioning, however, the difference was not significant (**Table 3**). A significant difference was observed in the mental health domain between females and males ($p = 0.005$) who were already established on their medications (Traditional NSAIDs or COX-2 Inhibitors) at the time of the questionnaire administration as well as in the mental component summary ($p = 0.042$).

An independent t-test was performed to compare the HRQoL in patients taking traditional NSAIDs with those taking selective COX-2 inhibitors (**Table 4**). Patients on NSAIDs had higher scores of HRQoL than those on selective COX-2 inhibitors in all domains except for physical functioning domain but the difference was not significant. However, there was a significant difference in the domain of mental health in favour for NSAIDs over COX-2 inhibitors ($p = 0.02$). Meloxicam 7.5 mg once daily was associated with better HRQoL in the domains of general health than celecoxib 200 mg once daily ($p = 0.053$) and in the domain of mental health. Diclofenac was better than celecoxib in bodily pain domain ($p = 0.025$).

Patients with knee OA showed significant difference in the mental health domain between traditional NSAIDs group and selective COX-2 inhibitors ($p = 0.047$) in favour of NSAIDs. Patients with spine OA who were on traditional NSAIDs had better domains of SF-36 except for the vitality when compared with patients with knee OA. Significant difference was also found in favour for NSAIDs in patients with OA in more than one joint in the domains of role physical ($p = 0.025$) and bodily pain ($p = 0.014$) between NSAIDs and selective COX-2 Inhibitors respectively.

Patients with comorbidities scored lower in all domains of SF-36 compared to those without, with significant difference noticed in the role physical domain ($p = 0.001$). Presence of musculoskeletal comorbidity was highly correlated with increased bodily pain ($r = 0.291$) ($p = 0.018$). Patients with other musculoskeletal disorders did not show to be different from those without, except when they were treated with celecoxib, there was a significant difference in the domain of bodily pain, where patient with other musculoskeletal disorders showed better HRQoL compared to those without ($p = 0.009$) (**Table 5**).

4. Discussion

The present study, to the best of our knowledge, is the first known study to examine the effects of different classes of analgesics associated with osteoarthritis on HRQoL of Arabic population. The use of the Medical Outcomes Study SF-36 questionnaire which was used in previous studies in patient with arthritis and it has been shown to has good responsiveness to changes in patients with rheumatic conditions compared with other longer instruments [16] [17], can be considered a strength of the present study. Unlike other instruments used to measure the functional impact of OA such as Western Ontario and MacMaster Universities Osteoarthritis (WOMAC), SF-36 is a multidimensional instrument and allow more global insight and assessment on different components of quality of life particularly in OA patients where comorbidities are common.

Females scored lower in all domains of SF-36 compared to males except for the domain of social functioning, where they showed to have similar quality of life. Many studies have shown that there are differences in HRQoL between the two genders [10] [15] [18] [19]. In general, mental health domains and mental health component

Table 2. Frequencies of types of medications prescribed.

Types of Medications	Frequency		Total	Percent
	Females (n = 151)	Males (n = 49)	Females & Males	(n = 200)
Traditional NSAID's	(n = 69) 45%	(n = 24) 49.0%	93	46.5%
	(n = 62) 31.0%	(n = 19) 38.3%	81	40.5%
Meloxicam 7.5 mg	(n = 3) 1.5%	(n = 2) 4.1%	5	2.5%
Diclofenac 50 mg				
Naproxen 200 mg	(n = 1) 0.7%	(n = 0)	1	0.5%
Ibuprofen 400 mg				
Piroxicam 20 mg	(n = 1) 0.7%	(n = 0)	1	0.5%
	(n = 3) 2.0%	(n = 2) 4.1%	5	2.5%
Selective COX-2 Inhibitors	(n = 81) 40.5%	(n = 26) 13.0%	107	53.5%

Table 3. SF-36 domains and gender (Mean ± SD).

SF-36 Scores	Female (n = 151)	Male (n = 49)
Physical Function	43.36 ± 20.23	49.32 ± 23.284
Role Physical	40.14 ± 26.36	44.50 ± 29.42
Bodily Pain	36.54 ± 16.26	39.67 ± 15.73
General Health	52.04 ± 17.80*	57.91 ± 20.16
Vitality	40.7 ± 18.46*	49.47 ± 22.21
Social Functioning	68.79 ± 27.11	68.87 ± 23.12
Role Emotional	81.00 ± 25.16	82.99 ± 23.87
Mental Health	76.07 ± 17.18**	84.00 ± 15.53
Physical Component	34.62 ± 10.90	34.76 ± 9.77
Mental Component	52.50 ± 9.83*	55.74 ± 9.42

*Note: SF-36 = Short Form-36, NS = Not significant; *$p \leq 0.05$; **$p \leq 0.01$; ***$p \leq 0.001$.*

Table 4. SF-36 Scores and types of medications prescribed (NSAID's Vs. Coxibs). (Mean ± SD).

SF-36 Scores	Traditional NSAIDs (n = 93)	Selective COX-2 Inhibitors (n = 107)
Physical Function	43.65 ± 20.49	45.83 ± 21.68
Role Physical	43.80 ± 27.90	38.96 ± 26.37
Bodily Pain	39.19 ± 17.33	35.67 ± 14.94
General Health	55.75 ± 18.27	51.50 ± 18.60
Vitality	42.71 ± 18.87	42.96 ± 20.57
Social Functioning	69.75 ± 26.15	67.99 ± 26.21
Role Emotional	80.91 ± 25.16	75.70 ± 27.06
Mental Health	80.86 ± 14.82*	75.54 ± 18.57
Physical Component	35.21 ± 10.51	34.16 ± 10.72
Mental Component	54.08 ± 9.85	52.62 ± 9.76

*Note: SF-36 = Short Form-36, NS = Not significant; *$p \leq 0.05$; **$p \leq 0.01$; ***$p \leq 0.001$.*

Table 5. SF-36 domains and presence of comorbidities. (Mean ± SD).

SF-36 Domains	Presence of Comorbidity	Mean	N	Mean
	Non-Musculoskeletal Disorders		**Musculoskeletal Disorders**	
Physical Function	Yes (n = 135)	44.24 ± 21.60	Yes (n = 46)	48.58 ± 21.43
	No (n = 65)	46.02 ± 20.17	No (n = 154)	43.69 ± 20.96
Role Physical	Yes (n = 135)	36.75 ± 26.11***	Yes (n = 46)	42.39 ± 26.83
	No (n = 65)	50.48 ± 27.04	No (n = 154)	40.86 ± 27.29
Bodily Pain	Yes (n = 135)	36.20 ± 15.95	Yes (n = 46)	41.73 ± 14.55**†
	No (n = 65)	39.61 ± 16.45	No (n = 154)	35.98 ± 16.41
General Health	Yes (n = 135)	51.40 ± 18.73	Yes (n = 46)	54.90 ± 15.97
	No (n = 65)	57.80 ± 17.44	No (n = 154)	53.05 ± 19.25
Vitality	Yes (n = 135)	43.03 ± 20.18	Yes (n = 46)	45.38 ± 19.15
	No (n = 65)	42.46 ± 18.99	No (n = 154)	42.09 ± 19.92
Social Functioning	Yes (n = 135)	67.96 ± 26.38	Yes (n = 46)	72.82 ± 24.33
	No (n = 65)	70.57 ± 25.71	No (n = 154)	67.61 ± 2 6.60
Role Emotional	Yes (n = 135)	78.20 ± 26.31	Yes (n = 46)	81.34 ± 24.03
	No (n = 65)	77.94 ± 26.37	No (n = 154)	77.16 ± 26.89
Mental Health	Yes (n = 135)	77.55 ± 17.65	Yes (n = 46)	78.55 ± 17.09
	No (n = 65)	78.98 ± 15.99	No (n = 154)	77.85 ± 17.16
Physical Component	Yes (n = 135)	34.17 ± 11.86	Yes (n = 46)	35.64 ± 9.90
	No (n = 65)	35.65 ± 7.35	No (n = 154)	34.35 ± 10.82
Mental Component	Yes (n = 135)	52.99 ± 9.99	Yes (n = 46)	53.85 ± 9.31
	No (n = 65)	53.93 ± 9.46	No (n = 154)	53.13 ± 9.97

Note: *SF-36 = Short Form -36, NS = Not significant*; $^{*}p \leq 0.05$; $^{**}p \leq 0.01$; $^{***}p \leq 0.001$; †: Only with Celecoxib.

(mental health, role emotional, social functioning & vitality) were better and less affected than physical health domains (physical functioning, role physical and bodily pain) for both genders, confirming the findings of the previous studies [10] [11].

We found significant difference between females and males in the domains of general health, mental health and Mental Component Summary. This can be explained by previous findings that emphasized on the biological and psychological differences between women and men [18]. This is can be of clinical importance since OA is more common in women than men. Our findings also suggest that females received analgesics more frequently than males, more specifically celecoxib. Previous conducted studies showed that there is a difference in prescribing patterns between the two genders, and they showed that women were significantly more likely to be prescribed an NSAID than men [6] [20].

Our results also suggest that compared to COX-2 inhibitors, NSAIDs treated patients scored higher on all domains of SF-36 except physical functioning, but the difference was not significant. However, we found significant difference between the two groups in the domain of mental health favoring NSAIDs. We found one study that conducted direct comparison between traditional NSAIDs and selective COX-2 inhibitors in terms of measuring HRQoL [12]. The study assessed the functional status and HRQoL of elderly osteoarthritis patients and showed improvement of HRQoL for both groups, on traditional NSAIDs naproxen and on celecoxib but could not find any significant difference between the two groups, confirming our results [12].

In terms of individual NASIDs, we found that meloxicam 7.5 mg once daily, showed to have better effect when compared to celecoxib 200 mg once daily in the domains of general health and mental health. We also found significant difference between diclofenac 50 mg twice daily and celecoxib 200 mg once daily in the domain of bodily pain where diclofenac had better effect than celecoxib. We found no difference between meloxicam 7.5 mg once daily and the other NSAIDs used in the present study. This can be explained by the fact that meloxicam was the most traditional NSAIDs prescribed in our study and that other NSAIDs were marginally prescribed limiting our ability to detect any significant differences. That was the most common prescribing trend followed in the study setting despite the fact that meloxicam was shown to be marginally inferior to other traditional NSAIDs for providing pain relief & for the symptomatic treatment of OA [21] [22]. Even though, we can attribute such trend in prescribing to the findings of different clinical trials that showed that meloxicam is associated with fewer endoscopic gastrointestinal ulcers and clinical and complicated upper gastrointestinal (UGI) events than non-selective NSAIDs, and thus more tolerated and accepted by the patients, although only the difference in clinical upper gastrointestinal events (peptic ulcer) reached statistical significance [21] [22].

With respect to the selective COX-2 inhibitors, celecoxib and etoricoxib are the only two medications in this class available in the UAE market. However, celecoxib was the only one available in the study hospital setting. We found that celecoxib was only better than NSAIDs in osteoarthritis patients with other comorbid musculoskeletal disorders. The difference was noticed only in the domain of bodily pain. This is probably can be explained by that such group of patients apparently required more analgesics and they were the most to benefit from their medications especially with an analgesic that is well tolerated by the patients . That was once reported in one of the studies but the effect was shown for NSAIDs [3], however, in that study, they did not include patients on selective COX-2 inhibitors which may explain the variances. *Erich* and co-workers reported that rofecoxib (COX-2 Inhibitors ,withdrawn 2004) treatment increased physical and mental HRQoL domain scores on the SF-36 when compared with placebo and they claimed that the improvements in mental health with rofecoxib use primarily resulted from effective treatment of OA (*i.e.*, reduction in pain and improvement in physical function) [11].

Our findings also suggest that females had more comorbidities compared to males, and they scored lower in all domains of HRQoL, especially the role physical domain where they showed significant difference. These results are independent of the fact that we have recruited more females than males and has been considered statistically. Studies focusing on comorbidity in OA patients showed that chronic conditions, such as hypertension, cardiovascular diseases, obesity, respiratory diseases and diabetes can be found alongside OA [23]. Previous studies showed that an increased prevalence of comorbidities was linked to a poorer HRQoL (SF-36 and WOMAC) [3] [6] [10]. On the other hand, one study showed no significant association between presence of comorbidity and HRQoL domains except for social functioning domain [6].

5. Limitations

A limitation of the present study that might has a potential impact on the results and that should be addressed in future studies is the rather heterogeneous sample of patients with regard to OA site; enrollment of a minority of patients with shoulder & foot OA, thus limiting the generalizability of the results to these groups of patients. Future studies to investigate whether a specific site of OA would have any substantial effects on patients' HRQoL are encouraged.

6. Conclusion

Because there is no disease modifying treatments for osteoarthritis, reducing the pain severity and improving the HRQoL become the main goals of the disease management [16] [24]. Females were found to have poorer HRQoL compared to their male peers. Our findings suggest that NSAIDs-treated patients did not differ significantly from celecoxib-treated patients in all domains of the SF-36 except for the mental health domain. Mental health domains were shown to be better compared to physical health domains including physical functioning and bodily pain. Meloxicam 7.5 mg once daily was associated with better HRQoL in the domains of general health and mental health compared to celecoxib.

Acknowledgements

The authors acknowledge the valuable support and collaboration of Dr. Assam Yahya, Senior Consultant Orthopaedic Surgeon and the head of Joint and Reconstruction Unit at Al Qassimi Hospital and Dr. Dalia Moustafa Abo-Raya, Specialist Clinical Pharmacist, Deputy Head Drug Information Department at Al Qassimi Hospital in performing this study at Al-Qassimi Hospital—Sharjah—United Arab Emirates.

References

[1]   Bryant, D. and Alldred, A. (2007) Rheumatoid Arthritis and Osteoarthritis. In: Walker, R. and Whittlesea, C., Eds., *Clinical Pharmacy and Therapeutics*, 4th Edition, Churchill Livingstone, China, 759-773.

[2]   Majani, G., Giardini, A. and Scotti, A. (2005) Subjective Impact of Osteoarthritis Flare-Ups on Patients' Quality of Life. *Health and Quality of Life Outcomes*, **3**, 14. http://dx.doi.org/10.1186/1477-7525-3-14

[3]   Rabenda, V., Burlet, N., Ethgen, O., Raeman, F., Belaiche, J. and Reginster, J. (2005) A Naturalistic Study of the Determinants of Health Related Quality of Life Improvement in Osteoarthritic Patients Treated with Non-Specific Non-Steroidal Anti-Inflammatory Drugs. *Annals of the Rheumatic Diseases*, **64**, 688-693. http://dx.doi.org/10.1136/ard.2004.026658

[4]   Geba, G., Weaver, A., Polis, A., Dixon, M., Schnitzer, T., *et al.* (2002) Efficacy of Rofecoxib, Celecoxib, and Acetaminophen in Osteoar Thritis of the Knee. *JAMA: The Journal of the American Medical Association*, **287**, 64-71. http://dx.doi.org/10.1001/jama.287.1.64

[5]   Breedveld, F. (2004) Osteoarthritis—The Impact of a Serious Disease. *Rheumatology*, **43**, i4-i8. http://dx.doi.org/10.1093/rheumatology/keh102

[6]   Zakaria, Z., Bakar, A., Hasmoni, H., Rani, F. and Kadir, S. (2009) Health-Related Quality of Life in Patients with Knee Osteoarthritis Attending Two Primary Care Clinics in Malaysia: A Cross-Sectional Study. *Asia Pacific Family Medicine*, **8**, 10. http://dx.doi.org/10.1186/1447-056X-8-10

[7]   Wiklund, I. (1999) Quality of Life in Arthritis Patients Using Nonsteroidal Anti-Inflammatory Drugs. *Canadian Journal of Gastroenterology*, **13**, 129.

[8]   Weiner, D. (2007) Office Management of Chronic Pain in the Elderly. *The American Journal of Medicine*, **120**, 306-315. http://dx.doi.org/10.1016/j.amjmed.2006.05.048

[9]   Bijlsma, J., Berenbaum, F. and Lafeber, F. (2011) Osteoarthritis: An Update with Relevance for Clinical Practice. *The Lancet*, **377**, 2115-2126. http://dx.doi.org/10.1016/S0140-6736(11)60243-2

[10]   Briggs, A., Scott, E. and Steele, K. (1999) Impact of Osteoarthritis and Analgesic Treatment on Quality of Life of an Elderly Population. *Annals of Pharmacotherapy*, **33**, 1154-1159. http://dx.doi.org/10.1345/aph.18411

[11]   Dominick, K.L., Ahern, F.M., Gold, C.H. and Heller, D.A. (2004) Health-Related Quality of Life and Health Service Use among Older Adults with Osteoarthritis. *Arthritis Care & Research*, **51**, 326-331. http://dx.doi.org/10.1002/art.20390

[12]   Lisse, J., Espinoza, L., Zhao, S., Dedhiya, S. and Osterhaus, J. (2001) Functional Status and Health-Related Quality of Life of Elderly Osteoarthritic Patients Treated with Celecoxib. *The Journals of Gerontology: Series A: Biological Sciences and Medical Sciences*, **56**, M167-M175. http://dx.doi.org/10.1093/gerona/56.3.M167

[13]   Brazier, J., Harper, R., Walters, S., Munro, J. and Sanith, M. (1999) Generic and Condition-Specific Outcome Measures for People with Osteoarthritis of the Knee. *Rheumatology*, **38**, 870-877. http://dx.doi.org/10.1093/rheumatology/38.9.870

[14]   Arthritis.ae. Emirates Arthritis Foundation (2013) http://www.arthritis.ae/index.php

[15]   Rosemann, T., Laux, G. and Szecsenyi, J. (2007) Osteoarthritis: Quality of Life, Comorbidities, Medication and Health Service Utilization Assessed in a Large Sample of Primary Care Patients. *Journal of Orthopaedic Surgery and Research*, **2**, 12. http://dx.doi.org/10.1186/1749-799X-2-12

[16]   Bakas, T., Mclennon, S., Carpenter, J., Buelow, J., Otte, J., Hanna, K., Ellett, M., Hadler, K. and Welch, J. (2012) Systematic Review of Health-Related Quality of Life Models. *Health and Quality of Life Outcomes*, **10**, 134. http://dx.doi.org/10.1186/1477-7525-10-134

[17]   Angst, F., Aeschlimann, A., Steiner, W. and Stucki, G. (2001) Responsiveness of the WOMAC Osteoarthritis Index as Compared with the SF-36 in Patients with Osteoarthritis of the Legs Undergoing a Comprehensive Rehabilitation Intervention. *Annals of the Rheumatic Diseases*, **60**, 834-840.

[18]   Woo, J., Lau, E., Lee, P., Kwok, T., Lau, W., Chan, C., Chiu, P., Li, E., Sham, A. and Lam, D. (2004) Impact of Osteoarthritis on Quality of Life in a Hong Kong Chinese Population. *The Journal of Rheumatology*, **31**, 2433-2438.

[19]   Leveille, S., Zhang, Y., Mcmullen, W., Kelly-Hayes, M. and Felson, D. (2005) Sex Differences in Musculoskeletal Pain in Older Adults. *Pain*, **116**, 332-338. http://dx.doi.org/10.1016/j.pain.2005.05.002

[20]   Dominick, K.L., Ahern, F.M., Gold, C.H. and Heller, D. (2003) Gender Differences in NSAID Use among Older

Adults with Osteoarthritis. *Annals of Pharmacotherapy*, **37**, 1566-1571. http://dx.doi.org/10.1345/aph.1C418

[21] Chen, Y., Jobanputra, P., Barton, P., Bryan, S., Fry-Smith, A., Harris, G. and Taylor, R. (2008) Cyclooxygenase-2 Selective Non-Steroidal Anti-Inflammatory Drugs (Etodolac, Meloxicam, Celecoxib, Rofecoxib, Etoricoxib, Valdecoxib and Lumiracoxib) for Osteoarthritis and Rheumatoid Arthritis: A Systematic Review and Economic Evaluation. NIHR Evaluation, Trials and Studies Coordinating Centre (UK).

[22] Yocum, D., Fleischmann, R., Dalgin, P., Caldwell, J., Hall, D. and Roszko, P. (2000) Safety and Efficacy of Meloxicam in the Treatment of Osteoarthritis: A 12-Week, Double-Blind, Multiple-Dose, Placebo-Controlled Trial. *JAMA Internal Medicine*, **160**, 2947-2954. http://dx.doi.org/10.1001/archinte.160.19.2947

[23] Van Dijk, G.M., Veenhof, C., Schellevis, F., Hulsmans, H., Bakker, J.P., Arwert, H., Dekker, J.H., Lankhorst, G.J. and Dekker, J. (2008) Comorbidity, Limitations in Activities and Pain in Patients with Osteoarthritis of the Hip or Knee. *BMC Musculoskeletal Disorders*, **9**, 95. http://dx.doi.org/10.1186/1471-2474-9-95

[24] Centers for Disease Control and Prevention (2000) Measuring Healthy Days: Population Assessment of Health-Related Quality of Life. Centers for Disease Control and Prevention, Atlanta.

List of Abbreviations

BMI: Body Mass Index
COX-2: Cyclo-oxygenase 2
EAF: Emirates Arthritis Foundation
HRQoL: Health Related Quality of Life
NSAIDs: Nonsteroidal Anti-inflammatory Drugs
OA: Osteoarthritis
SF-36: Short Form-36
SPSS: Statistical Package for Social Science
SD: Standard Deviation.
UGI: Upper Gastrointestinal
UAE: United Arab Emirates
WHO: World Health Organization.
WOMAC: Western Ontario and MacMaster Universities Osteoarthritis 14

9

Formulation Development of Generic Omeprazole 20 mg Enteric Coated Tablets

Christopher Oswald Migoha[1,2], Eliangiringa Kaale[2], Godliver Kagashe[3]

[1]Tanzania Food and Drugs Authority, Dar es Salaam, Tanzania
[2]Pharm R&D Lab, School of Pharmacy, Muhimbili University of Health and Allied Sciences, Dar es Salaam, Tanzania
[3]Department of Pharmaceutics , School of Pharmacy, Muhimbili University of Health and Allied Sciences, Dar es Salaam, Tanzania
Email: christophermigoha@yahoo.com

Abstract

Omeprazole is a potent proton pump inhibitor with powerful inhibition of secretion of gastric juice. Oral site-specific drug delivery systems have recently attracted a great interest for the local treatment of bowel disease and for improving systemic absorption of drugs which are unstable in the stomach. However, microenvironment in the gastrointestinal tract and varying absorption mechanisms cause hindrance for the formulation and optimization of oral drug delivery. The objective of the study was to develop and optimize enteric coating process for omeprazole tablets. Different batches of core tablets were sub coated, one set sub coated with opadry and another with a mixture of light magnesium oxide, magnesium stearate and absolute alcohol omeprazole magnesium. Seal coating was applied by using opadry to achieve certain weight gain and to protect omeprazole from acidic coating polymers. A comparative dissolution test was performed. The variation of thickness and diameter were observed to be minimal with a weight gain of 3% - 4% of enteric polymer. Disintegration test showed that in each tested batch the enteric coated layer remained intact in 0.1N HCl for 2 hours and when exposed to alkaline media of phosphate buffer pH 6.8, it dissolved within few minutes. Dissolution release was 98.8% to 102.4% within two hours when the product was exposed to phosphate buffer pH 6.8 after 2 hours. The similarity and dissimilarity factors were calculated and observed to be 54 to 61 and 4 to 5 respectively. Therefore a simple and good enteric coating process was developed and tested with potential for transfer this technology into local pharmaceutical industries using cheap and easily available materials.

Keywords

Omeprazole Magnesium, Enteric Coating, Tablets, Kollicoat (Methacrylic Acid/Ethyl Acrylate

Copolymers) (MAE)

1. Introduction

Omeprazole, 5-methoxy-2(((4-methoxy-3,5-dimethyl-2-pyridinyl)methyl)sulfinyl)-1H-benzimidazole (**Figure 1**), is a potent inhibitor of gastric acid secretion. It shows powerful inhibitory action against secretion of gastric juice and is used in treatment of duodenal and gastric ulcers [1]. However, omeprazole is susceptible to degradation/transformation in acid reacting and neural media [1].

The *in vitro* degradation of omeprazole is catalyzed by acidic compounds and is stabilized in mixtures with alkaline compounds. Moisture and organic solvents also affect the stability of omeprazole. From the data of stability studies of omeprazole, it is obvious that an oral dosage form must be protected from contact with acid gastric juice in order to reach the small intestine without degradation [1]-[3].

Human pharmacological studies showed that the rate of release of omeprazole from solid dosage form could influence the total extent of absorption of omeprazole to the general circulation [2]. A fully bioavailable dosage form of omeprazole must release the active drug rapidly in the proximal part of gastrointestinal canal [2].

The pharmaceutical dosage form with property of protecting omeprazole from contact with gastric acid must be developed, that is core. The core must be enteric coated. The core developed must be alkaline in nature as most of available acid compounds will not favor stability of omeprazole [4].

Coating polymer, such as Eudragit L 30, hydroxyl propyl methyl cellulose phthalate, cellulose acetate phthalate and acryl EZE® (Aqueous Acrylic Enteric System), to achieve 5% weight gain may be considered [5]. This is due to the fact that they permit the dissolution of the coating and the active drug contained in the core once in the proximal part of the small intestine. They also allow some diffusion of water of gastric acid through them into the cores, at the time when the dosage form resides in the stomach before it is emptied into the small intestine [5] [6].

It is expected that the diffused water of gastric juice will dissolve parts of the core in the close proximity of the enteric coating layer and form an alkaline solution in the coated dosage form. The alkaline solution is expected to interfere with the enteric coating and eventually dissolve it [6].

2. Materials and Methods

2.1. Equipments

The equipments include: Tabular mixer (Analytical Technology, Bangalore, India), Korsh EK 01 tablet press machine (Germany), auto coater (Glatt, Germany), Monsanto type tablet hardness tester (IEC, Mumbai, India), Roche Fribilator (electro lab, Bangalore, India), single pan balance (Shimadzu,AX200, Japan), Disintegration Apparatus USP (Elecrolab, Bangalore, India), graduated cylinder (Fisher Scientific, Germany), sieve analyzer (Endecott's, Germany), glass bottles (Fisher Scientific, Germany), HPLC (Shimazdu, Japan), ERWEKA TBH machine (Heusenstamm, Germany), Dissolution Test Apparatus (Elecro Lab, TDT-08L, Mumbai, India.

2.2. Materials

The materials include: Omeprazole magnesium (Metrochem API Private Limited, Hyderabad, India), Sodium laurl sulphate (LOBA Chemie Pvt. Ltd., Mumbai, India), Lactose (OXFORD Laboratories, Mumbai, India), Avicel ph 102 (Shandong Liaocheng Ehua Medicine Co. Ltd., Shandong, China), Maize starch (OXFORD Laboratories,

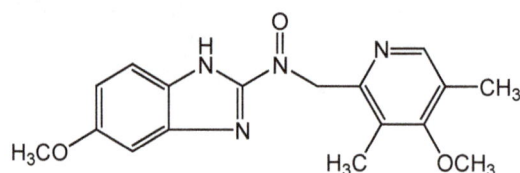

Figure 1. Structure of Omeprazole.

Mumbai, India), Water aerosil 200 (Shandong Liaocheng Ehua Medicine Co. Ltd., Shandong, China) and Magnesium stearate (Hozhou Zhanwang Pharmaceutical Co. Ltd., Huzhou, China), Kollicoat® MAE Polymers (BASF, Germany). Other reagents and solvents were procured commercially and were of pharmaceutical and analytical grade. Application of the entire materials (Active ingredient and excipients) has been described in **Table 1**.

In vitro analysis of the prepared tablets was carried out as per the requirements of enteric coated tablets as specified in official pharmacopoeia [7].

2.3. Experimental Methods

2.3.1. Preparation of Core Tablets

Since omeprazole magnesium is moisture sensitive material, all the processing steps including weighing, mixing, direct compression and coating was carried out at 30°C ± 2°C and 60% ± 5% RH [8].

The materials for preparation of core tablets for three different as listed in **Table 2** were accurately weighed and then sodium laurly sulphate was sieved through 0.5 mm sieve. Omeprazole magnesium, sodium laurly sulphate and maize starch together were placed in a tubular mixer and mixed for 10 minutes. Another mixture of maize starch, Lactose and water aerosil 200 were place in a tubular mixer and mixed for 10 minutes and then the two mixtures together with magnesium stearate was sieved through 0.8 sieves and mixed for 5 minutes. Thereafter the mixtures were compressed in Korsh EK 01 Tablet press machine using 9 mm-R15 punch to form tablets. Three batches were prepared for each formulation.

Table 1. Formulation ingredients of Omeprazole 20 mg enteric coated tablets.

Category	Ingredients	Application
Core Tablets Ingredients		
	Omeprazole Magnesium	Active
	Sodium Lauryl Sulphate	Lubricant
	Tablottose (Lactose)	Binder
	Avicel ph 102	Disintegrant
	Maize starch	Diluent
	Water Aerosil 200	Glidant
	Magnesium Stearate	Lubricant
Sub Coating I Ingredients		
	OPADRY White (HPMC)	
	Phosphate Buffer pH	
Sub Coating II Ingredients		
	Cellular Powder	Water Insoluble Polymer
	Light Magnesium Oxide	Stabilizer/Alkalizer
	Magnesium Stearate	Anti-Sticking Agent
	Absolute Alcohol	Solvent
Enteric Coating Ingredients		
	Kollicoat MAE 30 DP*	Enteric Coating Polymer
	Propylene Gycol	Plasticizer
	Water	Solvent

*Kollicoat MAE 30 DP is Methacrylic acid copolymer.

2.3.2. In Process Quality Control (IPQC) of Core Tables

Before sub coating of core tablets, IPQC tests was conducted. The parameters tested were weight variation, thickness, diameter, hardness, friability and disintegration time as per USP Pharmacopoeia [7].

2.3.3. Sub Coating of Core Tablets

Sub coating was done for the purpose of acting as moisture barrier to core tablet and preventing interaction between acidic labile omeprazole and acidic enteric coating material. Two sets of sub coating materials were considered (**Sub coating I and Sub coating II**) as depicted in **Table 1** and **Table 2**. The Sub Coating material for I was prepared by weighed 2.5 mg of OPADRY and dissolved it in phosphate buffer pH 7.4 to obtain 0.25% w/v of OPADRY solution. The obtained solution was atomized from the top of the apparatus for coating of tablets with coating parameters shown in **Table 3**. The materials for preparation of **Sub coating II** were dispensed as depicted in **Table 1** and **Table 2** and dissolved in absolute alcohol. The mixture was stirred for 45 minutes till homogenous suspension was obtained and sifted through 0.5 sieve then sub coating was done as per set parameters in **Table 3**. The sub coating for those tablets was done in Glatt auto coater.

2.3.4. Enteric Coating of Sub-Coated Tablets

Enteric coating of sub coated tablets was done after accurately weighed ingredients of coating materials as depicted in **Table 1** and **Table 2**. Propylene glycol was first dissolved in specified amount of water followed by stirring. Then Kollicoat MAE 30 DP was added while stirring. Machine parameters were as in **Table 4**. Sub

Table 2. Formulations details of Omeprazole 20 mg enteric coated tablets.

Formulations	OME 001	OME 002	OME 003	OME 004	OME 005	OME 006
Core Tablets Ingredients (mg)						
Omeprazole Magnesium	20.0	20.0	20.0	20.0	20.0	20.0
Sodium Lauryl Sulphate	2.0	2.0	1.9	2.0	1.9	2.1
Tablottose (Lactose)	76.0	76.0	76.0	76.0	76.0	76.0
Avicel ph 102	60.0	60.0	60.0	60.0	60.0	60.0
Maize starch						
Water Aerosil 200	0.6	0.6	0.6	0.6	0.6	0.6
Magnesium Stearate	1.4	1.4	1.4	1.4	1.4	1.4
Sub Coating 1 Ingredients						
OPADRY White (HPMC)	0.008	0.008	0.008	0.008	0.008	0.008
Phosphate Buffer pH	QS	QS	QS	QS	QS	QS
Sub Coating II Igredients						
Cellulose Powder	0.96	0.96	0.96	0.96	0.96	0.96
Light Magnesium Oxide	0.77	0.77	0.77	0.77	0.77	0.77
Magnesium Stearate	0.77	0.77	0.77	0.77	0.77	0.77
Absolute Alcohol	QS	QS	QS	QS	QS	QS
Enteric Coating Material						
Kollicoat MAE 30 DP[*]	70%	70%	70%	70%	70%	70%
Propylene glycol	4.2%	4.2%	4.2%	4.2%	4.2%	4.2%
Water	25.8%	25.8%	25.8%	25.8%	25.8%	25.8%

[*]Kollicoat MAE 30 DP is Methacrylic acid copolymer.

Table 3. Process Parameters to be controlled during sub coating.

Process Parameters	Formulation I	Formulation II
Pan speed	2 RPM	2 RPM
Inlet air temperature	40°C ± 5°C	50°C ± 5°C
Outlet air temperature	30°C ± 5°C	40°C ± 5°C
Air volume	360 m²/h	360 m²/h
Nozzle diameter	1.0 mm	1.0 mm
Atomizing air pressure	2.0 bar	2.0 bar
Spraying rate	1.5 ml/min	1 gm/min
Coating level	3%	3%

Table 4. Process parameters to be controlled during enteric coating.

Process Parameters	Set Limit
Pan speed	2 RPM
Inlet air temperature	50°C ± 5°C
Outlet air temperature	30°C ± 5°C
Air volume	360 m²/h
Nozzle diameter	1.0 mm
Atomizing air pressure	2.0 bar
Spraying rate	30 - 35 g/min (1.5 ml/Min)
Coating level	3% - 4%

coated tablets were pre heated in coating pan for 10 minutes at 40°C ± 5°C. The tablets were coated in Glatt auto coater to achieve 3% to 4% weight gain.

2.3.5. Evaluation of Coated Tablets

Enteric coated tablets of omeprazole were evaluated for weight variation, Thickness, Diameter, Hardness, Friability and Disintegration time as per USP Pharmacopoeia. The formulations assessed by content uniformity test and dissolution testing by USP Type I Basket apparatus at 100 RPM in 900 ml of 0.1 N HCl for 120 minutes and afterwards in phosphate buffer of 6.8 for 60 minutes [7].

3. Results and Discussion

All of the studied physical properties were within the acceptable range with narrow variation and complied with the pharmacopoeia specifications for both core and coated tablets. The parameters tested were diameter, hardness, friability and weight variation. The shape and the size of tablets for all batches were found to be within the acceptable limit. For core tablets diameter for all tablets range between 9.37 to 9.39 mm and hardness of all formulations lies within the range of 66 to 68 N. All formulations passes friability test as the percentage weight loss was within pharmacopeia limit, *i.e.* NMT 1%. The weight variation and drug content of all the formulations were found to be within the acceptable limit.

For coated tablets, three batches were taken and each was divided into two batches, *i.e.* OME 001, OME 002 & OME 003 divided into OME 001A, OME 001B, OME 002A, OME 002B, OME 003A and OME 003B. Where the A ones were of sub-coated I and of B were of sub-coated II. There was a weight gain of 3% - 4% of the enteric polymer. The thickness and diameter of 20 coated tablets from each formulation was determined using ERWEKA TBH machine and average value were calculated and evaluated as per USP 30. The hardness of tablets ranges from 67 N to 73 N. The variation of thickness and diameter was observed to be minimal. The percentage of friability of tablets ranges from 0.339% to 0.468% which was in acceptable range. The percentage of drug content of the formulated tablets when assayed was 100.1% to 105.9% which is within specification. Results showed no significant differences. Results for evaluation of core tablets are summarized in **Table 6**.

3.1. In Process Quality Control (IPQC) Tests for Core Tablets

Tablets were prepared by direct compression technique. The results of in process quality control tests are listed in **Table 5** and they show that the product was firm enough to withstand handling without breaking and not so hard that the disintegration time can be prolonged. Therefore all batches are considered to be optimized core tablets for further experiment.

3.2. Evaluation of Coated Tablets

The friability results of coated tablets indicate good mechanical resistance of tablets. Results showed no significant differences. Results for evaluation of coated tablets are summarized in **Table 6**.

Disintegration Test show that in all six tablets in each tested batch the enteric coated layer remained intact in 0.1N HCl for 2 hours but there were few signs of cracking and little swelling observed. The enteric coating layer of tablets started to imbibe the alkaline media of phosphate buffer pH 6.8 and completely removed approximately at 30 minutes and afterwards tablets were completely dissolved within 50 minutes.

3.3. *In Vitro* Drug Release

The *in vitro* dissolution of all formulated batches (*i.e.* OME 001A, OME 002A, OME 003A, OME 001B, OME 002B & OME 003B) was studied in 0.1N HCl for 2 hours and 1 hour in phosphate buffer pH 6.8. The results observed showed that for all batches there was physical resistance to the acid medium with few signs of cracking and swelling and the drug released after two hours was found to be within specified limit (**Table 7** and **Figure 2**).

Table 5. Evaluation test of Omeprazole core tablets.

Batches	Diameter (mm)	Thickness (mm)	Friability (%)	Hardness (N)	Weight uniformity (mg)	Assay (%)	Disintegration time (Min)
OME 001	9.37 ± 0.03	4.28 ± 0.11	0.369	66.75	221.55 ± 6	105.2 ± 1.1	NMT 5
OME 002	9.37 ± 0.03	4.28 ± 0.14	0.387	59.9	221.55 ± 5	104.5 ± 1.1	NMT6
OME 003	9.38 ± 0.05	4.28 ± 0.11	0.339	67	221.55 ± 5	105.2 ± 1.1	NMT 5
OME 004	9.38 ± 0.05	4.28 ± 0.11	0.350	70	221.55 ± 5	105.9 ± 0.1	NMT 7
OME 005	9.37 ± 0.03	4.28 ± 0.11	0.386	68	221.55 ± 6	99 ± 1.1	NMT6
OME 006	9.37 ± 0.03	4.28 ± 0.11	0.370	60	221.55 ± 7.	99 ± 1.1	NMT 5

NB: All values are expressed as mean ± SD (n = 20).

Table 6. Evaluation test of Omeprazole enteric coated tablets.

IPQC Parameters	OME 001A	OME 001B	OME 002A	OME 002B	OME00 3A	OME 00 3B
Diameter (mm)	9.4 ± 0.05	9.42 ± 0.05	9.38 ± 0.05	9.3 ± 0.05	9.41 ± 0.06	9.48 ± 0.06
Thickness (mm)	5.77 ± 0.11	5.78 ± 0.11	6.02 ± 0.10	6.0 ± 0.10	5.97 ± 0.11	5.90 ± 0.11
Friability (5)	0.369	0.387	0.339	0.350	0.468	0.384
Hardness (N)	69	70	67	73	68	72
Weight uniformity	229.6 ± 10	231.3 ± 10	231.1 ± 10	231.9 ± 10	231.8 ± 10	231.7 ± 10
Assay (%)	105.2 ± 1.1	104.5 ± 0.0	105.5 ± 0.1	105.9 ± 0.1	100.1 ± 0.3	100.1 ± 0.3

NB: All values are expressed as mean ± SD (n = 20).

Table 7. Drug release profile.

% Drug Release	OME 001A	OME 002A	OME 003A	OME 001B	OME 002B	OME 003B
0.1N HCl within 2 Hrs	0.00	0.00	0.00	0.00	0.00	0.00
Phosphate buffer pH 6.8 after 2 Hrs						
02:10	34.07	22.18	23.08	68.9	70.2	93.0
02:20	52.99	35.88	37.07	78.8	79.23	95.0
02:40	72.03	52.78	53.57	90.25	91.45	98.3
02:50	86.5	77.05	78.68	98.9	99.1	101.3
03:00	98.8	99.1	99.1	100.82	101.3	102.4

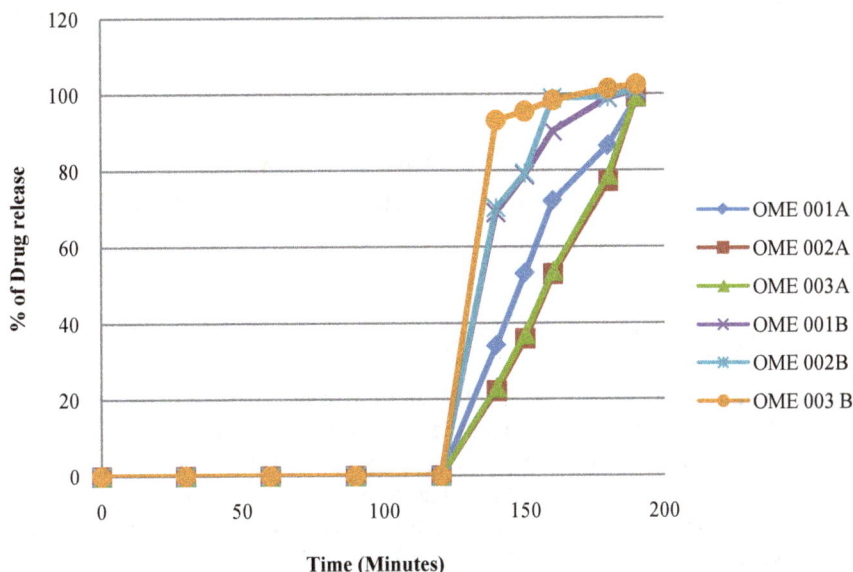

Figure 2. Drug release profile of formulated omeprazole enteric coated tablets in 0.1N HCL and phosphate buffer 6.8.

Therefore all batches were selected as optimized batches because they have shown better drug release even though the formulation sub coated with opadry solution has a better dissolution profile *i.e.* OME 001 - 003A and consumed less concentration of enteric coating polymer.

3.4. Comparison of Developed Generic Omeprazole Magnesium Enteric Coated with Marketed Products

The selected batches *i.e.* OME 001 and OME 002 were compared with Pilorsec capsules 20 mg and Losec Mups 20 mg. Pilorsec capsules was dropped from the study after the capsules dissolved immediately in the acid and noted that omeprazole powder and sodium bicarbonate was present in the capsules without any protection. The disintegration time and release profile of selected formulations and Losec is given in **Table 8**. From the results it was concluded that the formulated generic products had similar disintegration profile, drug content and percentage release with marketed product.

3.5. Similarity and Dissimilarity Studies

The Similarity Factor (F_2 value) and Dissimilarity Factor (F_1) were calculated using equation of similarity by using a simple model independent approach to compare dissolution profile between Formulated products OME 001A & OME 002B and marketed product Losec MUPS 20 mg [9]. The equations used were as follows:

Table 8. Dissolution test profile of prepared formulations with Losec Mups 20 mg.

Time (Minutes)	0	30	60	90	120	130	140	150	160	180	190
OME 001A	0	0	0	0	0	58	85.9	94.5	98.4	99.8	101.1
OME 001B	0	0	0	0	0	45	87	96	99	99.5	100.82
Losec Mups	0	0	0	0	0	72	88.2	96	98.7	99.3	100

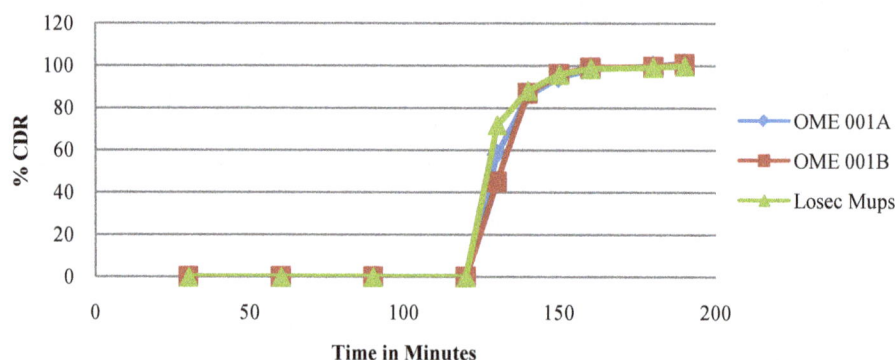

Figure 3. Comparative release profile between Losec Mups, OME 001A & OME 001B.

1) $F_1 = \left\{ \left[S_{t=1}^{n}\left(R_t - T_t\right) \right] / \left[S_{t=1}^{n} R_t \right] \right\} * 100$

2) $F_2 = 50\log\left\{ \left[1 + (1/n) S^{t=1n}\left(R_t - T_t\right)^2 \right]^{-0.5} * 100 \right\}$

By using the formula [10], F_2 value was calculate and found to be 61 for OME 001A and 54 for comparison with OME 002B. Therefore the F_2 values ensure the sameness or equivalence of two curves. The respective F_1 values were found to be 4 and 5 respectively. Using the mean dissolution values from the two curves at each time interval the different factor F_1 and similarity Factor F_2 were calculated using the above equations, the results showed that the curves were similar to F_1 which were close to zero *i.e.* between 0 and 15 and F_2 values close to 100 as the values were greater than 50 (**Figure 3**).

4. Conclusion

A simple and good enteric coated omeprazole magnesium tablets with potential for transfer into local industries in Tanzania was developed and tested. Opadry white coating (HPMC) (**Sub-coating I**) and a mixture of cellulose powder, light magnesium oxide, magnesium stearate and absolute alcohol (**Sub-coating II**) were used for sub-coating. The enteric coating was successfully done by using Kollicoat® Methacrylic acid AE 30 DP (Methacrylic acid/ethyl acrylate copolymers) which is an aqueous dispersion.

Acknowledgements

Migoha C.O is thankful to Tanzania Food & Drugs Authority for sponsoring the programme and for providing necessary facilities to carry out analysis work at its laboratory, also the School of Pharmacy for providing required facilities to carry out formulation development of the product.

Conflict of Interests

The authors declare that they have no conflict of interests regarding the publication of this article.

References

[1]   Blanchi, A., Delchier, J.C., Soule, J.C., Payen, D. and Bader, J.P. (1982) Control of Acute Zollinger-Ellison Syndrome with Intravenous Omeprazole. *Lancet*, **2**, 1223-1224.

[2]   Wurster, D.E. (1957) U.S Patent 2,799,241. Wisconsin Almini Research Foundation.

[3]   Wurster, D.E. (1959) Air-Suspension Technique of Coating Drug Particles. A Preliminary Report. *Journal of the American Pharmaceutical Association*, **48**, 451-454. http://dx.doi.org/10.1002/jps.3030480808

[4]   Hardman, J.G., Limburd, L.E., Molinoff, P.B., Ruddon, R.W. and Gilman, A.G. (Eds.) (1996) Goodman & Gilman's The Pharmacological Basis of Therapeutics. 9th Edition, McGraw-Hill, New York.

[5]   Nair, A.B., Gupta, R., Kumria, R., Jacob, S. and Attimarad, M. (2010) Formulation and Evaluation of Enteric Coated Tablets of Proton Pump Inhibitors. *Journal of Basic and Clinical Pharmacy*, **1**, 215-221.

[6]   Mäder, K., Bräunig, K., Meyer, K. and Kolter, K. (2005) Development and Stability Studies of Enteric Omeprazole Formulations Based on Kollicoat® MAE Polymers. BASF Aktiengesellschaft, Development Pharma Ingredients, Ludwigshafen.

[7]   United States Pharmacopoeia (USP) 30NF25.

[8]   http://www.pharmpedia.com/Tablet:Tablet_coating

[9]   Mukharya, A., Chaudhary, S., Bheda, A., Mulay, A., Mansuri, N. and Laddh, N. (2011) Stable and Bioequivalent Formulation Development of Highly Acid Labile Proton Pump Inhibitor: Rabeprazole. *International Journal of Pharmaceutical Research and Innovation*, **2**, 1-8.

[10]   FDA (2000) Guidance for Industry: Waiver of *in Vivo* Bioavailability and Bioequivalence Studies for Immediate-Release Solid Oral dosage Forms Based on a Biopharmaceutics Classification System.

10

Partitioning Behavior of Gemifloxacin in Anionic, Cationic and Nonanionic Surfactants. Calculation of Dermal Permeability Coefficient

Theophilus C. Onyekaba[1], Chukwudinma C. Achilefu[2], Chika J. Mbah[2*]

[1]Department of Pharmaceutical Chemistry, Faculty of Pharmaceutical Sciences, Delta State University, Abraka, Nigeria
[2]Department of Pharmaceutical and Medicinal Chemistry, Faculty of Pharmaceutical Sciences, University of Nigeria, Nsukka, Nigeria
Email: [*]cjmbah123@yahoo.com

Abstract

Transdermal delivery acts as an alternative to oral delivery of drugs and possibly provids also an alternative to hypodermic injection. Transdermal delivery when compared to oral route has a variety of advantages namely: avoiding the degradation of drugs in the stomach environment, providing steady plasma levels, avoiding first-pass metabolism, increaseing patient compliance, easy to use, non-invasive and inexpensive, increasing the therapeutic index with a simultaneous decrease in drug side effects. Despite these advantages, one of the greatest challenges to transdermal delivery is that only a limited number of drugs are amenable to administration by this route. Gemifloxacin, a broad spectrum fourth generation quinolone antibacterial agent has pharmacokinetic characteristics (particularly its low maximum plasma concentration, obtained following repeat oral dose of 320 mg) that makes it a potential target for transdermal delivery. The objective of the study was to explore the possibility of surfactants (anionic, cationic and nonionic) acting as dermal enhancers of gemifloxacin assuming that the drug is to be formulated into topical or transdermal pharmaceutical dosage form. To accomplish the objective, gemifloxacin was partitioned between chloroform and surfactants containing varying concentrations of sodium lauryl sulfate, cetyltrimethylammonium bromide, polysorbate-20 and polysorbate-80. The data obtained were used to estimate the dermal permeability coefficient. The partitioning was carried out by shake flask method at room temperature. It was observed that all the surfactants decreased the partition behavior of gemifloxacin when compared to that of water alone. Sodium lauryl sulfate produced the most decreasing partition effect at the highest concentration studied (2% w/v). The permeability coefficient (K_p) was estimated from the partition coefficient data and the molecular weight of the drug. As permeability coefficient is an important descriptor for evaluating dermal absorption of drugs employed in clinical treatment of various dermal accessible ailments, the results of the study suggest that the investigated surfactants might not be potential transdermal enhancers of gemifloxacin.

Keywords

Gemifloxacin, Surfactants, Partition Coefficient

1. Introduction

Gemifloxacin, 7-[{4Z}-3-(Aminomethyl)-4-(methoxyimino)-1-pyrrolidinyl]-1-cyclopropyl-6-fluoro-4-oxo-1,4-dihydro-1,8-naphthyridine-3-carboxylic acid, is a broad spectrum fourth generation quinolone antibacterial agent. Clinically, the drug is used to treat acute bacterial exacerbation of chronic bronchitis, mild to moderate pneumonia. Its mechanism of action involves the inhibition of DNA synthesis through the inhibition of DNA gyrase and topoisomerase IV, enzymes essential for bacterial growth [1] [2]. The pharmacokinetics of gemifloxacin indicates that the mean maximal plasma concentration (C_{max}) is 1.61 ± 0.51 μg /ml following repeat oral dose of 320 mg. It was therefore, envisaged that the dose could be significantly reduced while achieving the required maximum plasma concentration, if transdermal route is considered an alternative. Transdermal drug delivery has made many important contributions in disease therapies and the successful use of topical formulations depends on understanding the drug transport through the dermal barriers. The stratum corneum (the outermost layer of the epidermis, about 10 - 40 um thick) provides the most barrier to the absorption into the circulation of most drugs deposited on the skin surface [3] [4]. Surfactants (amphiphilic molecules composed of a hydrophilic moiety known as the head and a hydrophobic moiety known as the tail) have been reported to be drug carriers or dermal absorption enhancers [5]-[7]. Dermal absorption enhancers are often required in transdermal formulations to amongst other things reduce the drug dose and invariably the adverse effects of the drug. Partitioning of drug through biological membranes is responsible for the pharmacological activity of the drug [8] [9]. Partition coefficient has been reported to be a good descriptor in evaluating dermal absorption of compounds [10]. Another study has also reported that the rate of penetration into the skin (dermal absorption) can be quantitatively determined by use of the permeability coefficient [11] [12]. Other study has shown that dermal permeability coefficient depends on the partition coefficient and molecular weight of the compound [13]. Furthermore, dermal permeability coefficient has been found to be an easy parameter in evaluating the usage and effectiveness of topical drugs [14]. Against this background, the present study was aimed at investigating the dermal enhancement potentials of anionic, cationic and nonionic surfactants on gemifloxacin by studying the partition characteristics of the drug in micellar solutions and using the data obtained to calculate the dermal permeability coefficient.

2. Materials and Methods

Gemifloxacin (Oscient Pharmaceuticals, USA), sodium lauryl sulfate, cetyltrimethylammonium bromide, polysorbate-20 and polysorbate-80 (Sigma-Aldrich, USA), chloroform (Fisher Scientific, USA) and other chemicals were of analytical grade.

2.1. Standard Solution

The stock solution of gemifloxacin (10 μg/ml) was prepared in methanol. Aliquots (1.0 - 6.0 μg/ml) of the standard stock solution were pipette into a 10 ml volumetric flask and diluted to volume with methanol.

2.2. Partition Coefficient Measurement

The chloroform/water partition coefficient was measured by a shake-flask method [15]. To 5 ml of chloroform (saturated with different micellar solutions) containing 100 µg of gemifloxacin was added 5 ml of aqueous micellar solution (saturated with chloroform). The flasks were capped and agitated at room temperature for 2 h to achieve complete equilibration. After that, the aqueous phases were separated and the concentrations were determined by measuring the UV absorbance at a maximum wavelength of 265 nm. The partition coefficient of gemifloxacin was calculated using this equation [16]

$$P = \frac{(C_1 - C_w) V_w}{C_w V_o}$$

where P = partition coefficient; C_1 = total concentration of gemifloxacin; C_w = concentration of gemifloxacin in aqueous phase; V_w = volume of the aqueous phase; V_o = volume of the organic phase.

3. Results and Discussion

The regression equation describing the Beer's plot of absorbance versus concentration of gemifloxacin reference standard is: $A = 0.0685\, C + 0.0971$ ($R^2 = 0.9998$). The partition coefficient results of gemifloxacin are presented in **Table 1**.

The results show that all the surfactants used in the investigation decreased the partition coefficient of gemifloxacin. Sodium lauryl sulfate gave the most decreasing effect. For instance, at the highest concentration of surfactant (2.0% w/v) investigated, the logarithm of the partition coefficients of gemifloxacin are 1.904, 1.826, 1.812 and 1.770 for polysorbate-80, polysorbate-20, cetylmethylammonium bromide and sodium lauryl sulfate respectively. The overall decrease in the logarithm of partition coefficient of the drug at increasing surfactant concentrations could be due to the polar nature of the drug. For sodium lauryl sulfate, the decrease is probably associated more with alkaline pH of the surfactant solution (rather than micellar effect), which might have contributed to the ionization of the carboxylic acid group present in the drug, thus greater affinity the drug has for the aqueous phase than the organic phase. Ion association could be used more to explain the decreasing results observed with the cationic surfactant than the micellar effect. The positive charge on the cationic surfactant has the potential of forming ion pair with the primary amino group in the drug. However, for the nonionic surfactants, the decreasing effect is most likely to be due to the degree of entrapment of the drug in the micelles of the surfactant. The entrapment theory could be substantiated because it was observed that polysorbate-80 showed more decreasing effect than polysorbate-20. The plots of logarithm partition coefficient versus concentration of the surfactant are shown in **Figure 1**. A decrease linear relationship was observed for each surfactant. The correlation coefficients are −0.7785, −0.8711, −0.9472 and −0.9350 for polysorbate-80, polysorbate-20, cetylmethylammonium bromide and sodium lauryl sulfate respectively.

In this investigation, only two molecular descriptors namely hydrophobicity (represented by log P) and molecule size (represented by molecular weight) were used to study the efficacy of predicting K_p values. The results of the calculated permeability coefficients of gemifloxacin for various concentrations of the surfactants using the equation of Potts and Guy, are shown in **Table 2**.

Table 1. Effect of Sodium lauryl sulfate, Cetylmethylammonium bromide, Polysorbate-20 and Polysorbate-80 on the partition coefficient of Gemifloxacin.

Concentration of surfactant	Logarithm Partition Coefficient of Gemifloxacin			
	Sodium lauryl sulfate	Cetylmethylammonium bromide	Polysorbate-20	Polysorbate-80
0.00	2.283	2.283	2.283	2.283
0.05	1.958	2.018	2.106	2.192
0.10	1.936	1.980	2.042	2.096
0.20	1.895	1.955	1.988	2.013
0.50	1.861	1.912	1.948	1.963
1.0	1.813	1.870	1.903	1.921
2.0	1.770	1.812	1.826	1.904

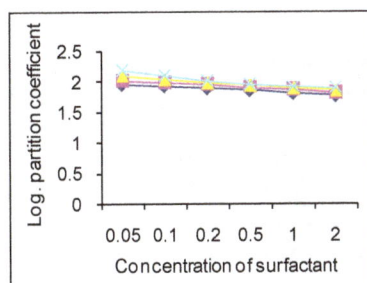

×------× = Polysorbate-80;   Δ------Δ = Polysorbate-20
□------□ = Cetylmethylammonium chloride   □------□ = Sodium lauryl sulfate

Figure 1. Plot of logarithm of partition coefficient of gemifloxacin versus concentration of surfactant.

Table 2. Effect of Sodium lauryl sulfate, Cetylmethylammonium bromide, Polysorbate-20 and Polysorbate-80 on the Permeability Coefficient of Gemifloxacin.

Concentration of surfactant	Logarithm Partition Coefficient of Gemifloxacin			
	Sodium lauryl sulfate	Cetylmethylammonium bromide	Polysorbate-20	Polysorbate-80
0.00	−3.4743	−3.4743	−3.4743	−3.4743
0.05	−3.7050	−3.6624	−3.5999	−3.5389
0.10	−3.7206	−3.6894	−3.6454	−3.6070
0.20	−3.7498	−3.7072	−3.6837	−3.6660
0.50	−3.7741	−3.7377	−3.7121	−3.7015
1.0	−3.8080	−3.7675	−3.7441	−3.7050
2.0	−3.8385	−3.8087	−3.7987	−3.7434

The equation is: $\log K_p = -2.72 + 0.71 \log P - 0.0061$ MW, where K_p is the permeability coefficient, P is the partition coefficient and MW is the molecular weight of the compound. Potts and Guy equation, was used to predict (calculate) K_p values because previous studies had demonstrated the equation to be a highly effective mathematical model for K_p determination. However, in order to confirm the applicability of the equation to this investigation, the calculated logarithm of permeability coefficient of gemifloxacin was plotted against the logarithm of partition coefficient of the drug at one concentration level (2.0 % w/v) of the studied surfactants. Linear relationship was observed and regression equation defining the plot is $\log K_p = 0.7098 \log P - 1.0949$ ($R^2 = 0.9999$).

4. Conclusion

The results suggest that the studied surfactants might not be potential transdermal enhancers of gemifloxacin. The investigation also suggests that the skin-vehicle partition coefficient may not be significantly affected, if any of the studied surfactants is found present in any dermal or topical formulation of gemifloxacin.

References

[1] Hooper, D.C. (2001) Emerging Mechanisms of Fluoroquinolones Resistance. *Emerging Infectious Diseases*, **7**, 337-341. http://dx.doi.org/10.3201/eid0702.010239

[2] Oliphant, C.M. and Green, G.M. (2002) Quinolones: A Comprehensive Review. *American Family Physician*, **65**, 455-464.

[3] Montagna, W., Van Scott, E.J. and Stoughton, R.B. (1972) Pharmacology and the Skin. Appleton Century Crafts, New York.

[4] Rutter, N. (1987) Drug Absorption through the Skin; a Mixed Blessing. *Archives of Disease in Childhood*, **62**, 220-221.

http://dx.doi.org/10.1136/adc.62.3.220

[5]   Hwang, C.C. and Danti, A.G. (1983) Percutaneous Absorption of Flufenamic Acid in Rabbits. Effect of Dimethylsul-foxide and Various Nonionic Surface Active Agents. *Journal of Pharmaceutical Sciences*, **72**, 857-860.
        http://dx.doi.org/10.1002/jps.2600720805

[6]   Shen, W.W., Danti, A.G. and Bruscato, F.N. (1976) Effect of Nonionic Surfactants on Percutaneous Absorption of Sa-licyclic Acid and Sodium Salicylate in the Presence of Dimethylsulfoxide. *Journal of Pharmaceutical Sciences*, **65**, 1780-1783. http://dx.doi.org/10.1002/jps.2600651222

[7]   Mbah, C.J. and Okekearu, L. (2013) Propylene Glycol, Polysorbate-80 and Sodium Lauryl Sulfate as Potential Dermal Absorption Enhancers of Celecoxib. *Standard Scientific Research and Essays*, **1**, 32-35.

[8]   Hansch, C. and Dunn III, W.J. (1972) Linear Relationships between Lipophilic Character and Biological Activity of Drugs. *Journal of Pharmaceutical Sciences*, **61**, 1-19. http://dx.doi.org/10.1002/jps.2600610102

[9]   Bawden, D., Gymer, G.E., Marriott, M.S. and Tute, M.S. (1984) Quantitative Structure-Activity Relationships in a Group of Imidazole Antimycotic Agents. *The European Journal of Medicinal Chemistry*, **18**, 91-96.

[10]   Bunge, A.L. and Cleek, R. L. (1995) A New Method for Estimating Dermal Absorption from Chemical Exposure. Ef-fect of Molecular Weight and Octanol-Water Partitioning. *Pharmaceutical Research*, **12**, 88-95.
        http://dx.doi.org/10.1023/A:1016242821610

[11]   (1992) United States Environmental Protection Agency: Dermal Exposure Assessment: Principles and Applications. EPA/600/8-91/011 B.

[12]   Karinth, S., Schaller, K.H. and Drexler, H. (2005) Is Permeability Coefficient K_p a Reliable Tool in Percutaneous Ab-sorption Studies. *Archives of Toxicology*, **79**, 155-159. http://dx.doi.org/10.1007/s00204-004-0618-4

[13]   Potts, R.V. and Guy, R.H. (1992) Predicting Skin Permeability. *Pharmaceutical Research*, **9**, 663-669.
        http://dx.doi.org/10.1023/A:1015810312465

[14]   Gennaro, A.R. (1995) Remington: The Science and Practice of Pharmacy. 19th Edition, Mack Publishing Company, Easton.

[15]   Wang, F.A. (2001) Molecular Thermodynamics and Chromatographic Retention. China Meteorology Press, Beijing.

[16]   Johansen, M. and Bundgaard, H. (1980) Prodrugs as Drug Delivery Systems XI. Solubility, Dissolution and Partition Behaviour of N-Mannich Bases and N-Hydroxymethyl Derivatives. *Arch. Pharm. Chem. Sci. Edu.*, **8**, 141-151.

11

Natural Products Modulate the Multifactorial Multidrug Resistance of Cancer

Safaa Yehia Eid[1,2], Mahmoud Zaki El-Readi[1,2,3*], Sameer Hassan Fatani[1],
Essam Eldin Mohamed Nour Eldin[1], Michael Wink[2*]

[1]Department of Biochemistry, Faculty of Medicine, Umm Al-Qura University, Makkah, Kingdom of Saudi Arabia
[2]Institute of Pharmacy and Molecular Biotechnology, Heidelberg University, Heidelberg, Germany
[3]Department of Biochemistry, Faculty of Pharmacy, Al-Azhar University, Assiut, Egypt
Email: *mzreadi@uqu.edu.sa, *wink@uni-heidelberg.de

Abstract

Multidrug resistance (MDR) is a critical problem in cancer chemotherapy. Cancer cells can develop resistance not only to a single cytotoxic drug, but also to entire classes of structurally and functionally unrelated compounds. Several mechanisms can mediate the development of MDR, including increased drug efflux from the cells by ABC-transporters (ABCT), activation of metabolic enzymes, and defective pathways towards apoptosis. Many plant secondary metabolites (SMs) can potentially increase sensitivity of drug-resistant cancer cells to chemotherapeutical agents. The present thesis investigates the modulation of MDR by certain medicinal plants and their active compounds. The inhibition of ABCTs (P-gp/MDR1, MRP1, BCRP) and metabolic enzymes (GST and CYP3A4), and the induction of apoptosis are useful indicators of the efficacy of a potential medicinal drug. The focus of this study was the possible mechanisms of drug resistance including: expression of resistance proteins, activation of metabolic enzymes, and alteration of the apoptosis and how to overcome their resistance effect on cancer cells. The overall goal of this review was to evaluate how commonly used medicinal plants and their main active secondary metabolites modulate multidrug resistance in cancer cells in order to validate their uses as anticancer drugs, introduce new therapeutic options for resistant cancer, and facilitate the development of their anticancer strategies and/or combination therapies. In conclusion, SMs from medicinal plants exhibit multitarget activity against MDR-related proteins, metabolic enzymes, and apoptotic signaling, this may help to overcome resistance towards chemotherapeutic drugs.

Keywords

Multidrug Resistance (MDR), ABC-Transporters (ABCT), Metabolic Enzymes, Apoptosis,

---

*Corresponding authors.

CytochromeP3A4 (CYP3A4), Glutathione-S-Transferase (GST)

1. Cancer

Cancer is the second leading cause of death, after heart disease, killing about every fifth or sixth person in western countries. Every year, more than 8.2 million cancer deaths are reported worldwide. Of the 14.1 million new cases each year, more than half occur in developing countries and 32.5 million persons are alive with cancer [1]. WHO predicts 23.6 million cases in 2030, 68% of which to be occurring in developing countries.

Cancer is defined as a disease in which normal tissue is invaded by abnormally dividing cells. Left untreated, it will spread throughout the body and becomes fatal. Chemotherapy (the use of cytotoxic agents to slow the progression of this uncontrolled cell division) is the major treatment when cancer is well established within the patient [2]. Resistance to anticancer drugs is a major problem in chemotherapy with 30% - 80% of cancer patients developing resistance to chemotherapeutical drugs [3]. Thus, counteracting drug resistance is crucial to providing the best treatment.

2. Multifactorial Multidrug Resistance

Cancer cells can not only develop resistance to one drug, but also to entire classes of drugs with similar mechanisms of action. After such resistance is established, some cells even become cross resistant to drugs, which are structurally and mechanistically unrelated; this phenomenon is known as multidrug resistance (MDR). This might explain why the treatment with multiple agent combinations addressing different targets is not effective. The main lines of cellular defense reactions involve:

- Decreased drug accumulation by enhanced cellular elimination, decreased uptake, and inactivation by intracellular metabolism (**Figure 1**). One example of the developmental resistance mediated by reduced drug uptake is water-soluble drugs that "piggyback" on transporters and carriers that bring nutrients into the cell [4] [5].

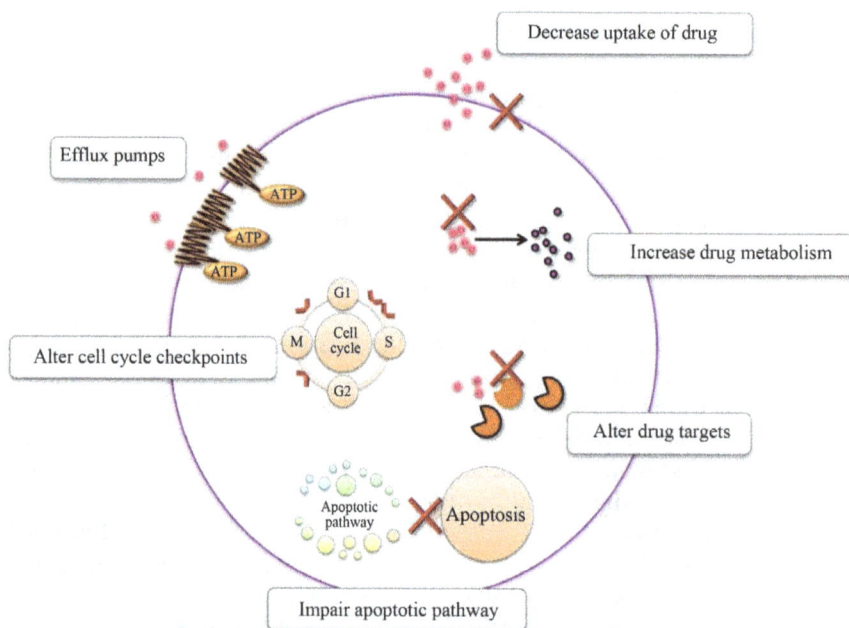

Figure 1. Cellular causes of drug resistance. Cells may develop resistance to anticancer drugs by increasing efflux pumps activity (like as ATP-dependent transporters) to remove the drug, reduced drug influx (e.g., by "piggyback" on intracellular carriers), activating detoxifying proteins (*i.e.* cytochrome P450 mixed-function oxidases), repairing their own DNA damage, disrupting apoptotic signalling pathways, or altered cell cycle checkpoints [6].

- Impaired drug delivery can result from poor absorption, increased drug metabolism, or increased excretion, resulting in lower levels of the drug in the blood and reduced diffusion of drugs from the blood into the tumor mass [7] [8]. The various causes of drug resistance can work simultaneously, increasing the resistance in a multifactorial manner. For example, the simultaneously induction of CYP3A4 and MDR1 was observed [9]. This type of multidrug resistance can be induced after exposure to any drug. Recent evidence indicates that certain nuclear receptors, such as PXR, might be involved in mediating this response to environmental stress while also acting in regulating metabolic enzymes and ABC transporters [10].
- Activation of DNA repair, due to genetic and epigenetic alterations and affecting drug sensitivity.
- Alteration or modification of the drug targets.
- Resistance resulting from defective apoptotic pathways. This might occur as a result of malignant transformation; for example, in tumors with mutable nonfunctional p53 [11].

Alternatively, cells may acquire changes in apoptotic pathways during exposure to chemotherapy, such as an alteration of ceramide levels or changes in the cell-cycle machinery, which activate checkpoints and prevent initiation of apoptosis [6] [12]. In addition, cancer cells, which survive cytotoxic drugs, are likely to be heterogeneous due to their mutated phenotypes. All these causes are involved multifactorial multidrug resistance (**Figure 1**) [6].

Current research is centering on how to combat this multifactorial resistance. Thus, we must study multiple means of drug resistance to develop the potent treatment options. Different types of cellular MDR have been identified [13]. They have been broadly classified into, cellular, and noncellular mechanisms, as detailed below.

3. Noncellular Resistance Mechanisms

Noncellular cytotoxic resistance mechanisms, such as *in vivo* tumor growth [14], environmental factors [15], or tumor geometry [16] are also worth further study, but are not the focus of this study.

4. Cellular Mechanisms of Multidrug Resistance

Detailed studies have been devoted to the cellular mechanisms of drug resistance. It is easy to generate *in vitro* models with cytotoxic drugs. Cellular mechanisms are categorized in terms of alterations in the biochemistry of malignant cells. Such mechanisms can be further classified into two major categories:

1) transport-based classical MDR phenotypes and 2) nonclassical MDR phenotypes.

4.1. Transport-Based Classical MDR Mechanisms

The biological membrane is a lipid bilayer into which numerous proteins are embedded, including transporter proteins. The activities of these transporters are important determinants for the pharmacokinetics and pharmacodynamics of many drugs. Considerable knowledge about these transporters has been gained over the past decade, including their functional characteristics, substrate specificities, and their specialized tissue distribution and subcellular localization [17]. This section will highlight the role of these transporters in MDR.

Classical multidrug resistance exerts increased drug efflux and lowers intracellular drug concentrations. ATP-dependent efflux pumps, belonging to ATP-binding cassette (ABC) transporters (largest family of transmembrane proteins), express broad drug specificity. Today, there are 48 identified human ABC genes. These are divided into seven distinct subfamilies (ABCA-ABCG) based on of their domain organization and sequence homology [18]. ABC transporters are responsible for the ATP-dependent movement of a wide variety of xenobiotics (including cytotoxic drugs), lipids, and metabolic products across the plasma and intracellular membranes [19] [20]. The cytotoxic drugs that are most frequently associated with classical MDR are hydrophobic, amphipathic natural products, such as microtubule-stabilizing taxanes (paclitaxel and docetaxel), vinca alkaloids (vinorelbine, vincristine, and vinblastine), anthracyclines (doxorubicin, daunorubicin, and epirubicin), epipodophyllotoxins (etoposide and teniposide), antimetabolites (methotrexate, fluorouracil, 5-azacytosine, 6-mercaptopurine, and gemcitabine) topotecan, and the RNA transcription inhibitor actinomycin-D [21].

4.1.1. P-Glycoprotein/Multidrug Resistance 1 (P-gp/MDR1)

Two highly hydrophobic integral membrane domains (each of which spans the membrane six times by alpha helices) and two hydrophilic nucleotide binding domains (NBDs) make up the four distinct parts of MDR1 (**Figure 2**).

Structure   Examples

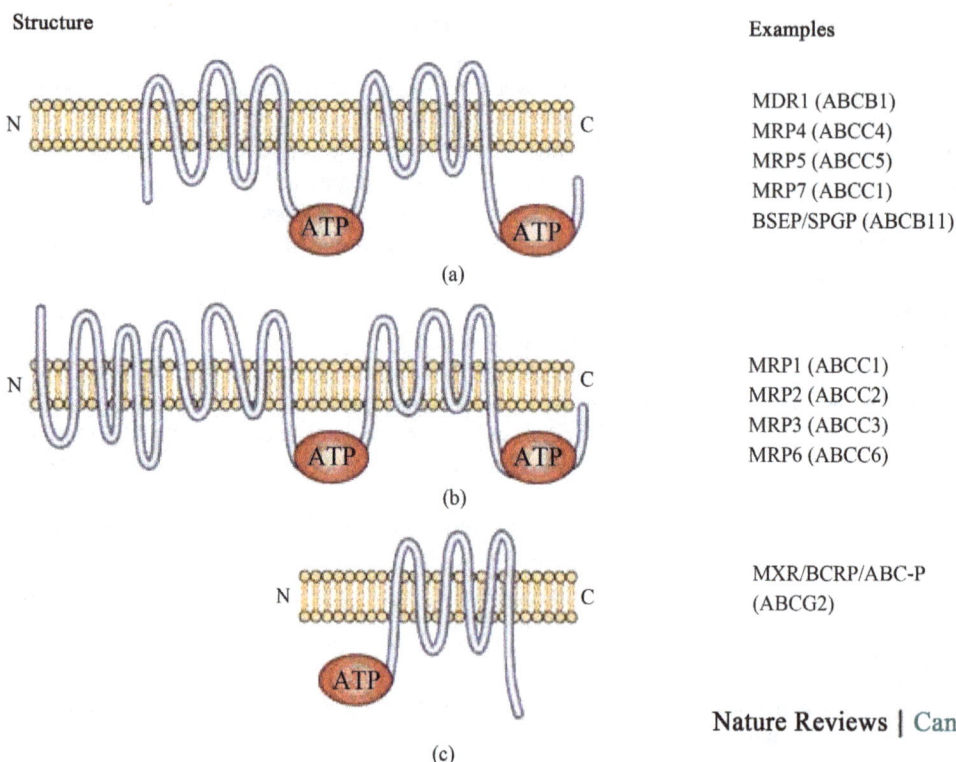

MDR1 (ABCB1)
MRP4 (ABCC4)
MRP5 (ABCC5)
MRP7 (ABCC1)
BSEP/SPGP (ABCB11)

(a)

MRP1 (ABCC1)
MRP2 (ABCC2)
MRP3 (ABCC3)
MRP6 (ABCC6)

(b)

MXR/BCRP/ABC-P
(ABCG2)

Nature Reviews | Cancer

(c)

Figure 2. The structures of three categories of ABC transporter known to confer drug resistance. Sample (a) shows ABC transporters (such as MDR1, MRP4, etc), which have 12 transmembrane domains and 2 ATP-binding sites. (b) Depicts those ABC transporters which have 2 ATP-binding domains and a domain consisting of five transmembrane segments at the amino-terminal end; there is a total of 17 transmembrane domains in these transporters (MRP1-6). Finally, (c) shows a "half-transporter" ABCG2. This half transporter, which is believed to function by homodimerizing or heterodimerizing, contains only one ATP-binding region and six transmembrane domains [22].

A 2.5-nm resolution structure of this broad-spectrum multidrug efflux pump was recently obtained by electron microscopy and single particle image analysis. This shows a large central pore, ~5 nm in diameter, which closes at the inner (cytoplasmic) side of the membrane.A gap may be present in the protein ring, which may allow substrates to access the central pore from the lipid phase [3] [19] (**Figure 3**).

4.1.2. Mechanism of the Efflux Pump

MDR1 efficiently removes cytotoxic drugs and many commonly used pharmaceuticals from the lipid bilayer. For many years, the model for drug resistance conferred by MDR1 has been a relatively simple one. Cytotoxic drugs are actively transported out of cells that express MDR1 against a concentration gradient, thereby reducing intracellular drug accumulation and inhibiting drug-mediated cell death (**Figure 3**) [23].

Initial mechanistic models define efflux of drugs by MDR1 hypothesized that MDR1 forms a hydrophilic pathway, and drugs are transported from the cytosol to the extracellular media through the middle of a pore, thereby shielding the substrate from the hydrophobic lipid phase (**Figure 3(a)**).

In summary, in order to transport one drug molecule, two ATP hydrolysis events must occur. The hydrophobic substrates that are either neutral or positively charged bind to the transmembrane domains in order to stimulate the ATPase activity of P-gp/MDR1 and cause substrate to be released to either the outer leaflet of the membrane or extracellular space. Then the transporter is required to be "reset" by hydrolysis so that it can bind substrate again. These two events complete in the catalytic cycle [24].

It appear that P-gp aids in MDR by intercepting a drug as it moves through the lipid membrane then "flipping" the drug so that it effluxes from the cells through the outer leaflet into the extracellular space (**Figure 3(b)**) [23]. This "flippase" function has also been observed in several related ABC molecules, leading to the assumption

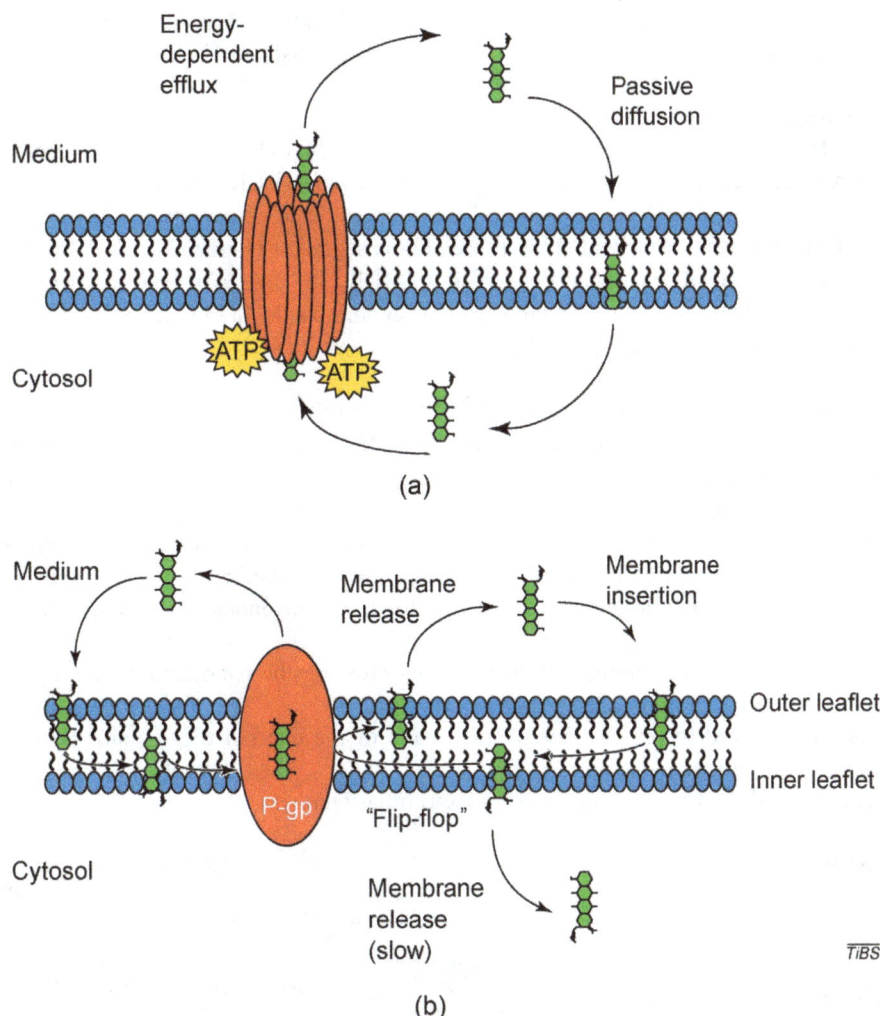

Figure 3. Possible mechanisms of action for drug efflux by P-glycoprotein/MDR1 (P-gp/MDR1). (a) The "pump" model for drug transport. The three-dimensional structure of MDR1 consists of a single drug pore (shown in *red*). Chemotherapeutic drugs (*green*) diffuse through the lipid membrane and are transported out of the cell by P-gp in an ATP-dependent manner. (b) The "flippase" model for drug transport. A drug interacts with lipids of the membrane before it interacts with MDR1. The drug can then interact with MDR1 and is transported from the inner leaflet directly into the extracellular medium. Alternatively, drug intercalated into the inner leaflet of the lipid bilayer is "flipped" into the outer leaflet and released into the extracellular space. Movement of drug from the inner to the outer leaflet is a relatively quick process, whereas drug movement from the inner leaflet to the cytosol is relatively slow [23].

that they comprise a large, polymorphous drug-binding domain [23]. P-gp/MDR1 also binds with various hydrophobic compounds, making it simple to find potent P-gp/MDR1 inhibitors. Two such inhibitors being studied for their reversal effect on MDR are verapamil (a calcium channel blocker) and cyclosporine A (an immunosuppressant).

4.1.3. Multidrug Resistance Protein (MRP)

Multidrug resistant cells have been found which contain no P-gp/MDR, but instead the efflux pumps protein, multidrug-resistance-associated protein 1 (MRP1, or ABCC1) [25]. MRP1 works similarly to P-gp/MDR1, it transport transports glutathione and its conjugates, cotransports unconjugated glutathione, and recognizes both neutral and anionic hydrophobic natural products. Structurally, it is very similar to P-gp/MDR1 with an added amino terminal containing five-membrane spanning domains attached to the core (**Figure 2**) [26]. The discovery of MRP1 spurred further research, which led to the discovery of 8 additional members of the ABCC subfamily of transporters [27]. Many of these have a potential in fighting drug resistance [27].

4.1.4. Breast Cancer Resistance Protein (BCRP)

Mitoxantrone, is a chemotherapeutical agent, but poor substrate for MDR1 and MRP1. It is a selective substrate for ABCG2 protein, which called MXR (mitoxantrone-resistance gene), BCRP (breast cancer resistance protein) [28]. Structurally, BCRP is a homodimer of two half-transporters, each containing an ATP-binding domain at the amino-terminal end of the molecule and six transmembrane segments (**Figure 2**). The substitution of even a single amino acid can change substrate specificity of P-gp/MDR1 [21]. As observed in ABCG2 gene cloning from resistant cells encoded proteins by substituted arginine at amino acid 482 by threonine or glycine led to increase the ability to transport doxorubicin [29] [30].

4.1.5. ABC Transporters in Normal Cells and Their Physiological Function

MDR1 is found in both tumor cells (where it contributes to MDR) and normal cells. It is generally found in cell tissues with excretory (kidney, liver, adrenal gland) and barrier functions (intestine, blood brain barrier, placenta, testis and ovarian) [31] (**Figure 4**). These placements allow to suggesting that MDR1 has a role in detoxification and protection of the body against toxic drug and metabolites by secreting these compounds into bile, urine, and the intestinal lumen and by blocking their accumulation in the brain, testis, and fetus. The general function of ABC transporters is the protection of cells from many endogenous or exogenous toxins, as detailed below (**Figure 4**) [32]:

- P-gp/MDR1 plays a role in preventing cytotoxines from crossing the endothelium and attacking the brain [33].
- MRP proteins are localized to the basolateral membrane of the choroid plexus, and pump the metabolic waste products of CSF into the blood.
- MDR1 protects the testis by transporting toxins to the capillary lumen.

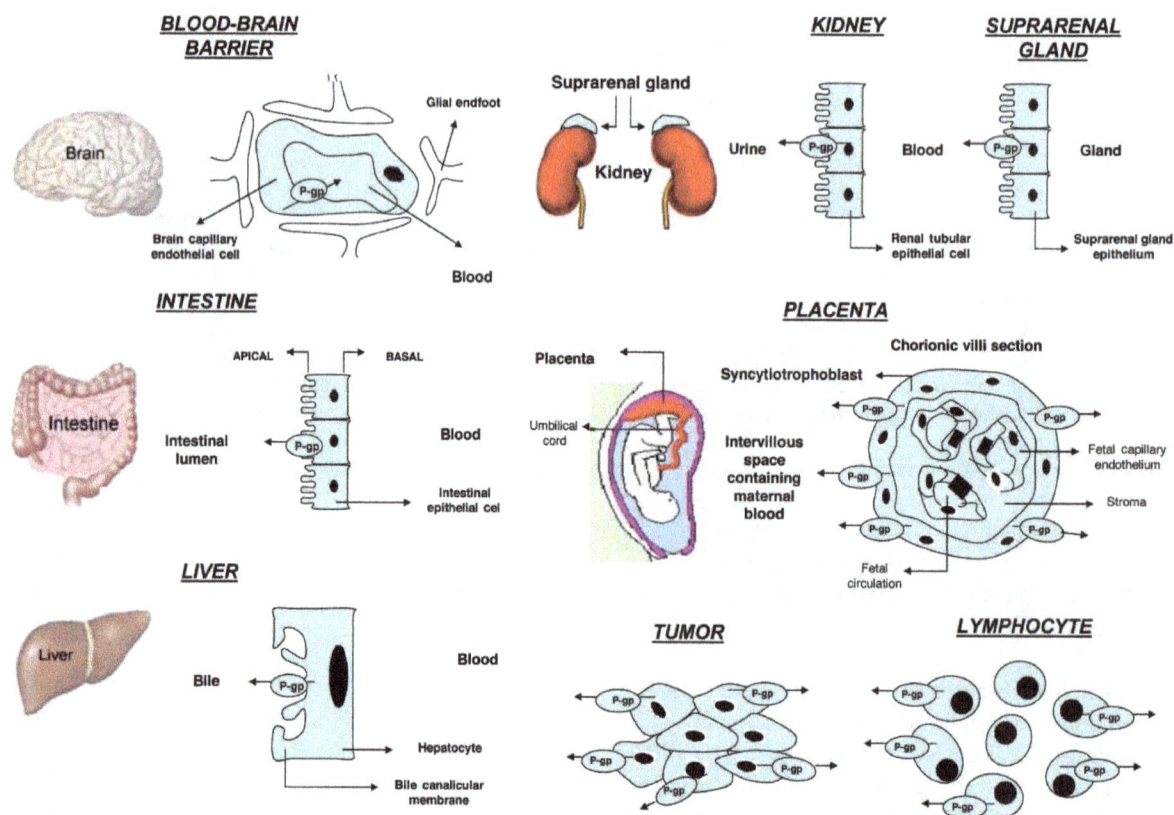

Figure 4. Schematic representations of the main sites of localization of P-gp/MDR1 in the body [32].

- MDR1 is localized on the apical syncytiotrophoblast surface in the placenta; it can protect the fetus from cationic xenobiotics [34].
- MRP and ABCG2 are also localized in the placenta [35] [36]; they appear have protecting functions for fetal blood [37]
- MDR1 protects the liver by transporting toxins into the bile [38].
- MDR1 is localized in apical membranes of inessential mucosal cells; it has a role in determining oral drug bioavailability [39].
- MRP1 is located in the basolateral membrane of mucosal cells; it transports substrates into the blood, rather than across the apical surface into the intestinal lumen [40].

The protective mechanism of ABC transporter-mediated extrusion of such toxic substances (natural drugs or metabolic waste products) causes cancer cells to be resistant to the toxic effects of many chemotherapeutic agents. ABC transporters not only protect vital tissue from toxins (as in the liver, GIT, and kidneys), they also actively excrete toxins. This function must be considered when determining the bioavailability of oral drugs. In short, ABC transporters effectively protect both normal and cancerous cells. Their protective properties must be circumvented in order to effectively destroy malignant cells.

4.1.6. ABC Transporters in Human Cancers

Early research into ABC transporters focused almost exclusively on P-gp because it is so highly expressed in colon, kidney, adrenocortical, and hepatocellular cancers [41]. Traditionally, research has focused on expression impairing response to chemotherapy, expression levels increasing, as tumor become more drug resistant. The idea was that tumors depending on P-gp expression for survival have the highest rates of MDR1 expression [22]. Initial hopes were that decreasing only P-gp expression could solve the multidrug resistance problem. It became clear that multiple factors (not solely MDR1) are involved when the aforementioned cancers failed to respond to drugs that are not P-gp substrates.

Patient's studies have shown a correlation between P-gp/MDR1 expression and drug resistance, being strongest in acute myelogenous leukemia (AML). MDR1 expression is present in approximately 30% of newly diagnosed leukemia patients and 50% of those in relapse [42] [43]. *In vivo* studies have shown that MDR1 expression reduces the intracellular accumulation of doxorubicin and that this can be counteracted by use of a MDR1 inhibitor [44] [45].

Research has also focused on MRP1 and LRP expression, however, unlike with MDR1 [46], there has not yet been an indication that these have an effect on prognosis, but observed a correlation between MDR1 expression and prognosis [43]. Interestingly, AML cells have been observed to have low expression levels of BCRP/MXR [47]. Treatment of colorectal cancer, the leading cause of cancer-related death in the western world, has not yet begun to accurate identify subgroups of patients whose differing forms of the disease will respond to varying treatments. The expression of proteins responsible for active processes in Caco-2 cells can also be induced by xenobiotics. This is probably due to the cancerous origin of Caco-2, since e.g. vinca alkaloids induce MDR1 in these cells, according to the concept of multidrug resistance [48].

Induction of many other phase I and phase II metabolic enzymes has also been reported [49]-[51]. The roles of several active uptake and efflux proteins and metabolic enzymes (as well as the interplay between them) should be studied in order to better understand MDR in Caco-2 cells. Past studies have focused primarily on the easily observable *in vitro* flavonoids. Pharmacokinetic models of Caco-2 cells have recently been construed [52] [53].

4.1.7. ABC-Transporter Substrates

MDR1 transports a broad range of substrates, which include several pharmacologically distinct agents used not only for chemotherapy but also for hypertension, allergy relief, infections, immunosupression, neurology, and inflammation.

The structure-activity relationship of these substrates is not clear, though it appears lipophilicity and hydrogen bonds correlate proportionally to the affinity of MDR1 [54]. Since the substrates appear to be freely diffused into the cells, they can be found by looking for MDR1 in the plasma membrane, as it appears from *in vitro* testing that MDR1 recognizes its substrates before they enter the cytoplasm [55]. Studies find that many substrates of MDR1 are also substrates of drug-metabolizing enzymes, such as CYP3A4. This overlap may be to some extent a result of a coordinated regulation of tissue expression of CYP3A4 and MDR1 (both of which are located in close proximity on the same chromosome) in organs such as the liver and intestine [56]. However, such overlap is not always present; some MDR1 substrates, such as digoxin, fexofonadine, celiprolol, and tarlinolol do not significantly interact with CYP enzymes and others, such as midazolam, are not transported by MDR1 [56]-[58].

4.1.8. ABC-Transporter Inhibitors

Historically research has focused on the ABC superfamily when searching for the reasons of chemotherapy failure. Only a small number of transporters obtained from patients at diagnosis have been investigated. These studies confirmed that MDR1 is relevant in several cancers; however, the relevance of other transporters is not yet clear [59]. As research in this area continues, developing ABC transport inhibitors appears to be a useful addition to chemotherapy.

Many studies have tried to combat MDR by inhibiting MDR transporters, suppressing MDR mechanisms, or circumventing MDR mechanisms. There are many MDR modulators belonging to several chemical classes, including calcium channel blockers, calmodulin inhibitors, coronary vasodilators, indole alkaloids, quinolines, hormones, cyclosporines, surfactants, and antibodies [60]. These have risks associated with needing very high doses of toxic drugs in order to produce needed results [61]. To minimize these risks, new analogs of these early chemosensitizing agents were tested and developed with the goal of finding patent MDR1 modulators, which require less toxicity. Other avenues to explore are: using anticancer drugs which are not substrates of ABC transporters (such as alkylating drugs, antimetabolites, and anthracycline modified drugs) [62] [63]. Such compounds are called MDR inhibitors, MDR modulators, MDR reversal agents, or chemosensitizers and they may inhibit one or more transporters. Excellent examples of chemosensitizers (e.g. limonin) are included in this study [64].

Chemosensitization involves the co-administration of an MDR1 inhibitor (MDR modulator) with an anticancer drug in order to cause enhanced intracellular anticancer drug accumulation via impairing the MDR1 function. Many early chemosensitizing agents were themselves substrates for MDR1 and worked by keeping the MDR pump too busy effluxing the inhibitor to fully efflux the cytotoxic drugs [21]. There are advantages of using chemosensitizing agents when they exhibit affinity for the same substrates and interfering with other enzyme systems and transporters [61] [65].

MDR1 inhibitors, like MDR1 substrates, show no relation between their chemical structures or pharmacological actions and their inhibitory effects. Reports indicate a strong correlation between physicochemical parameters and MDR1 inhibition. An MDR1 modulator is considered a good candidate if it possesses a log p value of 2.92 or higher, a molecular axis of 18 or more atoms in length, one or more tertiary basic nitrogen atoms, and high energy in its highest occupied orbit [66].

Inhibition of MDR1 could potentially result from the blockage of specific recognition of the substrate, binding to ATP, ATP hydrolysis, or coupling of ATP hydrolysis to translocation of the substrate. Most reversing agents block MDR1 by acting as competitive or noncompetitive inhibitors [67] and by binding either to drug interaction sites, [68] or to other modulator binding sites, leading to allosteric changes. Competitive modulators compete as a substrate with the cytotoxic agent for transport by the pump. This limits the efflux of the cytotoxic agent, increasing its intracellular concentration.

Noncompetitive inhibition of the MDR1 transporter binds with high affinity to the pump but is not itself a substrate. This induces a conformational change in the protein, thereby preventing ATP hydrolysis and transport of the cytotoxic agent out of the cell, resulting in an increased intracellular concentration. MDR modulators such as verapamil are substrates of MDR1, which inhibit the transport function in a competitive manner without interrupting the catalytic cycle of MDR1 [69]. Cyclosporin A, as one of the reversing agents, inhibits MDR1 function by interfering with both substrate recognition and ATP hydrolysis [70]. Because ATP hydrolysis is required for transport, modulators that inhibit ATPase activity are unlikely to be transported by MDR1 [71]. Verapamil inhibits the function of MDR1, making malignant cells more susceptible to cytotoxic drugs [72]. Besides the functional inhibitory effect on MDR1 and down-regulate the MDR1 gene in leukemic cell lines [73]. In this thesis, verapamil was used to inhibit MDR1 as a positive control.

Clinical trials helped to unravel the problems associated with combining together with an MDR inhibitor. The first factor to be determined before a clinical trial is to identify the ABC transporter protein involved in drug resistance. The second factor is to monitor the plasma concentrations and *in vivo* effectiveness of the tested MDR inhibitor. The pharmacokinetic interaction between the anticancer drug(s) and the MDR inhibitor must be searched and avoided to prevent a reduction in anticancer drug dosage [74].

4.2. Nonclassical MDR Phenotypes

Mechanisms of drug resistance involving membrane-associated protein pumps, although the most thoroughly characterized, are not the only means by which drug resistance can arise within tumor cells. Clinical studies investigating other drug-resistance mechanisms (called non-classical MDR), are fewer in number, but are no less important. These non-transport mechanisms affect multiple drug classes. This type of resistance can be caused by the altered activity of specific enzyme systems (such as cytochrome P450 (CYP3A4) and glutathione-S-transferase (GST)), which can decrease the cytotoxic activity of drugs in a manner independent of intracellular drug concentrations. In addition, changes in the balance of proteins that control apoptosis can also reduce chemosensitivity since most anticancer drugs are exert their cytotoxicity via apoptotic processes. This section outlines some of these MDR mechanisms and their role in the overall MDR phenomenon.

4.2.1. Cytochrome P450

Since it is estimated that the enzyme CYP (cytochrome P-450) metabolizes (in full or in part) over half of all therapeutic drugs, it is essential that we gain a clear understanding of how CYP3A4 gene expression is regulated. Changes in the hepatic expression of CYP3A4 can significantly impact drug metabolism and thus the pharmacokinetics of medications [75].

CYP's main function is catalyzing the metabolic conversion of xenobiotics. Catalyzing helps convert those to polar derivatives (which can be easily excreted) or causes them to become more desirable substrates, which further then biotransformation of phase II enzymes or drug transporters. To clarify, in phase I, a lipophilic molecule is made more hydrophilic by introducing hydroxyl groups by cytochrome P450 oxidases (CYP); other CYPs. They cleave N-methyl, O-methyl, or methylene groups in order to obtain a more hydrophilic or more readily accessible substrate. In phase II, the hydroxylated compounds are conjugated with polar molecules, such as glutathione, sulfate, and glucuronic acid. These conjugates are eliminated via the kidneys and urine.

Several chemomodulating agents inhibit cytochrome P-4503A (CYP3A) activity in addition to inhibiting MDR proteins. Some drugs (such as tamoxifen, methoxymorpholinyl doxorubicin, cyclophosphamide and ifosfamide) requiring activation by CYP3A4 may have a reduced therapeutic effect even when MDR1 inhibition enhances their intracellular accumulation.

On the other hand, some drugs that depend on CYP3A4 for excretion can build up to overly toxic a mounts and the dose may need to be reduced. Therefore, it is essential to understand how CYP3A4 interacts with MDR1 inhibitors when using them in combination with cytotoxic drugs. In addition, reversal agents, which have MDR1 inhibition effects, also inhibit cytochrome P-450 3A (CYP3A) activity [56]. Herbs or drugs may inhibit CYPs by three mechanisms: competitive inhibition, noncompetitive inhibition, and mechanism-based inhibition [76].

Competitive inhibition may occur between drug and herbal/drug, which are metabolized by the same CYPs enzyme. Noncompetitive inhibition is caused by the binding to the haem portion of the CYPs enzyme this occurs by herbal/drug, which containing electrophilic groups (e.g. hydrazine or imidazole). The formation of a complex between CYPs and herbal/drug metabolites is the main cause of the mechanism-based inhibition of CYPs. Ever since the initial cloning of this receptor, the implications of PXR mediated gene regulation in drug, metabolism and drug-drug interactions were recognized. PXR was first postulated to regulate CYP3A gene expression in both human and rodents [77] (**Figure 5**).

On the other hand, PXR participates in the modulating metabolic processes and the regulation of drug transporters responsible for both efflux and uptake of endogenous and exogenous chemicals [78].

Mechanisms involving PXR regulation of efflux transporters tend to be more commonly studied, given that efflux transporters are often postulated as the major blockades for drugs to achieve therapeutic concentrations by crossing barriers such as the blood-brain barrier into the central nervous system, or the placenta during pregnancy [80] (**Figure 5**).

4.2.2. Glutathione-S-Transferease (GST)

Another component of MDR is the catalytic glutathione-S-transferase (GSTs). Several resistant cell lines have been shown to overexpress GST [81]. GSTs are detoxification enzymes conjugated of glutathione to the electrophilic center of various drugs and resulting in excretion of polar molecules. GSTs are able to metabolized cisplatin, doxorubicin, and melphalan and protecting the cells from environmental or oxidative stress [82].

There are two intracellular pools of GST, one residing in the cytosol and the other in the microsomal com-

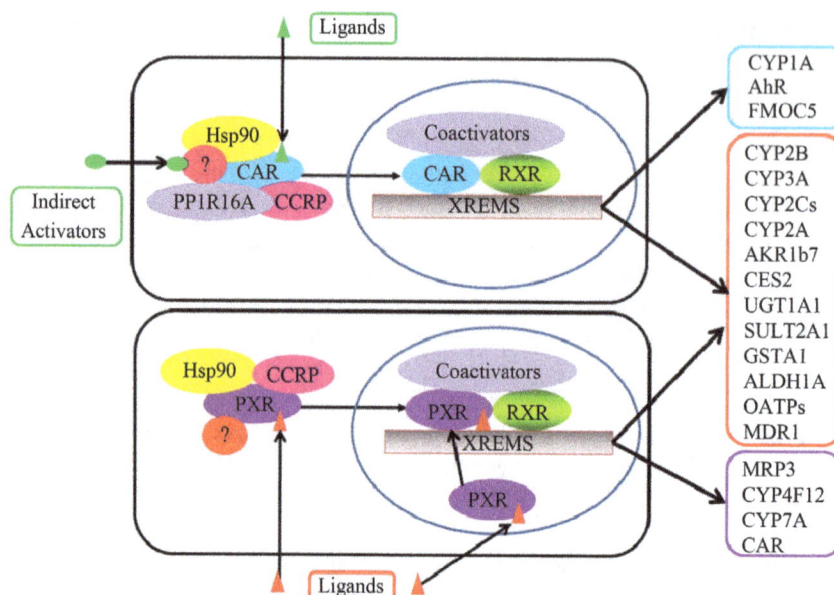

Figure 5. Schematic illustration of the activation mechanisms and target genes of CAR and PXR. Activation of PXR is purely ligand dependent. CAR and PXR shared target genes are grouped in a *red* box, CAR-specific targets in a *blue* box, and PXR-specific targets in a *purple* box [79].

partment. Cytosolic GSTs are composed of 23-29-kDa subunits which may be homo or hetero-dimers [83]. In contrast, microsomal GSTs are trimeric and composed of identical 17-kDa subunits [84]. Among its various activities, GST plays an important role in protecting cells from reactive epoxides [85]. This is believed to occur via the catalytic addition of GSH to the epoxide moiety, as observed by the metabolism of aflatoxin B1 to an 8,9-epoxide which is detoxified by GST [86]. GST is the predominant enzyme found in ovarian carcinoma and several studies have been performed to determine whether levels of this enzyme have prognostic significance, where the levels of GSTs were correlated to a poor response to chemotherapy.

The first linkage between PXR and GSTs observed in rat GSTA2, GSTA2 expression was suppressed at nanomolar concentration of DEX (GR activation) in cultured hepatocytes, but induced by DEX at micromolar (PXR activation) concentrations or RU486, which is a GR antagonist and PXR agonist [87] (**Figure 5**). More recently, studies have focused on the inhibition of apoptosis as the so-called de novo mechanism of drug resistance.

4.2.3. Apoptosis
In the last few years, clinical trials using plant-derived drugs for prevention and/or treatment of tumors have become increasingly widespread in cancer therapy. The search for novel agents designed to induce cell cycle arrest and apoptosis in cancer cells is being seriously pursued. The ability of tumor cells to evade apoptosis plays a significant role in their resistance to conventional therapeutic regimens [88]. Apoptosis describes the terminal morphological and biochemical events seen in programmed cell death (PCD). Apoptotic cells are characterized by morphological changes including: cellular shrinkage, plasma and nuclear membrane blebbing, organelle re-localization and compaction, nuclear DNA condensation with or without fragmentation, and hypersegmentation of nuclear chromatin of irregular size. These nuclear structures may then bud from the rapidly blebbing cell surface to form "apoptotic bodies" [89].

Three mechanisms are known to be involved in the apoptotic process: 1) a receptor-ligand mediated mechanism, 2) a mitochondrial pathway and 3) a mechanism in which the endoplasmic reticulum plays a central role (**Figure 6**). All three mechanisms activate caspases, which are responsible for the characteristic morphological changes observed during apoptosis. Cell death marked by cellular swelling is called oncosis. Necrosis cell deaths various from apoptosis in several ways. Necrosis results from direct injury, which usually begins at the cell surface. Early lysis of the plasma membrane is exhibited by necrotic cells before any significant alterations in

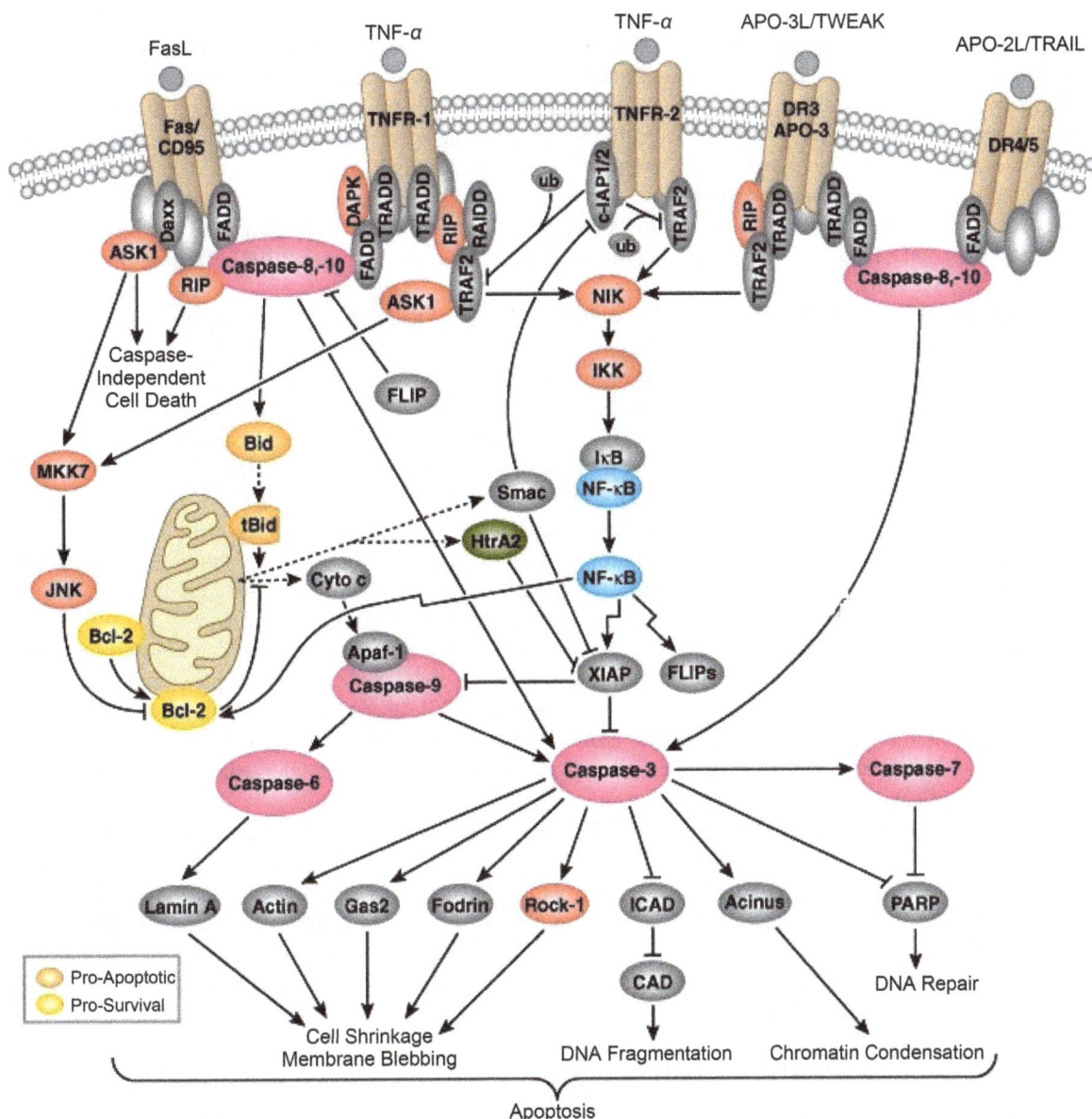

Figure 6. Apoptosis can be induced through the activation of death receptors including Fas, TNFαR, DR3, DR4, and DR5 by their respective ligands. Specialized adaptor proteins are recruited as a result. Caspase cascades are also, activated. Fas trimerization is induced by the binding of FasL leading to the initiation (via the adaptor protein FADD) of caspase-8. Then, oligomerzes activated by autocatalysis. This activation stimulates apoptosis in two parallel cascades, which can bind directly and activate caspase-3 or cleave Bid. Next, truncated Bid (tBid) induces cytochrome c release by translocation to mitochondria, which sequentially activating caspase-9 and -3. TNFαR and DR3 (which can deliver pro-or anti-apoptotic signals) encourage apoptosis by use of TRADD/FADD (adapter proteins) and activating caspase-8. TNF-α interacts with TNFαR, which may result in the activation of a NF-κB pathway via NIK/IKK. The expression of prosurvival genes (such as FLIP, which can directly inhibit caspase 8 activation, and NF-κB) is induced by the activation of NF-κB. Additionally FasL and TNF-α, Bcl-2 (by phosphorylation), may activate JNK (via ASKI/MKK7).

nuclear morphology. Necrotic cells also have different surface futures than apoptotic cells. Necrotic cells are characterized by swelling and lysing, in contrast apoptotic cells have intense cell surface zeioticblebbing [90]. Genetically, mutation disturbs apoptosis. It believed that defects in apoptotic pathways contribute to several human diseases, including neurodegenerative disorders to malignancy. A high frequency of apoptosis in spontaneously regressing tumors and in tumors treated with cytotoxic anticancer agents, has been shown in multiple studies [91].

Thus, we can conclude that anticancer agents may induce apoptotic cell death. It follows that even after the drug-target interaction and cellular responses can have an impact on drug-induced cell death [92] as shown in **Figure 6**. The caspase-cascade system plays a vital role in the induction, transduction, and amplification of intracellular apoptotic signals. Caspases, closely associated with apoptosis, are aspartate-specific cysteine proteases and members of the interleukin-1β-converting enzyme family. The activation and function of caspases, involved in the delicate caspase-cascade system, are regulated by various kinds of molecules, such as the inhibitor of apoptosis protein, Bcl-2 family proteins, Ca^{2+}, and calpain [93]. Not all caspases are involved in apoptosis. The caspases that have been well described are caspase-3,-6,-7,-8, and caspase-9 [94]. Caspase-3 is a key factor in apoptosis execution.

Apoptosis is believed to be started when mitochondrial damage leads to a release of cytochrome C and the activation of Apaf-1, when in turn activates the caspase machinery responsible for executing apoptosis. The chain of events causing this mitochondrial damage begins when procaspase-3 activated (by caspase-3,-8,-9,-10, cysteine protease protein of molecular mass 32 KDa, granzyme B, etc.). Caspase-3 downstream substrates include various components of the cytoskeleton as well as: procaspase-3, procaspase-6, procaspase-9, DNA protein kinase (DNA-PK), protein kinase C (PKCγ), poly(ADP-ribose) polymerase (PARP), D4-GDP-dissociation inhibitor for the Rho family GTPases (D4-GDI) [95] (**Figure 6**).

It is important that we have this understanding of how apoptosis works because it has effects on tumorgenisis and cancer treatment. Inhibiting apoptosis can make cancer cells more resistant to treatment with chemotherapy and radiotherapy, the cells often increase survival proteins to protect themselves and inhibit apoptosis. On the other hand, apoptosis defects have been shown to increase the number of neoplastic cells.

Two hypotheses can propose the interplay between MDR expression and apoptosis inhibition. First, the expressing of a large molecule (such as MDR1) might disturb the content and context of plasma membrane, thereby interfering with DISC formation. Briefly, the ligation of cell death receptor molecules (e.g. Fas or TNF receptor), recruit the adapter proteins, which followed by the formation of death inducing signaling complex (DISC). This in turn triggers the caspase cascade. It is important to note that interfering with this DISC formation may significantly inhibit subsequent caspase formation.

Second hypothesis is that MDR expression alters intracellular pH (pHi), which contributes to MDR1 gaining resistance to several forms of caspase-dependant cell death stimuli resulting in lower drug concentrations. Briefly, as MDR1-correlates to an increase in pHi, and the transmembrane partitioning or intracellular sequestration is altered. This happens at the intracellular acidification stage, which often precedes apoptosis. Increasing the intracellular pHi can inhibit DNA fragmentation, and decrease the normal sensitivity of cells to inducing the apoptosis as response to Fas cross-linking or serum starvation and cells becoming resistant to caspase-dependent-death stimuli [23] [96] [97].

5. Plant-Derived Natural Products

Throughout history, humankind has used natural products found in plants, animal, microorganisms, etc. to treat disease. Increasingly, scientists are investigating the active ingredients in natural remedies (called secondary metabolites), to further develop effective drug treatments. Much work remains to be done as it is estimated that only 5% - 15% of the approximately 250,000 known plant species have been studied for their bioactive SMS [98]. Interestingly, even as production of and demand for synthetic drugs has been increasingly high, 80% of the world' s population rely primarily on traditional herbal medicines [99].

6. Cancer and Natural Products

Increased cancer mortality and the high cost of treatment spur a continued search for better anticancer drugs. In recent decades, natural compounds have attracted considerable attention as cancer chemopreventive agents and as cancer therapeutics [100]. Some of the most effective cancer treatments to date are natural products, or compounds derived from natural products.The first natural product used as an anticancer compound was when podophyllotoxin was islolated from *Podophyllumpeltatum* in 1947. Later, etoposide and teniposide (chemical derivative), vinca alkaloid (vinblastine and vincristine), andpaclitaxel (Taxol®), were discovered as active principleof *Taxusbrevifolia* [101]. Natural products and their synthetic derivatives comprise over 77% (63/81) of the approved anticancer drug candidates developed between 1981 and 2006 (**Figure 7**) [102]. This combined per-

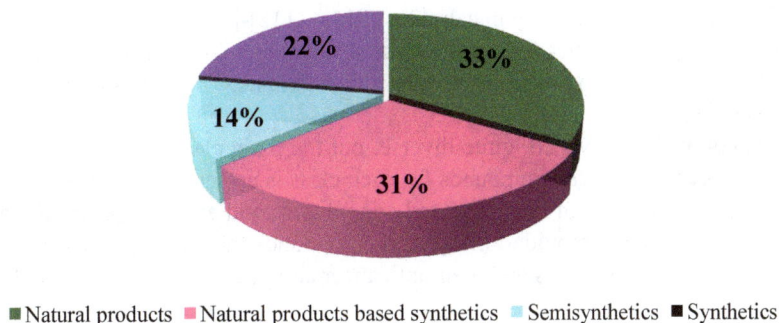

Figure 7. Role of natural products in anticancer.

■ Natural products ■ Natural products based synthetics ■ Semisynthetics ■ Synthetics

centage highlights the importance of natural products to drug development.

Our laboratory's focus is on isolation, identification, and investigation of the biological activities of interests in natural product uses against cancer. There are three main reasons why our laboratory workers believe researches into natural compounds is worthwhile:

First, natural compounds that show anticancer potential fit into the mechanism-based approach as perfectly as a hand fits into a glove. There is solid evidence that these compounds inhibit cancer by interfering with one, or more, of the mechanisms that researchers now feel are central to cancer progression.

Second, although the future does look bright for eventual success in the fight against cancer, we are not there yet. Much work remains to be done. As a science, the field of natural compound research can contribute to a greater understanding of cancer and a faster development of successful therapies.

Third, we must study natural compounds because they are already being used in cancer treatment (and in the treatment of other diseases). For better or for worse, hundreds of thousands if not millions, of patients around the world are experimenting with natural compounds in their efforts to heal themselves of cancer. Researchers estimate that anywhere from 10 to 80 percent of US, European, Australian, and Mexican cancer patients use some form of complementary medicine as part of their overall therapy [103]. For many of these patients, the use of natural compounds is an essential part of the complementary approach. For example, two studies in the United States have reported that roughly 40% - 60% of cancer patients who use some combination of complementary medicine including herbs, vitamins, and/or antioxidants [103] [104]. Most of these patients are using natural compounds without the guidance of their oncologist, or any real guidance from scientific studies. Because the popularity of using natural compounds in cancer treatment appears to be growing rather than declining, we are compelled to study natural compounds so that we can properly guide the public.

On the other hand, the new mechanism-based approach informs us that many different events contribute to the eventual success of a cancer. Any single drug can, at best target a small number of these events, leaving the rest to occur uninterrupted. Moreover, we know that cancer cells have some ability to adapt or resistant to therapy. We can imagine that a cancer cell can adapt better to one, or a few, interrupted events than to many.

To overcome this problem, it is necessary to use multiple compounds in combination. Natural compounds are ideally suited for this type of application; they are active at reasonable concentrations, and yet their mild nature allows a variety of large combinations to be used safely [105].

Thus, we studied traditional herbs, which are currently in widespread use. We focused on 3 plant families: *Chelidoniummajus* (Papaveraceae) [106], *Fallopia japonica* (Polygonaceae) (in preparation)*, and *Citrus jambhiri* (and *Citrus pyriformis*) (Rutaceae) [64]. Our previous investigations were focused on their SMs such as flavonoids, limonoids, steroids, polyphenols, and alkaloid looking at their possible modulation effect on multidrug resistance in cancer cells in order to validate their traditional use [64] [107]-[110] [111]. The following section highlights the chemistry and anticancer activity (especially the interaction with multidrug resistance proteins) and the resulting effect of these secondary metabolites on cancer.

7. Plant Secondary Metabolites

In the last century, thorough phytochemical investigations were conducted on these herbal drugs using simple and/or modern techniques of isolation and structure elucidation with the aim of finding substances responsible for the claimed medicinal effects.

This has led to a focus on plants secondary metabolites (SMs) [112]-[114]. Secondary metabolites are derived biosynthetically from primary metabolites (e.g., carbohydrates, amino acids, lipids, and acetyl-CoA) and are not directly involved in the growth, development, or reproduction of plants. Thousands of newly isolated secondary metabolites are discovered each year.

The chemical structures of these SMs are quite diverse, but the main classes of these SMs can be easily distinguished. An estimation of the isolated compounds for each class is presented in **Table 1**.

The screening of anticancer activity of these isolated compounds, and even the parent extracts, has generated as immense body of information and provided many lead compounds that could be modified for better activity. The major classes of secondary metabolites and their anticancer activities are highlighted in the next section.

7.1. Phenolics

Phenolic compounds constitute one of the most numerous groups in the plant kingdom with over 800 identified to date. Phenolics are characterized by the absence of nitrogen atoms and having at least one aromatic ring with one or more hydroxyl groups attached [116]. They range from simple, low molecular weight, single aromatic-ringed compounds to large and complex tannins and can be divided into 10 general classes (based on the number and arrangement of their carbon atoms). They are commonly found conjugated to sugars and organic acids. The most abundantly occurring polyphenols in plants are phenolic acids, flavonoids, stilbenes and lignans, of which flavonoids and phenolic acids account for 60% and 30%, respectively, of dietary polyphenols.

Flavonoids

Over 4000 varieties of flavonoids have been identified to date, making these universally distributed natural plants pigments, one of the most numerous and widespread of all. Additionally, 6500 different flavonoids have been identified from plant sources of which at least 400 appear to be prenylated [117]. Flavonoids are divided

Table 1. Approximate numbers of known secondary metabolites from higher plants [115].

Type of secondary metabolites	Estimated number[*]
Nitrogen-containing SMs	
Alkaloids	21,000
Non-protein amino acids (NPAAs)	700
Amines	100
Cyanogenic glycosides	60
Glucosinolates	100
Alkylamides	150
Lectins, peptides, polypeptides	2000
SMs without nitrogen	
Monoterpenes (C_{10})[**]	2500
Sesquiterpenes (C_{15})[**]	5000
Diterpenes (C_{20})[**]	2500
Triterpenes, steroids, saponins (C_{30}, C_{27})[**]	5000
Tetraterpenes (C_{40})[**]	500
Flavonoids, tannins	5000
Phenylpropanoids, lignin, coumarins, lignans	2000
Polyacetylenes, fatty acids, waxes	1500
Polyketides	750
Carbohydrates, simple acids	400

[*]Approximate number of known structures, [**]Total number of all terpenoides exceeds 33,000 at present.

into various classes according to their molecular structure; depend on the oxidation level of the central ring (ring C), however, all share a common carbon skeleton of diphenylpropanes (C_6-C_3-C_6; *i.e.*, two benzene rings joined by a linear three-carbon chain that forms an oxygenated heterocycle). The main groups are flavanols, flavones, flavanones, flavonols, isoflavones and anthocyanidins (**Figure 8**).

Flavonoid compounds are particularly abundant in fruits (especially in *Citrus*), vegetables, nuts, stems, flowers, wine, and tea. They constitute an important part of the human diet with an average of 200 mg consumed daily in the Western diet [118] [119].

The basic flavonoid skeleton can have numerous substituents. Hydroxyl groups are usually present at the 4', 5, and 7 positions. Sugars are very common with the majority of flavonoids, existing naturally as glycosides. While both sugars and hydroxyl groups increase the water solubility of flavonoids, other substituents, such as methyl groups and isopentyl units, make flavonoids lipophilic [120]. Generally, modifications such as hydroxylation, methylation, and glycosylation are also possible in either of the two aromatic rings. These structural modifications have a great impact on the anticancer activity of these SMs through their effect on the solubility and bioavailability of these compounds.

Anticancer activity of flavonoids: Recently, much research has focused on the anti-cancer properties of flavonoids. Epidemiological studies suggest an association between flavonoid intake and a reduced risk of certain cancers [121]. Flavonoids appear to work with no or little toxicity as large doses of these compounds (up to 500 mg/kg) have been administered to animals, with little or no toxicity reported [122]. There is a long history of human consumption of flavonoids.

Many flavonoids are substrates of the most pharmacologically relevant ABC transporters, P glycoprotein/MDR1, MRP, and BCRP [123] [124] but so far scientific effort has focused on the modulation of the transporter by flavonoids [125]. Whereas some flavonoids were shown to inhibit MDR1-mediated transport processes by directly interacting with the vicinal ATP- and steroid-binding sites [126], others (like (–) epicatechin from green tea) were shown to activate MDR1 by a heterotropic allosteric mechanism [127].

To clarify, MDR1 possesses at least two positively cooperative sites for drug binding, with the H site preferring Hoechst 33,342 to rhodamine 123 and the R site preferring rhodamine 123 to Hoechst 33,342. Binding to one of these sites has been shown to stimulate binding to the other site and transport activity. Therefore, the conflicting reports regarding flavonoid-MDR1 interactions might be explained by the different binding properties

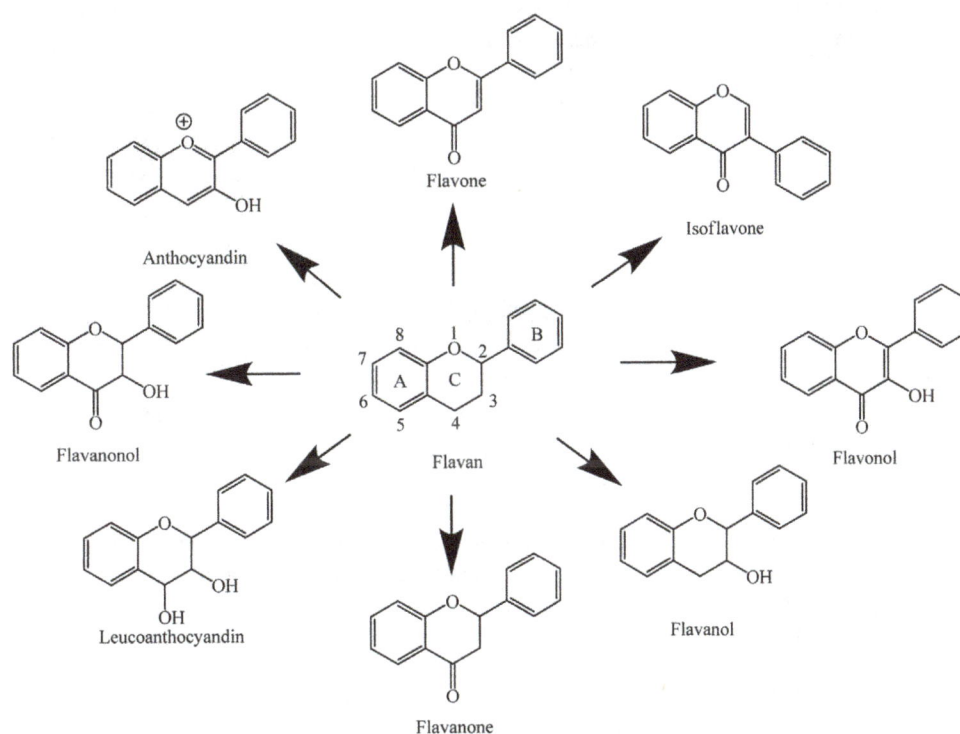

Figure 8. Generic structures of the major flavonoids subclasses.

of the model substrates used [128]. Thus, polyphenols might be potential agents for modulating the bioavailability of MDR1 substrates at the intestine and the multidrug resistance phenotype associated with expression of this transporter in cancer cells [129]. In any case, the majority of studies have indicated that many flavonoids have an inhibitory activity on MDR1-mediated transport [130].

Citrus flavonoids are shown to have anti-carcinogenic effects. Nobiletin (5,6,7,8,3',4'-hexamethoxyflavone), a polymethoxyflavonoids in citrus fruit, showed strong inhibitory effects on tumor promotion in mice and the growth of human prostate carcinoma cells [131]. Therefore, citrus phytochemicals are considered promising chemopreventive agents. Likewise, the ingestion of citrus fruit has been reported to be beneficial for the reduction of certain types of human cancer [132].

However, further studies of the absorption, distribution, metabolism, and excretion of citrus phytochemicals in the human body are needed to clarify the inhibitory effects of these compounds at the site of drug action, in the tumor tissues and cancer cells. We have recently reported the inhibitory effects of several isolated compounds from citrus on the functions of MDR1 using MDR1-mediated multidrug-resistant human caco-2 and CEM/ADR5000 cells [64]. Recently, reported state to grapefruit juice, compounds in orange juice can inhibit MDR1 [133]. Our results are comparable to this study in that the transport of Rho123, a substrate of MDR1, in Caco-2 cells was inhibited by citrus flavonoids [64].

Furthermore, increasing *in vitro* and *in vivo* evidence has indicated that the pharmacokinetic interaction of drugs with herbal products containing flavonoids may be attributable not only to the modulation of drug transporters such as MDR1 but also to metabolizing enzymes such as several CYP450s, esterases, glucuronidases, oxidases, and other enzymes [134]-[136]. One well-documented food-interaction is the altered oral bioavailability of many marketed drugs from co-administered grapefruit juice and citrus fruit [134] [137]. The *citrus* appear to inhibit the MDR1 and CYP3A4, thus changing the drug absorption in the small intestine [137]. The enhancement of the detoxification pathway for the elimination of toxic electrophiles by the Phase-II enzymes; glutathione *S*-transferase (GST), may cause of citrus anticarcinogenic effect. To that end, the effects of citrus flavonoids (hesperidin, naringin, and crude flavonoids mixture) were investigated in various mice tissues. *Citrus* flavonoids showed the most significant induction of GST in the stomach. The GST induction by the flavonoids appeared to be tissue-specific and related to the structures of the compounds. The enhanced level of phase-II enzymes by citrus flavonoids suggests their importance in chemoprevention.

Finally, the observed antiproliferative properties of flavonoids suggest that these compounds may induce apoptosis by modulating different key targets involved in both apoptotic pathways. However, little is known regarding the precise mechanism of flavonoid-induced apoptosis, and only recently has interest started to focus on flavonoids' potential to interact with intracellular signaling pathways. Many genes participate in the regulation of the apoptotic process, and activation of caspases is a central effector mechanism. For example in different cell lines, many isoflavonoids increased the activity and levels of caspase-3 and caspase-9, in concentration and time dependent manner [138]-[142].

7.2. Terpenoids

The term terpenoids is widely used to describe a diverse and widespread class of natural products derived from a common biosynthetic pathway [143]. C_5 isopentenoid units constitute the main building block in more than 30,000 reported individual members [144]. Classification of terpenoids is based on the number of the isoprenoid units. Terpenoids with two isoprene units are called monoterpenes, while those containing three to six isoprene units are called sesquiterpenes, diterpenes, sesterterpenes, and triterpenes, respectively [145].

7.2.1. Limonoids

Limonoids are a group of highly oxygenated triterpenoids. Hundreds of limonoids have been isolated from various plants yet, their occurrence in the plant kingdom is confined to only plant families the Rutales, Meliaceae, and Rutaceae [146]. Limonoids are stereochemically homogenous compounds, with a prototypical structure either containing or derived from a precursor with a 4,4,8-trimethyl-17-furanylsteroid skeleton [146]. All naturally occurring citrus limonoids contain a furan ring attached to the D-ring, at C-17, as well as oxygen containing functional groups at C-3, C-4, C-7, C-16, and C-17 [146]. Citrus fruits and their closely related genera contain about 36 limonoidaglycones and 17 limonoidglucosides [147]. Citrus limonoids and their glucosides, the water-soluble triterpenoid compounds that occur naturally in citrus fruit and citrus juice in amounts comparable to vitamin C, can be reclaimed from citrus processing and citrus seeds as by-products in large quantities [146]. Limonin, the first characterized compound of this group of phytochemicals, has been known as a constituent of *Citrus* since 1841 (**Figure 9**) [148].

Anticancer activity of limonoids: Many studies revealed that the limonoids present in citrus fruits and their juice have cancer chemopreventive property. *In vitro* limonoids inhibit the growth of estrogen receptor-negative and -positive human breast cancer cells. Limonoids have also been found to target and stop neuroblastoma cells [149]. The decreased colon tumor-genesis associated with ingesting orange juice may be explained by the potential chemopreventive effect of limonin, hesperidin, and other flavonoids [150]. The citrus limonoidsobacunone, limonin, nomilin and their glucosides, and some aglycones inhibit chemically induced carcinogenesis and a series of human cancer cell lines, with remarkable cytotoxicity against lung, colon, oral and skin cancer in animal test system and human breast cancer cells [151]-[153]. Pure limoninglucoside and limonin, (its water insoluble relative lacking glucose) have been found to possess significant antitumor properties in animal tests and with human cells [147].

Nutritional research on the health benefits of chemicals present in plant foods suggest that citrus limonoids possess substantial anticancer activity and they are also free of any toxic effects in animal models [146]. Moreover, limonoid have shown a modifying effect on the development of aberrant crypt foci. These compounds also have ability to induce specific carcinogen-metabolizing enzymes, glutathione-*S*-transferase and quinine reductase in the liver and mucosa of the small intestine to detoxify chemical carcinogenesis. Studies show that the activity of phase II enzyme glutathione-*S*-transferase in the liver of rats, fed diets containing limonin and nomilin, increased significantly in a dose dependent manner. While simultaneously, the limonoidsnomilin and limonin were found to have no significant affect on the phase I enzyme cytochrome P450 [146]. The data from these studies suggest that certain rings in the limonoid nucleus may be critical to antineoplastic activity.

The structure-activity relationships of limonoids, showing that limonoids with an intact apoeuphol skeleton, a 14, 15 b epoxide, and a reactive site such as either a 19 - 28 lactol bridge or a cyclohexanone "A" ring, are biologically very active. In addition, α-,β-unsaturated ketone in ring "A" has been proposed as a common feature that is primarily responsible for their biological activity and absence of these structural features resulting in reduced activity [154] (**Figure 9**).

7.2.2. Sterols

Phytosterol is a general term widely used to describe a particular subclass of natural products possessing the steroidal nucleus. These steroids represent a large group of natural SMs widely occurring in plants and animals possessing a basic cyclopentanoperhydrophenanthrene skeleton (**Figure 10**).

Plant steroids comprise sterols, steroid saponins, steroid alkaloids, cardiac glycosides, pregnanes, estranes and ectysteroids [145]. They are all considered as triterpenes which have lost a minimum of three methyl groups during their biosynthesis [155].

Anticancer activity of sterols: Cholesterol is an essential structural component of animal cell membranes. Plant sterols play analogues roles in plants. The major dietary phytosterols are β-sitosterol and stigmasterol. Their contents are high in edible oils, seeds, and nuts. Steroids, in general have a wide range of biological activities [156] [157]. Epidemiologic and experimental studies also suggest that dietary plant sterols play a role in cancer protection (such as colon, breast, and prostate) [158]. In contrast to cholesterol, β-sitosterol is poorly absorbed from the intestine, and its concentration in the blood and tissues of normal mammals is uniformly low.

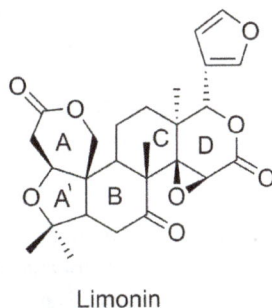

Limonin

Figure 9. Chemical structure of the *Citrus*limonoid, limonin.

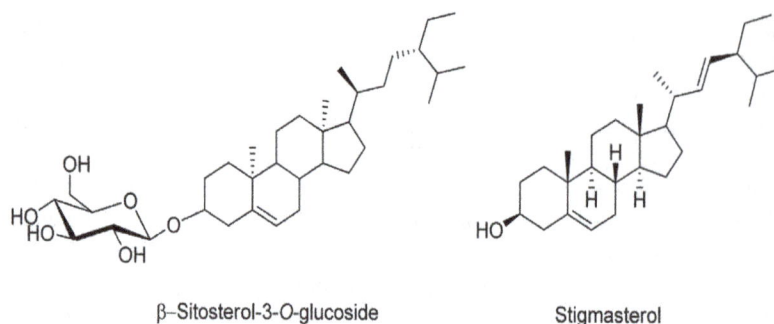

β–Sitosterol-3-O-glucoside   Stigmasterol

Figure 10. Chemical structures of the major phytosterols.

ABCG5 and ABCG8, which are present almost exclusively in the small intestine and liver, are considered functional transporters for the efflux of plant sterols and stanols as well as cholesterol. In addition to ABCG5 and ABCG8, it has been reported that other ABC transporters, ABCA1 and ABCB4, are implicated in lipid homeostasis. ABCA1 mediates the efflux of cholesterol and phospholipids to form high-density lipoprotein [159]. ABCB4 (MDR2), highly homologous with MDR1 (MDR1), functions in the secretion of phosphatidylcholine into bile ducts from hepatocytes [160]. Therefore, it is conceivable that MDR1 also interacts with membrane lipids.

Foods supplemented with plant sterols, and dietary supplements and/or herbal remedies containing phytosterols have been widely used, often conveniently with prescribed medications. However, little attention has been paid to the interactions between drugs and food and the effects of food components on the function of drug transporters, such as MDR1 and MRP1, have not fully investigated. We reported that the anticancer activity of citrus sterols related to their ability to reverse multidrug resistance (MDR1) in leukemia and human colon carcinoma, which endogenously expresses MDR1. Furthermore, Citrus sterols reversed doxorubicin resistance in both cell lines [64]. Phytosterol glycosides could interact with the cell biomembrane due to their structural similarity with cholesterol, resulting in increasing the fluidity of the cell membrane and leading to leakage of electrolytes and metabolites or even cell death [161]. Additionally, we reported that β-sitosterol-O-glucoside is more effective than stigmasterol in interacting with cell membrane proteins and in reversal of doxorubicin resistance [64]. The pharmacological activity of phytosterols has been shown to be mediated by the antagonism of the nuclear receptor and a ligand for multiple nuclear receptors [162]. Brobst *et al.* showed that phytosterols activate the estrogen receptor an isoform, progesterone receptor, and pregnane X receptor (PXR, NR1I2) [162]. They also showed that phytosterol-mediated activation of PXR induces the expression of drug-metabolizing enzyme cytochrome P450 (CYP) CYP3A gene. PXR is known to be activated by a variety of drugs, xenobiotics, and bile acids, and is a key regulator of human CYP3A4 and MDR1 genes [78].

7.3. Alkaloids

Alkaloids, a cyclic compound containing nitrogen in a negative oxidation state which is of limited distribution in living organisms, represent a very extensive group of secondary metabolites [163]. Over 21,000 alkaloids have been identified with diverse structures, distribution in nature, and important biological activities [164]. Alkaloids provide chemical defense against herbivores or predators. Strong physiological effects and the selectivity of some alkaloids present opportunities for utilizing the alkaloids in human medicine. During evolution, the constitution of alkaloids has been modulated so that they usually contain more than one active functional group allowing them to interact with several molecular targets. Therefore, a pleiotropic effect is a common term in alkaloids and other SM [114] [115] [165] (**Figure 11**).

Isoquinoline Alkaloids

The isoquinolines, one of the largest groups of alkaloids, skeletons are a basic building block of various types of alkaloids including benzylisoquinolines, protopines, benzo[c]phenanthridines, protoberberines, and others. Isoquinolines, alkaloids are biogenetically derived from tyrosine. Sanguinarine (SA), chelidonine (CH) (**Figure 11**), and chelerythrine (CHE), benzo[c]phen-anthridine alkaloids, have been isolated from *Sanguinariacanadensis*,

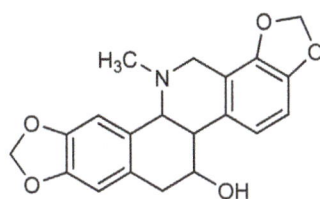

Chelidonine

Figure 11. Chemical structures of the isoquinoline alkaloid, chelidonine.

Chelidoniummajus, and *Macleyacordata* that are known to exert a wide spectrum of biological activities, e.g. from antimicrobial, antifungal, anti-inflammatory, adrenolytic, sympatholytic, and local anaesthetic as well as showing cytotoxicity against various human normal and cancer cell lines [166].

Anticancer activity of isoquinoline alkaloids: Benzylisoquinoline alkaloids, which are found in several herbal products, such as golden seal (*Hydrastiscanadensis*), *Berberis*and Oregon grape root (*Mahoniaaquifolia*), have been shown to interact with MDR1 and have the potential for drug-diet interactions [167] [168]. For example, Fu *et al.* (2001) screened potential MDR modifiers from a series of naturally occurring benzylisoquinoline alkaloids that were isolated from natural plants using resistance tumor cells. Many of these natural compounds showed potent activities to decrease the tumor cells resistance to MDR1 substrates, (such as doxorubicin and vincristine) and increased intracellular drug accumulation of [3H] vincristine. Their results suggest that the mechanism of these compounds to reverse MDR was probably linked to increased intracellular drug accumulation by inhibiting the activity of MDR1 [167].

He and Liu (2002) screened various IQAs to examine their effect on the functional activity of MDR1 in cultured bovine brain capillary endothelial cells (BCEC). All compounds tested increased the intracellular accumulation of MDR1 substrate (Rho123) in a concentration-dependent manner. The rank order of these agents in increasing Rh123 accumulation in endothelial cells was as follows: tetrandrine > vincristine > *dl*-tetrahydropalmatine > dauricine > azithromycin > berbamine > daurisoline > berberine = doxorubicin > *l*-te-trahydropalmatine [169] [170].

Möller *et al.* reported that emetine reversed efflux pump function and up regulated the expression of MDR1 in resistance cells. This indicating that emetine acts as competitive substrate for MDR1 but not for MRP1 [171]. This was the first research showing that chelidonine inhibited the ABC transporters in Caco-2 cells, interacted with metabolic enzymes phase I and phase II and induced apoptosis in resistance cells, which indicating that chelidonine may be an active MDR inhibitor.

Extensive studies of the interaction of IQAs (36 compounds) with the most important human CYP enzymes have been performed. Overall, there were clear differences in the ability of these alkaloids to inhibit individual CYP forms [172] [173].

In addition, IQAs exert cell growth-inhibitory effects via the induction of apoptosis in a variety of cancer cells [106] [174] [175]. IQAs-mediated apoptosis has been found in human cancer through their activation of caspase-3 and depletion of GSH [106] [176]. IQAs were found to result in increased levels of cytochrome c and Apaf-1 and in a significant increase in the active form of caspases 3, 7, 8, and 9 in a dose-dependent manner in many cancer cells [174] [177]-[180].

8. Molecular Targets of Secondary Metabolites

The modulation of a molecular target will negatively influence its communication with other components of the cellular network, especially proteins (cross-talk of proteins), or elements, or signal transducers. Consequently, the metabolism and function of cells, tissues, organs, and eventually the whole organism will be affected. Although we know the structures of many SM, our knowledge concerning their molecular mode(s) of action is largely fragmentary and incomplete. SM with broad activities interacts mainly with proteins, biomembranes, and DNA/RNA [165] (**Figure 12**).

Conformational changes, associated with the lessening of protein activity can occur when a covalent or a noncovalent interaction modulates the three-dimensional protein structure. This conformational change is usual-

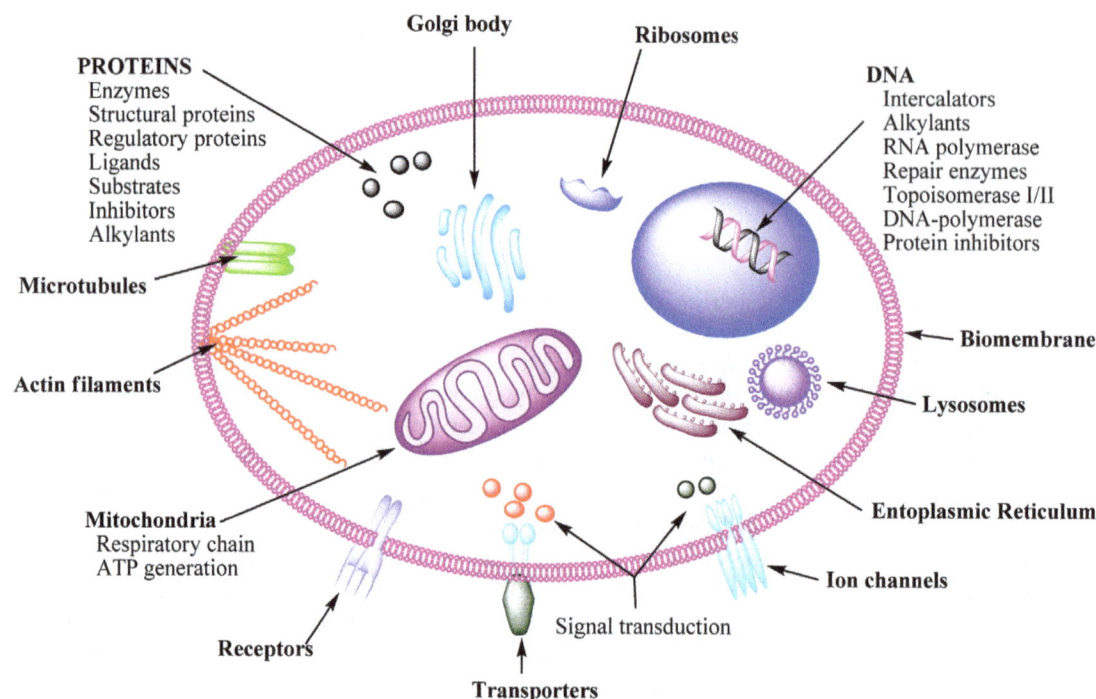

Figure 12. The main molecular targets of secondary metabolites in mammalian cells [165].

ly associated with a loss or reduction in the activity of a protein [165]. Covalent bond occur when double bond, epoxide, phenolic radicals, exocyclic or terminal methylene groups are activated by reactive functional groups of polyphenols. When physiological condition cause dissociation for OH groups of flavonoids, and other compounds with phenolic hydroxyl groups, changed it to phenolate anions, which can create hydrogen bonds with proteins or nucleic acids, positively charged amino acid residues (e.g. lysine, arginine, or histidine). Weaker non covalent bonds can be very powerful when they work together. These include: hydrogen bonds, ionic bonds, hydrophobic interactions and Vander Waal forces.

Nitrogen-containing compounds, such as alkaloids, usually have positively charged N-atoms (under physiological conditions) in their molecules that can form ionic bonds with negatively charged amino acid residues of aspartic and glutamic acid in proteins. Alkaloids are able to form covalent bonds with proteins and nucleic acids and noncovalent bonding. IQAs containing also OH groups which are crucial for the biological activity of phenolics. Both the covalent and non-covalent interactions will modulate the three-dimensional protein structure, *i.e.*, the conformation that is so important for their bioactivities. A conformational change is usually associated with a loss or reduction in the activity of a protein [165] [181].

The activity of IQAs related to their structure, the neutral form (pseudobase) of isoquinoline alkaloids (IQAs) can interact with proteins [182]; it is involved in the interactions with cellular biomacromolecules and may elicit a cytotoxic response [183]. IQAs interconvert between the cationic vs. neutral form; they penetrate the cell membrane in the form of nonpolar pseudobase [184]. The iminium bond, $C6 = N^+$ in the cationic form is susceptible to nucleophilic attack and plays a key role in inhibition of SH-proteins [185]. The binding of IQAs with human serum albumin and L-cysteine is radically weaker at pH 5.0 than at pH 7.4. In addition, IQAs forms *in vitro* DNA adducts via modification of the $C(11) = C(12)$ bond detectable by ^{32}P-postlabelling [186]. Although IQAs mediated DNA damage *in vitro* and *in vivo* has been published [187].

The cytotoxic effect of IQAs resulting from their molecular interactions with many important targets in a cancer cell include: DNA, RNA, and the associated enzymes and processes (*i.e.*, replication, repair, transcription, polymerase, topoisomerase, telomerase, protein biosynthesis, protein conformation, biomembranes, and membrane proteins.

In addition, the IQAs are intercalating compounds, it has planar, lipophilic characters, can disturbed the replication and transcription process by interact with base pairs and stabilize the DNA double helix, and inhibition of microtubule [165] [181]. Alkaloids with a planar and polycyclic structure (e.g. isoquinoline, quinoline, and indole) are good candidates for DNA intercalation. Protonable ring nitrogens can stabilize the alkaloid-DNA complex by binding to the negatively charged DNA surface [165].

Furthermore, terpenoids (lipophilic compounds) have ability to associate with other hydrophobic molecules in a cell (biomembranes or the hydrophobic core of many proteins and of the DNA double helix) [165] [181]. A major target for terpenoids, especially saponins or saponins like structure (e.g. β-sitosterol-O-glucoside) is the biomembrane. This structure can also change the fluidity of biomembranes and reducing their protective function as a permeation barrier [165] [181] (**Figure 13**).

For example, both saponins and sterol glycosides are amphiphilic molecules, which function as detergents and are active mostly in their mono-desmosidic forms. The monodesmosides are anchored with their lipophilic moiety in the lipophilic membrane bilayer after complexing with cholesterol, while the hydrophilic sugar part remains outside the cell and can interact with other glycoproteins or glycolipids (**Figure 13**). As a result, loss of the membrane integrity and fluidity occurs with the subsequent leakage of many polar molecules out of the cells or the entry of unwanted molecules into a cell. Such activity of many SMs can explain the cytotoxic effects against a wide range of cells (cancer, bacteria, and fungi) [188].

In addition, other lipophilic SMs such as mono- and sesquiterpenes can dissolve in biomembranes resulting in a disturbance of the close interaction between membrane lipids and proteins, thereby changing the conformation of membrane proteins leading to loss of function. These membrane proteins include ion channels, transporters for nutrients and intermediates, receptors, and proteins of signal transduction. This type of interaction between

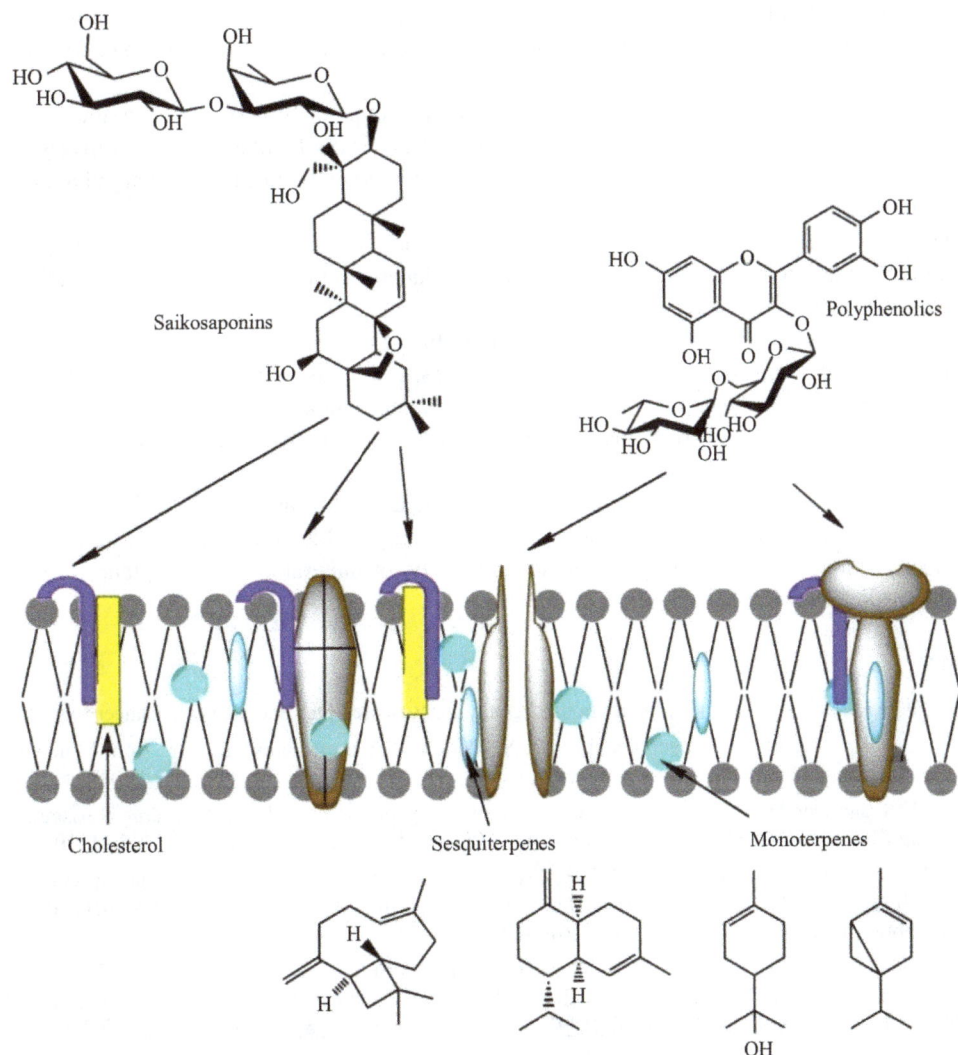

Figure 13. Interactions of some representative secondary metabolites with the cell membrane [161].

the SM and the biomembranes could explain the cytotoxic, antimicrobial and antiviral effects of many SMs [107] [109] [110] [161].

Plants extracts are a mixture of SMs, often both phenolics, terpenoids, and alkaloids. Thus, exhibit both covalent and noncovalent interactions. These activities are probably both additive and synergistic [165] [181].

9. Conclusions

Based on the overall study, it can concluded that certain natural products obtained from medicinal plants may serve as potent drugs for reversing multidrug resistance in cancer cells due to their ability to inhibit ABC-transporters, metabolic enzymes, and to induce apoptosis. In particular, the MDR modulatory activity of the crude extracts such as *C. majus* may be useful in cancer treatment, which would validate their traditional ethno-pharmacological uses in cancer formulas in China and Japan.

Plant extracts contain numerous and diverse secondary metabolites (SMs). Generally, it is difficult to attribute the biological and pharmacological activities of a multicomponent mixture, as plant extracts, to only a single compound of a multicomponent extract. Furthermore, SMs can unselectively affect many molecular targets in the cells.

Active SMs have shown the ideal character of MDR inhibitors or substrates, they have at least two hydrophobic centers containing more than two aromatic rings, which have more than two H-bond acceptors and at least one H-bond donor center. Therefore, under physiological conditions, the OH groups of resveratrol, emodin, and citrus flavonoids (polyphenols) change to phenolate ions and form ionic bonds with positively charged amino acid residues, such as those from lysine, arginine, and histidine in several proteins (e.g. ABCT, CYP3A4, and caspases).

Covalent bonds can be formed also with reactive functional groups of SM, such as epoxides (e.g. limonin), activated double bonds, and exocyclic or terminal methylene groups. Chelidonine has positively charged N-atoms (under physiological conditions) that can form also ionic bonds with negatively charged amino acid residues of glutamic and aspartic acid in proteins.

Chelidonine can be considered as a good candidate as a cytotoxic drug and for induction of apoptosis. One explanation could be that the protonated ring nitrogens with planar and polycyclic structure of chelidonine facilitate its penetration of the cell membrane, forming stable complexes with DNA by binding to the negatively charged DNA surface, leading to DNA intercalation, and inhibiting reverse transcriptase.

Non-covalent bonds, especially hydrogen bonds, ionic bonds, and hydrophobic interactions can be effective if they act cooperatively together. Both the covalent and non-covalent interactions will modulate the three-dimensional protein structure, resulting in conformational change, which is usually associated with a loss or reduction in the activity of a protein.

Finally, interference of different SMs/extracts with phase I, CYP3A4, and phase II, GST metabolizing enzymes can cause many serious interactions. Therefore, studies on possible herbal-herbal or herbal-drug interactions and standardization of drugs are very important, especially for integration and acceptance of plant extracts in conventional medicine as anti-cancer drugs.

References

[1]   Stewart, B.W. and Kleihues, P. (2014) International Agency for Research on Cancer. World Cancer Report 351, Lyon.

[2]   Altieri, F., Grillo, C., Maceroni, M. and Chichiarelli, S. (2008) DNA Damage and Repair: From Molecular Mechanisms to Health Implications. *Antioxidants & Redox Signaling*, **10**, 891-938. http://dx.doi.org/10.1089/ars.2007.1830

[3]   Velingkar, V.S. and Dandekar, V.D. (2010) Modulation of P-Glycoprotein Mediated Multidrug Resistance (MDR) in Cancer Using Chemosensitizers. *International Journal of Pharma Sciences and Research (IJPSR)*, **1**, 104-111.

[4]   Shen, D., Pastan, I. and Gottesman, M.M. (1998) Cross-Resistance to Methotrexate and Metals in Human Cisplatin-Resistant Cell Lines Results from a Pleiotropic Defect in Accumulation of These Compounds Associated with Reduced Plasma Membrane Binding Proteins. *Cancer Research*, **58**, 268-275.

[5]   Shen, D.W., Goldenberg, S., Pastan, I. and Gottesman, M.M. (2000) Decreased Accumulation of [^{14}C]Carboplatin in Human Cisplatin-Resistant Cells Results from Reduced Energy-Dependent Uptake. *Journal of Cellular Physiology*, **183**, 108-116. http://dx.doi.org/10.1002/(SICI)1097-4652(200004)183:1<108::AID-JCP13>3.0.CO;2-4

[6]   Chai, S., To, K.K. and Lin, G. (2010) Circumvention of Multi-Drug Resistance of Cancer Cells by Chinese Herbal Medicines. *Chinese Medicine*, **5**, 26. http://dx.doi.org/10.1186/1749-8546-5-26

[7]   Jain, R.K. (2001) Delivery of Molecular and Cellular Medicine to Solid Tumors. *Advanced Drug Delivery Reviews*, **46**, 149-168. http://dx.doi.org/10.1016/S0169-409X(00)00131-9

[8]   Pluen, A., Boucher, Y., Ramanujan, S., McKee, T.D., Gohongi, T., di Tomaso, E., *et al.* (2001) Role of Tumor-Host Interactions in Interstitial Diffusion of Macromolecules: Cranial vs. Subcutaneous Tumors. *Proceedings of the National Academy of Sciences of the United States of America*, **98**, 4628-4633. http://dx.doi.org/10.1073/pnas.081626898

[9]   Schuetz, E.G., Beck, W.T. and Schuetz, J.D. (1996) Modulators and Substrates of P-Glycoprotein and Cytochrome P4503A Coordinately Up-Regulate These Proteins in Human Colon Carcinoma Cells. *Molecular Pharmacology*, **49**, 311-318.

[10] Jiang, H., Chen, K., He, J., Pan, F., Li, J., Chen, J.F., *et al.* (2009) Association of Pregnane X Receptor with Multidrug Resistance-Related Protein 3 and Its Role in Human Colon Cancer Chemoresistance. *Journal of Gastrointestinal Surgery*, **13**, 1831-1838. http://dx.doi.org/10.1007/s11605-009-0964-x

[11] Lowe, S.W., Ruley, H.E., Jacks, T. and Housman, D.E. (1993) P53-Dependent Apoptosis Modulates the Cytotoxicity of Anticancer Agents. *Cell*, **74**, 957-967. http://dx.doi.org/10.1016/0092-8674(93)90719-7

[12] Liu, Y.Y., Han, T.Y., Giuliano, A.E. and Cabot, M.C. (2001) Ceramide Glycosylation Potentiates Cellular Multidrug Resistance. *FASEB Journal*, **15**, 719-730. http://dx.doi.org/10.1096/fj.00-0223com

[13] Fan, D., Beltran, P.J. and O'Brien, C.A., Eds. (1994) Reversal of Multidrug Resistance. CRC Press, Boca Raton.

[14] Huang, G. and Chen, L. (2010) Recombinant Human Endostatin Improves Anti-Tumor Efficacy of Paclitaxel by Normalizing Tumor Vasculature in Lewis Lung Carcinoma. *Journal of Cancer Research and Clinical Oncology*, **136**, 1201-1211. http://dx.doi.org/10.1007/s00432-010-0770-6

[15] Green, S.K., Frankel, A. and Kerbel, R.S. (1999) Adhesion-Dependent Multicellular Drug Resistance. *Anti-Cancer Drug Design*, **14**, 153-168.

[16] Durand, R.E. and Olive, P.L. (2001) Resistance of Tumor Cells to Chemo- and Radiotherapy Modulated by the Three-Dimensional Architecture of Solid Tumors and Spheroids. *Methods in Cell Biology*, **64**, 211-233. http://dx.doi.org/10.1016/S0091-679X(01)64015-9

[17] Litman, T., Druley, T.E., Stein, W.D. and Bates, S.E. (2001) From MDR to MXR: New Understanding of Multidrug Resistance Systems, Their Properties and Clinical Significance. *Cellular and Molecular Life Sciences CMLS*, **58**, 931-959. http://dx.doi.org/10.1007/PL00000912

[18] Dean, M., Hamon, Y. and Chimini, G. (2001) The Human ATP-Binding Cassette (ABC) Transporter Superfamily. *Journal of Lipid Research*, **42**, 1007-1017.

[19] Juliano, R.L. and Ling, V. (1976) A Surface Glycoprotein Modulating Drug Permeability in Chinese Hamster Ovary Cell Mutants. *Biochimica et Biophysica Acta*, **455**, 152-162. http://dx.doi.org/10.1016/0005-2736(76)90160-7

[20] Ueda, K., Cardarelli, C., Gottesman, M.M. and Pastan, I. (1987) Expression of a Full-Length cDNA for the Human "MDR1" Gene Confers Resistance to Colchicine, Doxorubicin, and Vinblastine. *Proceedings of the National Academy of Sciences of the United States of America*, **84**, 3004-3008. http://dx.doi.org/10.1073/pnas.84.9.3004

[21] Ambudkar, S.V., Dey, S., Hrycyna, C.A., Ramachandra, M., Pastan, I. and Gottesman, M.M. (1999) Biochemical, Cellular, and Pharmacological Aspects of the Multidrug Transporter. *Annual Review of Pharmacology and Toxicology*, **39**, 361-398. http://dx.doi.org/10.1146/annurev.pharmtox.39.1.361

[22] Gottesman, M.M., Fojo, T. and Bates, S.E. (2002) Multidrug Resistance in Cancer: Role of ATP-Dependent Transporters. *Nature Reviews Cancer*, **2**, 48-58. http://dx.doi.org/10.1038/nrc706

[23] Johnstone, R.W., Ruefli, A.A. and Smyth, M.J. (2000) Multiple Physiological Functions for Multidrug Transporter P-Glycoprotein? *Trends in Biochemical Sciences*, **25**, 1-6. http://dx.doi.org/10.1016/S0968-0004(99)01493-0

[24] Sauna, Z.E. and Ambudkar, S.V. (2000) Evidence for a Requirement for ATP Hydrolysis at Two Distinct Steps during a Single Turnover of the Catalytic Cycle of Human P-Glycoprotein. *Proceedings of the National Academy of Sciences of the United States of America*, **97**, 2515-2520. http://dx.doi.org/10.1073/pnas.97.6.2515

[25] Cole, S.P., Bhardwaj, G., Gerlach, J.H., Mackie, J.E., Grant, C.E., Almquist, K.C., *et al.* (1992) Overexpression of a Transporter Gene in a Multidrug-Resistant Human Lung-Cancer Cell-Line. *Science*, **258**, 1650-1654. http://dx.doi.org/10.1126/science.1360704

[26] Jedlitschky, G., Leier, I., Buchholz, U., Barnouin, K., Kurz, G. and Keppler, D. (1996) Transport of Glutathione, Glucuronate, and Sulfate Conjugates by the MRP Gene-Encoded Conjugate Export Pump. *Cancer Research*, **56**, 988-994.

[27] Borst, P., Evers, R., Kool, M. and Wijnholds, J. (2000) A Family of Drug Transporters: The Multidrug Resistance-Associated Proteins. *Journal of the National Cancer Institute*, **92**, 1295-1302. http://dx.doi.org/10.1093/jnci/92.16.1295

[28] Allikmets, R., Schriml, L.M., Hutchinson, A., Romano-Spica, V. and Dean, M. (1998) A Human Placenta-Specific ATP-Binding Cassette Gene (ABCP) on Chromosome 4q22 that Is Involved in Multidrug Resistance. *Cancer Research*,

58, 5337-5339.

[29] Honjo, Y., Hrycyna, C.A., Yan, Q.W., Medina-Perez, W.Y., Robey, R.W., van de Laar, A., *et al.* (2001) Acquired Mutations in the MXR/BCRP/ABCP Gene Alter Substrate Specificity in MXR/BCRP/ABCP-Overexpressing Cells. *Cancer Research*, **61**, 6635-6639.

[30] Komatani, H., Kotani, H., Hara, Y., Nakagawa, R., Matsumoto, M., Arakawa, H. and Nishimura, S. (2001) Identification of Breast Cancer Resistant Protein/Mitoxantrone Resistance/Placenta-Specific, ATP-Binding Cassette Transporter as a Transporter of NB-506 and J-107088, Topoisomerase I Inhibitors with an Indolocarbazole Structure. *Cancer Research*, **61**, 2827-2832.

[31] Thiebaut, F., Tsuruo, T., Hamada, H., Gottesman, M.M., Pastan, I. and Willingham, M.C. (1987) Cellular Localization of the Multidrug-Resistance Gene Product P-Glycoprotein in Normal Human Tissues. *Proceedings of the National Academy of Sciences of the United States of America*, **84**, 7735-7738. http://dx.doi.org/10.1073/pnas.84.21.7735

[32] Fletcher, J.I., Haber, M., Henderson, M.J. and Norris, M.D. (2010) ABC Transporters in Cancer: More than Just Drug Efflux Pumps. *Nature Reviews Cancer*, **10**, 147-156. http://dx.doi.org/10.1038/nrc2789

[33] Schinkel, A.H., Wagenaar, E., Mol, C.A. and van Deemter, L. (1996) P-Glycoprotein in the Blood-Brain Barrier of Mice Influences the Brain Penetration and Pharmacological Activity of Many Drugs. *Journal of Clinical Investigation*, **97**, 2517-2524. http://dx.doi.org/10.1172/JCI118699

[34] Cordon-Cardo, C., O'Brien, J.P., Boccia, J., Casals, D., Bertino, J.R. and Melamed, M.R. (1990) Expression of the Multidrug Resistance Gene Product (P-Glycoprotein) in Human Normal and Tumor Tissues. *Journal of Histochemistry & Cytochemistry*, **38**, 1277-1287. http://dx.doi.org/10.1177/38.9.1974900

[35] Jonker, J.W., Smit, J.W., Brinkhuis, R.F., Maliepaard, M., Beijnen, J.H., Schellens, J.H.M. and Schinkel, A.H. (2000) Role of Breast Cancer Resistance Protein in the Bioavailability and Fetal Penetration of Topotecan. *Journal of the National Cancer Institute*, **92**, 1651-1656. http://dx.doi.org/10.1093/jnci/92.20.1651

[36] Maliepaard, M., Scheffer, G.L., Faneyte, I.F., van Gastelen, M.A., Pijnenborg, A.C., Schinkel, A.H., *et al.* (2001) Subcellular Localization and Distribution of the Breast Cancer Resistance Protein Transporter in Normal Human Tissues. *Cancer Research*, **61**, 3458-3464.

[37] St-Pierre, M.V., Serrano, M.A., Macias, R.I., Dubs, U., Hoechli, M., Lauper, U., *et al.* (2000) Expression of Members of the Multidrug Resistance Protein Family in Human Term Placenta. *American Journal of Physiology-Regulatory, Integrative and Comparative Physiology*, **279**, R1495-R1503.

[38] Schinkel, A.H., Mayer, U., Wagenaar, E., Mol, C.A.A.M., van Deemter, L., Smit, J.J.M., *et al.* (1997) Normal Viability and Altered Pharmacokinetics in Mice Lacking Mdr1-Type (Drug-Transporting) P-Glycoproteins. *Proceedings of the National Academy of Sciences of the United States of America*, **94**, 4028-4033. http://dx.doi.org/10.1073/pnas.94.8.4028

[39] Zhou, S.F., Lim, L.Y. and Chowbay, B. (2004) Herbal Modulation of P-Glycoprotein. *Drug Metabolism Reviews*, **36**, 57-104. http://dx.doi.org/10.1081/DMR-120028427

[40] Evers, R., Zaman, G.J., Van Deemter, L., Jansen, H., Calafat, J., Oomen, L.C., *et al.* (1996) Basolateral Localization and Export Activity of the Human Multidrug Resistance-Associated Protein in Polarized Pig Kidney Cells. *Journal of Clinical Investigation*, **97**, 1211-1218. http://dx.doi.org/10.1172/JCI118535

[41] Goldstein, L.J., Galski, H., Fojo, A., Willingham, M., Lai, S.L., Gazdar, A., *et al.* (1989) Expression of Multidrug Resistance Gene in Human Cancers. *Journal of the National Cancer Institute*, **81**, 116-124. http://dx.doi.org/10.1093/jnci/81.2.116

[42] Dorr, R., Karanes, C., Spier, C., Grogan, T., Greer, J., Moore, J., *et al.* (2001) Phase I/II Study of the P-Glycoprotein Modulator PSC 833 in Patients with Acute Myeloid Leukemia. *Journal of Clinical Oncology*, **19**, 1589-1599.

[43] Leith, C.P., Kopecky, K.J., Chen, I.M., *et al.* (1999) Frequency and Clinical Significance of the Expression of the Multidrug Resistance Proteins MDR1/P-Glycoprotein, MRP1, and LRP in Acute Myeloid Leukemia: A Southwest Oncology Group Study. *Blood*, **94**, 1086-1099.

[44] Michieli, M., Damiani, D., Ermacora, A., Masolini, P., Raspadori, D., Visani, G., *et al.* (1999) P-Glycoprotein, Lung Resistance-Related Protein and Multidrug Resistance Associated Protein in *de novo* Acute Non-Lymphocytic Leukaemias: Biological and Clinical Implications. *British Journal of Haematology*, **104**, 328-335. http://dx.doi.org/10.1046/j.1365-2141.1999.01172.x

[45] Tidefelt, U., Liliemark, J., Gruber, A., Liliemark, E., Sundman-Engberg, B., Juliusson, G., *et al.* (2000) P-Glycoprotein Inhibitor Valspodar (PSC 833) Increases the Intracellular Concentrations of Daunorubicin *in Vivo* in Patients with P-Glycoprotein-Positive Acute Myeloid Leukemia. *Journal of Clinical Oncology*, **18**, 1837-1844.

[46] El-Sharnouby, J.A., Abou El-Enein, A.M., El Ghannam, D.M., El-Shanshory, M.R., Hagag, A.A., Yahia, S. and Elashry, R. (2010) Expression of Lung Resistance Protein and Multidrug Resistance-Related Protein (MRP1) in Pediatric Acute Lymphoblastic Leukemia. *Journal of Oncology Pharmacy Practice*, **16**, 179-188.

http://dx.doi.org/10.1177/1078155209351329

[47] Van Der Pol, M.A., Broxterman, H.J., Pater, J.M., Feller, N., van der Maas, M., Weijers, G.W., *et al.* (2003) Function of the ABC Transporters, P-Glycoprotein, Multidrug Resistance Protein and Breast Cancer Resistance Protein, in Minimal Residual Disease in Acute Myeloid Leukemia. *Haematologica*, **88**, 134-147.

[48] Laska, D.A., Houchins, J.O., Pratt, S.E., Horn, J., Xia, X.L., Hanssen, B.R., *et al.* (2002) Characterization and Application of a Vinblastine-Selected CACO-2 Cell Line for Evaluation of P-Glycoprotein. *In Vitro Cellular & Developmental Biology-Animal*, **38**, 401-410. http://dx.doi.org/10.1290/1071-2690(2002)038<0401:CAAOAV>2.0.CO;2

[49] Engman, H.A., Lennernas, H., Taipalensuu, J., Otter, C., Leidvik, B. and Artursson, P. (2001) CYP3A4, CYP3A5, and MDR1 in Human Small and Large Intestinal Cell Lines Suitable for Drug Transport Studies. *Journal of Pharmaceutical Sciences*, **90**, 1736-1751. http://dx.doi.org/10.1002/jps.1123

[50] Lampen, A., Ebert, B., Stumkat, L., Jacob, J. and Seidel, A. (2004) Induction of Gene Expression of Xenobiotic Metabolism Enzymes and ABC-Transport Proteins by PAH and a Reconstituted PAH Mixture in Human Caco-2 Cells. *Biochimica et Biophysica Acta*, **1681**, 38-46. http://dx.doi.org/10.1016/j.bbaexp.2004.09.010

[51] Muller, J., Sidler, D., Nachbur, U., Wastling, J., Brunner, T. and Hemphill, A. (2008) Thiazolides Inhibit Growth and Induce Glutathione-S-Transferase Pi (GSTP1)-Dependent Cell Death in Human Colon Cancer Cells. *International Journal of Cancer*, **123**, 1797-1806. http://dx.doi.org/10.1002/ijc.23755

[52] Dai, J.Y., Yang, J.L. and Li, C. (2008) Transport and Metabolism of Flavonoids from Chinese Herbal Remedy Xiaochaihu-Tang across Human Intestinal Caco-2 Cell Monolayers. *Acta Pharmacologica Sinica*, **29**, 1086-1093. http://dx.doi.org/10.1111/j.1745-7254.2008.00850.x

[53] Heikkinen, A.T., Monkkonen, J. and Korjamo, T. (2009) Kinetics of Cellular Retention during Caco-2 Permeation Experiments: Role of Lysosomal Sequestration and Impact on Permeability Estimates. *Journal of Pharmacology and Experimental Therapeutics*, **328**, 882-892. http://dx.doi.org/10.1124/jpet.108.145797

[54] Ecker, G., Huber, M., Schmid, D. and Chiba, P. (1999) The Importance of a Nitrogen Atom in Modulators of Multidrug Resistance. *Molecular Pharmacology*, **56**, 791-796.

[55] Litman, T., Skovsgaard, T. and Stein, W.D. (2003) Pumping of Drugs by P-Glycoprotein: A Two-Step Process? *Journal of Pharmacology and Experimental Therapeutics*, **307**, 846-853. http://dx.doi.org/10.1124/jpet.103.056960

[56] Kim, R.B., Wandel, C., Leake, B., Cvetkovic, M., Fromm, M.F., Dempsey, P.J., *et al.* (1999) Interrelationship between Substrates and Inhibitors of Human CYP3A and P-Glycoprotein. *Pharmaceutical Research*, **16**, 408-414. http://dx.doi.org/10.1023/A:1018877803319

[57] Marzolini, C., Paus, E., Buclin, T. and Kim, R.B. (2004) Polymorphisms in Human MDR1 (P-Glycoprotein): Recent Advances and Clinical Relevance. *Clinical Pharmacology & Therapeutics*, **75**, 13-33. http://dx.doi.org/10.1016/j.clpt.2003.09.012

[58] Milne, R.J. and Buckley, M.M.T. (1991) Celiprolol—An Updated Review of Its Pharmacodynamic and Pharmacokinetic Properties, and Therapeutic Efficacy in Cardiovascular Disease. *Drugs*, **41**, 941-969. http://dx.doi.org/10.2165/00003495-199141060-00009

[59] Szakacs, G., Paterson, J.K., Ludwig, J.A., Booth-Genthe, C. and Gottesman, M.M. (2006) Targeting Multidrug Resistance in Cancer. *Nature Reviews Drug Discovery*, **5**, 219-234. http://dx.doi.org/10.1038/nrd1984

[60] Krishna, R. and Mayer, L.D. (2001) Modulation of P-Glycoprotein (PGP) Mediated Multidrug Resistance (MDR) Using Chemosensitizers: Recent Advances in the Design of Selective MDR Modulators. *Current Medicinal Chemistry-Anti-Cancer Agents*, **1**, 163-174. http://dx.doi.org/10.2174/1568011013354705

[61] Krishna, R. and Mayer, L.D. (2000) Multidrug Resistance (MDR) in Cancer: Mechanisms, Reversal Using Modulators of MDR and the Role of MDR Modulators in Influencing the Pharmacokinetics of Anticancer Drugs. *European Journal of Pharmaceutical Sciences*, **11**, 265-283. http://dx.doi.org/10.1016/S0928-0987(00)00114-7

[62] Borowski, E., Bontemps-Gracz, M.M. and Piwkowska, A. (2005) Strategies for Overcoming ABC-Transporters-Mediated Multidrug Resistance (MDR) of Tumor Cells. *Acta Biochimica Polonica*, **52**, 609-627.

[63] Liscovitch, M. and Lavie, Y. (2002) Cancer Multidrug Resistance: A Review of Recent Drug Discovery Research. *Idrugs*, **5**, 349-355.

[64] El-Readi, M.Z., Hamdan, D., Farrag, N., El-Shazly, A. and Wink, M. (2010) Inhibition of P-Glycoprotein Activity by Limonin and Other Secondary Metabolites from Citrus Species in Human Colon and Leukaemia Cell Lines. *European Journal of Pharmacology*, **626**, 139-145. http://dx.doi.org/10.1016/j.ejphar.2009.09.040

[65] Theis, J.G.W., Chan, H.S.L., Greenberg, M.L., Malkin, D., Karaskov, V., Moncica, I., *et al.* (2000) Assessment of Systemic Toxicity in Children Receiving Chemotherapy with Cyclosporine for Sarcoma. *Medical and Pediatric Oncology*, **34**, 242-249. http://dx.doi.org/10.1002/(SICI)1096-911X(200004)34:4<242::AID-MPO2>3.0.CO;2-U

[66] Wang, R.B., Kuo, C.L., Lien, L.L. and Lien, E.J. (2003) Structure-Activity Relationship: Analyses of P-Glycoprotein

Substrates and Inhibitors. *Journal of Clinical Pharmacy and Therapeutics*, **28**, 203-228. http://dx.doi.org/10.1046/j.1365-2710.2003.00487.x

[67] Garrigos, M., Mir, L.M. and Orlowski, S. (1997) Competitive and Non-Competitive Inhibition of the Multidrug-Resistance-Associated P-Glycoprotein ATPase. Further Experimental Evidence for a Multisite Model. *European Journal of Biochemistry*, **244**, 664-673. http://dx.doi.org/10.1111/j.1432-1033.1997.00664.x

[68] Dey, S., Ramachandra, M., Pastan, I., Gottesman, M.M. and Ambudkar, S.V. (1997) Evidence for Two Nonidentical Drug-Interaction Sites in the Human P-Glycoprotein. *Proceedings of the National Academy of Sciences of the United States of America*, **94**, 10594-10599. http://dx.doi.org/10.1073/pnas.94.20.10594

[69] Ford, J.M. (1996) Experimental Reversal of P-Glycoprotein-Mediated Multidrug Resistance by Pharmacological Chemosensitisers. *European Journal of Cancer*, **32**, 991-1001. http://dx.doi.org/10.1016/0959-8049(96)00047-0

[70] Tamai, I. and Safa, A.R. (1991) Azidopine Noncompetitively Interacts with Vinblastine and Cyclosporin a Binding to P-Glycoprotein in Multidrug Resistant Cells. *Journal of Biological Chemistry*, **266**, 16796-16800.

[71] Loo, T.W. and Clarke, D.M. (1995) Covalent Modification of Human P-Glycoprotein Mutants Containing a Single Cysteine in Either Nucleotide-Binding Fold Abolishes Drug-Stimulated ATPase Activity. *Journal of Biological Chemistry*, **270**, 22957-22961. http://dx.doi.org/10.1074/jbc.270.39.22957

[72] Solary, E., Bidan, J.M., Calvo, F., Chauffert, B., Caillot, D., Mugneret, F., *et al.* (1991) P-Glycoprotein Expression and *in Vitro* Reversion of Doxorubicin Resistance by Verapamil in Clinical Specimens from Acute Leukaemia and Myeloma. *Leukemia*, **5**, 592-597.

[73] Muller, C., Goubin, F., Ferrandis, E., Cornil-Scharwtz, I., Bailly, J.D., Bordier, C., *et al.* (1995) Evidence for Transcriptional Control of Human Mdr1 Gene Expression by Verapamil in Multidrug-Resistant Leukemic Cells. *Molecular Pharmacology*, **47**, 51-56.

[74] Ozben, T. (2006) Mechanisms and Strategies to Overcome Multiple Drug Resistance in Cancer. *FEBS Letters*, **580**, 2903-2909. http://dx.doi.org/10.1016/j.febslet.2006.02.020

[75] Guengerich, F.P. (1991) Reactions and Significance of Cytochrome P-450 Enzymes. *Journal of Biological Chemistry*, **266**, 10019-10022.

[76] Zhou, S.F., Gao, Y.H., Jiang, W.Q., Huang, M., Xu, A.L. and Paxton, J.W. (2003) Interactions of Herbs with Cytochrome P450. *Drug Metabolism Reviews*, **35**, 35-98. http://dx.doi.org/10.1081/DMR-120018248

[77] Bertilsson, G., Heidrich, J., Svensson, K., Åsman, M., Jendeberg, L., Sydow-Bäckman, M., *et al.* (1998) Identification of a Human Nuclear Receptor Defines a New Signaling Pathway for CYP3A Induction. *Proceedings of the National Academy of Sciences of the United States of America*, **95**, 12208-12213. http://dx.doi.org/10.1073/pnas.95.21.12208

[78] Urquhart, B.L., Tirona, R.G. and Kim, R.B. (2007) Nuclear Receptors and the Regulation of Drug-Metabolizing Enzymes and Drug Transporters: Implications for Interindividual Variability in Response to Drugs. *Journal of Clinical Pharmacology*, **47**, 566-578. http://dx.doi.org/10.1177/0091270007299930

[79] Tolson, A.H. and Wang, H. (2010) Regulation of Drug-Metabolizing Enzymes by Xenobiotic Receptors: PXR and CAR. *Advanced Drug Delivery Reviews*, **62**, 1238-1249. http://dx.doi.org/10.1016/j.addr.2010.08.006

[80] Kimura, Y., Matsuo, M., Takahashi, K., Saeki, T., Kioka, N., Amachi, T. and Ueda, K. (2004) ATP Hydrolysis-Dependent Multidrug Efflux Transporter: MDR1/P-Glycoprotein. *Current Drug Metabolism*, **5**, 1-10. http://dx.doi.org/10.2174/1389200043489090

[81] Lewis, A.D., Forrester, L.M., Hayes, J.D., Wareing, C.J., Carmichael, J., Harris, A.L., *et al.* (1989) Glutathione S-Transferase Isoenzymes in Human Tumours and Tumour Derived Cell Lines. *British Journal of Cancer*, **60**, 327-331. http://dx.doi.org/10.1038/bjc.1989.280

[82] Green, J.A., Robertson, L.J. and Clark, A.H. (1993) Glutathione S-Transferase Expression in Benign and Malignant Ovarian Tumours. *British Journal of Cancer*, **68**, 235-239. http://dx.doi.org/10.1038/bjc.1993.321

[83] Mannervik, B. and Jensson, H. (1982) Binary Combinations of Four Protein Subunits with Different Catalytic Specificities Explain the Relationship between Six Basic Glutathione S-Transferases in Rat Liver Cytosol. *Journal of Biological Chemistry*, **257**, 9909-9912.

[84] Morgenstern, R., Depierre, J.W. and Jornvall, H. (1985) Microsomal Glutathione Transferase. Primary Structure. *Journal of Biological Chemistry*, **260**, 13976-13983.

[85] Kuzmich, S. and Tew, K.D. (1991) Detoxification Mechanisms and Tumor Cell Resistance to Anticancer Drugs. *Medicinal Research Reviews*, **11**, 185-217.

[86] Ramsdell, H.S. and Eaton, D.L. (1990) Mouse Liver Glutathione S-Transferase Isoenzyme Activity toward Aflatoxin B1-8,9-Epoxide and Benzo[A]Pyrene-7,8-Dihydrodiol-9,10-Epoxide. *Toxicology and Applied Pharmacology*, **105**, 216-225. http://dx.doi.org/10.1016/0041-008X(90)90183-U

[87] Falkner, K.C., Rushmore, T.H., Linder, M.W. and Prough, R.A. (1998) Negative Regulation of the Rat Glutathione

S-Transferase A2 Gene by Glucocorticoids Involves a Canonical Glucocorticoid Consensus Sequence. *Molecular Pharmacology*, **53**, 1016-1026.

[88] Kasibhatla, S. and Tseng, B. (2003) Why Target Apoptosis in Cancer Treatment? *Molecular Cancer Therapeutics*, **2**, 573-580.

[89] Schultehermann, R., Bursch, W., Graslkraupp, B., Török, L., Ellinger, A. and Müllauer, I. (1995) Role of Active Cell Death (Apoptosis) in Multi-Stage Carcinogenesis. *Toxicology Letters*, **82-83**, 143-148. http://dx.doi.org/10.1016/0378-4274(95)03550-8

[90] Collins, J.A., Schandl, C.A., Young, K.K., Vesely, J. and Willingham, M.C. (1997) Major DNA Fragmentation Is a Late Event in Apoptosis. *Journal of Histochemistry & Cytochemistry*, **45**, 923-934. http://dx.doi.org/10.1177/002215549704500702

[91] Bruckheimer, E.M. and Kyprianou, N. (2000) Apoptosis in Prostate Carcinogenesis—A Growth Regulator and a Therapeutic Target. *Cell and Tissue Research*, **301**, 153-162. http://dx.doi.org/10.1007/s004410000196

[92] Dive, C. and Hickman, J.A. (1991) Drug-Target Interactions: Only the First Step in the Commitment to a Programmed Cell Death? *British Journal of Cancer*, **64**, 192-196. http://dx.doi.org/10.1038/bjc.1991.269

[93] Launay, S., Hermine, O., Fontenay, M., Kroemer, G., Solary, E. and Garrido, C. (2005) Vital Functions for Lethal Caspases. *Oncogene*, **24**, 5137-5148. http://dx.doi.org/10.1038/sj.onc.1208524

[94] Thornberry, N.A. and Lazebnik, Y. (1998) Caspases: Enemies Within. *Science*, **281**, 1312-1316. http://dx.doi.org/10.1126/science.281.5381.1312

[95] Hajra, K.M. and Liu, J.R. (2004) Apoptosome Dysfunction in Human Cancer. *Apoptosis*, **9**, 691-704. http://dx.doi.org/10.1023/B:APPT.0000045786.98031.1d

[96] Gottlieb, R.A., Nordberg, J., Skowronski, E. and Babior, B.M. (1996) Apoptosis Induced in Jurkat Cells by Several Agents Is Preceded by Intracellular Acidification. *Proceedings of the National Academy of Sciences of the United States of America*, **93**, 654-658. http://dx.doi.org/10.1073/pnas.93.2.654

[97] Robinson, L.J., Roberts, W.K., Ling, T.T., Lamming, D., Sternberg, S.S. and Roepe, P.D. (1997) Human MDR 1 Protein Overexpression Delays the Apoptotic Cascade in Chinese Hamster Ovary Fibroblasts. *Biochemistry*, **36**, 11169-11178. http://dx.doi.org/10.1021/bi9627830

[98] Kinghorn, A.D., Balandrin, M.F., American Chemical Society, Division of Agricultural and Food Chemistry, *et al.* (1993) Human Medicinal Agents from Plants. American Chemical Society, Washington DC, xii, 356 p.

[99] Cordell, G.A. (2002) Natural Products in Drug Discovery—Creating a New Vision. *Phytochemistry Reviews*, **1**, 261-273. http://dx.doi.org/10.1023/A:1026094701495

[100] Nobili, S., Lippi, D., Witort, E., Donnini, M., Bausi, L., Mini, E. and Capaccioli, S. (2009) Natural Compounds for Cancer Treatment and Prevention. *Pharmacological Research*, **59**, 365-378. http://dx.doi.org/10.1016/j.phrs.2009.01.017

[101] Colegate, S.M. and Molyneux, R.J. (2008) Bioactive Natural Products: Detection, Isolation, and Structural Determination. 2nd Edition, CRC Press, Boca Raton, xiii, 605 p.

[102] Newman, D.J. and Cragg, G.M. (2007) Natural Products as Sources of New Drugs over the Last 25 Years. *Journal of Natural Products*, **70**, 461-477. http://dx.doi.org/10.1021/np068054v

[103] Richardson, M.A., Sanders, T., Palmer, J.L., Greisinger, A. and Singletary, S.E. (2000) Complementary/Alternative Medicine Use in a Comprehensive Cancer Center and the Implications for Oncology. *Journal of Clinical Oncology*, **18**, 2505-2514.

[104] Sparber, A., Jonas, W., White, J., Derenzo, E., Johnson, E. and Bergerson, S. (2000) Cancer Clinical Trials and Subject Use of Natural Herbal Products. *Cancer Investigation*, **18**, 436-439. http://dx.doi.org/10.3109/07357900009032815

[105] Boik, J. (2001) Natural Compounds in Cancer Therapy. Oregon Medical Press, Princeton, xiii, 521 p.

[106] El-Readi, M.Z., Eid, S., Ashour, M.L., Tahrani, A. and Wink, M. (2013) Modulation of Multidrug Resistance in Cancer Cells by Chelidonine and *Chelidonium majus* Alkaloids. *Phytomedicine*, **20**, 282-294. http://dx.doi.org/10.1016/j.phymed.2012.11.005

[107] Eid, S.Y., El-Readi, M.Z., Eldin, E.E., Fatani, S.H. and Wink, M. (2013) Influence of Combinations of Digitonin with Selected Phenolics, Terpenoids, and Alkaloids on the Expression and Activity of P-Glycoprotein in Leukaemia and Colon Cancer Cells. *Phytomedicine*, **21**, 47-61. http://dx.doi.org/10.1016/j.phymed.2013.07.019

[108] Eid, S.Y., El-Readi, M.Z. and Wink, M. (2012) Carotenoids Reverse Multidrug Resistance in Cancer Cells by Interfering with ABC-Transporters. *Phytomedicine*, **19**, 977-987. http://dx.doi.org/10.1016/j.phymed.2012.05.010

[109] Eid, S.Y., El-Readi, M.Z. and Wink, M. (2012) Digitonin Synergistically Enhances the Cytotoxicity of Plant Secondary Metabolites in Cancer Cells. *Phytomedicine*, **19**, 1307-1314. http://dx.doi.org/10.1016/j.phymed.2012.09.002

[110] Eid, S.Y., El-Readi, M.Z. and Wink, M. (2012) Synergism of Three-Drug Combinations of Sanguinarine and Other

Plant Secondary Metabolites with Digitonin and Doxorubicin in Multi-Drug Resistant Cancer Cells. *Phytomedicine*, **19**, 1288-1297. http://dx.doi.org/10.1016/j.phymed.2012.08.010

[111] Wink, M., Ashour, M.L. and El-Readi, M.Z. (2012) Secondary Metabolites from Plants Inhibiting ABC Transporters and Reversing Resistance of Cancer Cells and Microbes to Cytotoxic and Antimicrobial Agents. *Frontiers in Microbiology*, **3**, 130. http://dx.doi.org/10.3389/fmicb.2012.00130

[112] Wink, M. (1999) Introduction: Biochemistry, Role and Biotechnology of Secondary Metabolites. *Annual Plant Reviews*, **2**, 1-16.

[113] Wink, M. (2003) Evolution of Secondary Metabolites from an Ecological and Molecular Phylogenetic Perspective. *Phytochemistry*, **64**, 3-19. http://dx.doi.org/10.1016/S0031-9422(03)00300-5

[114] Wink, M. (2008) Plant Secondary Metabolism: Diversity, Function and Its Evolution. *Natural Product Communications*, **3**, 1205-1216.

[115] Wink M (1999) Introduction: Biochemistry, Role and Biotechnology of Secondary Metabolites. In: Wink, M., Ed., *Functions of Plant Secondary Metabolites and Their Exploitation in Biotechnology*, Academic, Sheffield, 1-16.

[116] Mann, J. (1994) Natural Products: Their Chemistry and Biological Significance. 1st Edition, Longman Scientific & Technical, Wiley, Harlow, Essex, England, New York, ix, 455 p.

[117] Harborne, J.B. and Williams, C.A. (2000) Advances in Flavonoid Research Since 1992. *Phytochemistry*, **55**, 481-504. http://dx.doi.org/10.1016/S0031-9422(00)00235-1

[118] Manach, C., Morand, C., Gil-Izquierdo, A., Bouteloup-Demange, C. and Rémésy, C. (2003) Bioavailability in Humans of the Flavanones Hesperidin and Narirutin after the Ingestion of Two Doses of Orange Juice. *European Journal of Clinical Nutrition*, **57**, 235-242. http://dx.doi.org/10.1038/sj.ejcn.1601547

[119] Vallejo, F., Larrosa, M., Escudero, E., Zafrilla, M.P., Cerdá, B., Boza, J., *et al.* (2010) Concentration and Solubility of Flavanones in Orange Beverages Affect Their Bioavailability in Humans. *Journal of Agricultural and Food Chemistry*, **58**, 6516-6524. http://dx.doi.org/10.1021/jf100752j

[120] Crozier, A., Clifford, M.N. and Ashihara, H. (2006) Plant Secondary Metabolites: Occurrence, Structure and Role in the Human Diet. Blackwell Pub., Oxford, Ames, Iowa, xii, 372 p.

[121] Cho, Y.A., Kim, J., Park, K.S., Lim, S.Y., Shin, A., Sung, M.K. and Ro, J. (2010) Effect of Dietary Soy Intake on Breast Cancer Risk According to Menopause and Hormone Receptor Status. *European Journal of Clinical Nutrition*, **64**, 924-932. http://dx.doi.org/10.1038/ejcn.2010.95

[122] Middleton, E., Kandaswami, C. and Theoharides, T.C. (2000) The Effects of Plant Flavonoids on Mammalian Cells: Implications for Inflammation, Heart Disease, and Cancer. *Pharmacological Reviews*, **52**, 673-751.

[123] Cao, J., Chen, X., Liang, J., Yu, X.Q., Xu, A.L., Chan, E., *et al.* (2007) Role of P-Glycoprotein in the Intestinal Absorption of Glabridin, an Active Flavonoid from the Root of *Glycyrrhiza glabra*. *Drug Metabolism and Disposition*, **35**, 539-553. http://dx.doi.org/10.1124/dmd.106.010801

[124] Wang, Y., Cao, J. and Zeng, S. (2005) Involvement of P-Glycoprotein in Regulating Cellular Levels of Ginkgo Flavonols: Quercetin, Kaempferol, and Isorhamnetin. *Journal of Pharmacy and Pharmacology*, **57**, 751-758. http://dx.doi.org/10.1211/0022357056299

[125] Cermak, R. and Wolffram, S. (2006) The Potential of Flavonoids to Influence Drug Metabolism and Pharmacokinetics by Local Gastrointestinal Mechanisms. *Current Drug Metabolism*, **7**, 729-744. http://dx.doi.org/10.2174/138920006778520570

[126] Conseil, G., Baubichon-Cortay, H., Dayan, G., Jault, J.M., Barron, D. and Di Pietro, A. (1998) Flavonoids: A Class of Modulators with Bifunctional Interactions at Vicinal ATP- and Steroid-Binding Sites on Mouse P-Glycoprotein. *Proceedings of the National Academy of Sciences of the United States of America*, **95**, 9831-9836. http://dx.doi.org/10.1073/pnas.95.17.9831

[127] Johnson, W.W., Wang, E.J., Barecki-Roach, M., *et al.* (2002) Allosteric Elevation of P-Glycoprotein Function by a Catechin in Green Tea. *Drug Metabolism Reviews*, **34**, 87.

[128] Morris, M.E. and Zhang, S. (2006) Flavonoid-Drug Interactions: Effects of Flavonoids on ABC Transporters. *Life Sciences*, **78**, 2116-2130. http://dx.doi.org/10.1016/j.lfs.2005.12.003

[129] Shapiro, A.B. and Ling, V. (1997) Positively Cooperative Sites for Drug Transport by P-Glycoprotein with Distinct Drug Specificities. *European Journal of Biochemistry*, **250**, 130-137. http://dx.doi.org/10.1111/j.1432-1033.1997.00130.x

[130] Di Pietro, A., Conseil, G., Perez-Victoria, J.M., Dayan, G., Baubichon-Cortay, H., Trompier, D., *et al.* (2002) Modulation by Flavonoids of Cell Multidrug Resistance Mediated by P-Glycoprotein and Related ABC Transporters. *Cellular and Molecular Life Sciences CMLS*, **59**, 307-322. http://dx.doi.org/10.1007/s00018-002-8424-8

[131] Tang, M., Ogawa, K., Asamoto, M., Hokaiwado, N., Seeni, A., Suzuki, S., *et al.* (2007) Protective Effects of Citrus

Nobiletin and Auraptene in Transgenic Rats Developing Adenocarcinoma of the Prostate (TRAP) and Human Prostate Carcinoma Cells. *Cancer Science*, **98**, 471-477. http://dx.doi.org/10.1111/j.1349-7006.2007.00417.x

[132] Ju-Ichi, M. (2005) Chemical Study of Citrus Plants in the Search for Cancer Chemopreventive Agents. *Yakugaku Zasshi*, **125**, 231-254. http://dx.doi.org/10.1248/yakushi.125.231

[133] Takanaga, H., Ohnishi, A., Yamada, S., Matsuo, H., Morimoto, S., Shoyama, Y., *et al.* (2000) Polymethoxylated Flavones in Orange Juice Are Inhibitors of P-Glycoprotein but Not Cytochrome P450 3A4. *Journal of Pharmacology and Experimental Therapeutics*, **293**, 230-236.

[134] Dresser, G.K. and Bailey, D.G. (2003) The Effects of Fruit Juices on Drug Disposition: A New Model for Drug Interactions. *European Journal of Clinical Investigation*, **33**, 10-16. http://dx.doi.org/10.1046/j.1365-2362.33.s2.2.x

[135] Evans, A.M. (2000) Influence of Dietary Components on the Gastrointestinal Metabolism and Transport of Drugs. *Therapeutic Drug Monitoring*, **22**, 131-136. http://dx.doi.org/10.1097/00007691-200002000-00028

[136] Ioannides, C. (2002) Topics in Xenobiochemistry. Pharmacokinetic Interactions between Herbal Remedies and Medicinal Drugs. *Xenobiotica*, **32**, 451-478. http://dx.doi.org/10.1080/00498250210124147

[137] Dahan, A. and Altman, H. (2004) Food-Drug Interaction: Grapefruit Juice Augments Drug Bioavailability—Mechanism, Extent and Relevance. *European Journal of Clinical Nutrition*, **58**, 1-9. http://dx.doi.org/10.1038/sj.ejcn.1601736

[138] Chen, A.C. and Donovan, S.M. (2004) Genistein at a Concentration Present in Soy Infant Formula Inhibits Caco-2BBe Cell Proliferation by Causing G2/M Cell Cycle Arrest. *Journal of Nutrition*, **134**, 1303-1308.

[139] Horie, N., Hirabayashi, N., Takahashi, Y., Miyauchi, Y., Taguchi, H. and Takeishi, K. (2005) Synergistic Effect of Green Tea Catechins on Cell Growth and Apoptosis Induction in Gastric Carcinoma Cells. *Biological and Pharmaceutical Bulletin*, **28**, 574-579. http://dx.doi.org/10.1248/bpb.28.574

[140] Kaneuchi, M., Sasaki, M., Tanaka, Y., Sakuragi, N., Fujimoto, S. and Dahiya, R. (2003) Quercetin Regulates Growth of Ishikawa Cells through the Suppression of EGF and Cyclin D1. *International Journal of Oncology*, **22**, 159-164.

[141] Kumi-Diaka, J., Sanderson, N.A. and Hall, A. (2000) The Mediating Role of Caspase-3 Protease in the Intracellular Mechanism of Genistein-Induced Apoptosis in Human Prostatic Carcinoma Cell Lines, DU145 and LNCaP. *Biology of the Cell*, **92**, 595-604. http://dx.doi.org/10.1016/S0248-4900(00)01109-6

[142] Nguyen, T.T., Tran, E., Nguyen, T.H., Do, P.T., Huynh, T.H. and Huynh, H. (2004) The Role of Activated MEK-ERK Pathway in Quercetin-Induced Growth Inhibition and Apoptosis in A549 Lung Cancer Cells. *Carcinogenesis*, **25**, 647-659. http://dx.doi.org/10.1093/carcin/bgh052

[143] Banthorpe, D. (1991) Classification of Terpenoids and General Procedures for Their Characterization. In: Charlwood, B. and Banthorpe, D., Eds., *Methods in Plant Biochemistry: Terpenoids*, Academic Press, London, 1-41.

[144] Davis, E. and Croteau, R. (2000) Cyclization Enzymes in the Biosynthesis of Monoterpenes, Sesquiterpenes, and Diterpenes. In: Leeper, F. and Vederas, J., Eds., *Topics in Current Chemistry: Biosynthesis: Aromatic Polyketides, Isoprenoids, Alkaloids*, Springer, Berlin, New York, 53-95.

[145] Gershenzon, J. and Kreis, W. (1999) Biochemistry of Terpenoids. In: Wink, M., Ed., *Biochemistry of Plant Secondary Metabolism, Annual Plant Reviews*, Sheffield Academic Press, CRC Press, Sheffield, Boca Raton, 222-299.

[146] Roy, A. and Saraf, S. (2006) Limonoids: Overview of Significant Bioactive Triterpenes Distributed in Plants Kingdom. *Biological & Pharmaceutical Bulletin*, **29**, 191-201. http://dx.doi.org/10.1248/bpb.29.191

[147] Manners, G.D., Jacob, R.A., Breksa III, A.P., Schoch, T.K. and Hasegawa, S. (2003) Bioavailability of Citrus Limonoids in Humans. *Journal of Agricultural and Food Chemistry*, **51**, 4156-4161. http://dx.doi.org/10.1021/jf0300691

[148] Berhow, M.A., Hasegawa, S., Manners, G.D., *et al.* (2000) Citrus Limonoids: Functional Chemicals in Agriculture and Food. American Chemical Society, Washington DC, xiii, 253 p.

[149] Poulose, S.M., Harris, E.D. and Patil, B.S. (2005) Citrus Limonoids Induce Apoptosis in Human Neuroblastoma Cells and Have Radical Scavenging Activity. *Journal of Nutrition*, **135**, 870-877.

[150] Miyagi, Y., Om, A.S., Chee, K.M. and Bennink, M.R. (2000) Inhibition of Azoxymethane-Induced Colon Cancer by Orange Juice. *Nutrition and Cancer—An International Journal*, **36**, 224-229. http://dx.doi.org/10.1207/S15327914NC3602_12

[151] Berhow, M.A., Omura, M., Ohta, H., Ozaki, Y. and Hasegawa, S. (1994) Limonoids in Seeds of 3 Citrus Hybrids Related to *Citrus ichangensis*. *Phytochemistry*, **36**, 923-925. http://dx.doi.org/10.1016/S0031-9422(00)90464-3

[152] Silalahi, J. (2002) Anticancer and Health Protective Properties of Citrus Fruit Components. *Asia Pacific Journal of Clinical Nutrition*, **11**, 79-84. http://dx.doi.org/10.1046/j.1440-6047.2002.00271.x

[153] Tanaka, T., Kohno, H., Tsukio, Y., Honjo, S., Tanino, M., Miyake, M. and Wada, K. (2000) Citrus Limonoids Obacunone and Limonin Inhibit Azoxymethane-Induced Colon Carcinogenesis in Rats. *BioFactors*, **13**, 213-218. http://dx.doi.org/10.1002/biof.5520130133

[154] Madyastha, K.M. and Venkatakrishnan, K. (2000) Structural Flexibility in the Biocatalyst-Mediated Functionalization

of Ring "A" in Salannin, a Tetranortriterpene from *Azadirachta indica*. *Journal of the Chemical Society, Perkin Transactions*, **1**, 3055-3062. http://dx.doi.org/10.1039/b004260i

[155] Dewick, P.M. (2009) Medicinal Natural Products: A Biosynthetic Approach. 3rd Edition, Wiley, Chichester, x, 539 p.

[156] Katan, M.B., Grundy, S.M., Jones, P., Law, M., Miettinen, T. and Paoletti, R. (2003) Efficacy and Safety of Plant Stanols and Sterols in the Management of Blood Cholesterol Levels. *Mayo Clinic Proceedings*, **78**, 965-978. http://dx.doi.org/10.1016/S0025-6196(11)63144-3

[157] Lichtenstein, A.H. and Deckelbaum, R.J. (2001) AHA Science Advisory. Stanol/Sterol Ester-Containing Foods and Blood Cholesterol Levels. A Statement for Healthcare Professionals from the Nutrition Committee of the Council on Nutrition, Physical Activity, and Metabolism of the American Heart Association. *Circulation*, **103**, 1177-1179. http://dx.doi.org/10.1161/01.CIR.103.8.1177

[158] Awad, A.B. and Fink, C.S. (2002) Phytosterols as Anticancer Dietary Components: Evidence and Mechanism of Action (Reprinted from Vol 130, Pg 2127, 2000). *Journal of Nutrition*, **132**, 2127-2130.

[159] Oram, J.F. and Vaughan, A.M. (2006) ATP-Binding Cassette Cholesterol Transporters and Cardiovascular Disease. *Circulation Research*, **99**, 1031-1043. http://dx.doi.org/10.1161/01.RES.0000250171.54048.5c

[160] Sarkadi, B., Homolya, L., Szakacs, G. and Váradi, A. (2006) Human Multidrug Resistance ABCB and ABCG Transporters: Participation in a Chemoimmunity Defense System. *Physiological Reviews*, **86**, 1179-1236. http://dx.doi.org/10.1152/physrev.00037.2005

[161] Wink, M. (2008) Evolutionary Advantage and Molecular Modes of Action of Multi-Component Mixtures Used in Phytomedicine. *Current Drug Metabolism*, **9**, 996-1009. http://dx.doi.org/10.2174/138920008786927794

[162] Brobst, D.E., Ding, X., Creech, K.L., Goodwin, B., Kelley, B. and Staudinger, J.L. (2004) Guggulsterone Activates Multiple Nuclear Receptors and Induces CYP3A Gene Expression through the Pregnane X Receptor. *Journal of Pharmacology and Experimental Therapeutics*, **310**, 528-535. http://dx.doi.org/10.1124/jpet.103.064329

[163] Roberts, M.F. and Wink, M. (1998) Alkaloids: Biochemistry, Ecology, and Medicinal Applications. Springer, New York, 1-7.

[164] Wink, M. (1998) A Short History of Alkaloids. In: *Alkaloids: Biochemistry, Ecology, and Medicinal Applications*, Springer, New York, 11-43.

[165] Wink, M. (2007) Molecular Modes of Action of Cytotoxic Alkaloids: From DNA Intercalation, Spindle Poisoning, Topoisomerase Inhibition to Apoptosis and Multiple Drug Resistance. *Alkaloids: Chemistry and Biology*, **64**, 1-47. http://dx.doi.org/10.1016/S1099-4831(07)64001-2

[166] Zdarilova, A., Malikova, J., Dvorak, Z., Ulrichová, J. and Šimánek, V. (2006) Quaternary Isoquinoline Alkaloids Sanguinarine and Chelerythrine. *In Vitro* and *in Vivo* Effects. *Chemické Listy*, **100**, 30-41.

[167] Fu, L.W., Deng, Z.A., Pan, Q.C. and Fan, W. (2001) Screening and Discovery of Novel MDR Modifiers from Naturally Occurring Bisbenzylisoquinoline Alkaloids. *Anticancer Research*, **21**, 2273-2280.

[168] Jakubikova, J., Duraj, J., Hunakova, L., Chorvath, B. and Sedlak, J. (2002) PK11195, an Isoquinoline Carboxamide Ligand of the Mitochondrial Benzodiazepine Receptor, Increased Drug Uptake and Facilitated Drug-Induced Apoptosis in Human Multidrug-Resistant Leukemia Cells *in Vitro*. *Neoplasma*, **49**, 231-236.

[169] He, L. and Liu, G.Q. (2002) Effects of Various Principles from Chinese Herbal Medicine on Rhodamine123 Accumulation in Brain Capillary Endothelial Cells. *Acta Pharmacologica Sinica*, **23**, 591-596.

[170] Wakusawa, S., Nakamura, S., Tajima, K., Miyamoto, K., Hagiwara, M. and Hidaka, H. (1992) Overcoming of Vinblastine Resistance by Isoquinolinesulfonamide Compounds in Adriamycin-Resistant Leukemia Cells. *Molecular Pharmacology*, **41**, 1034-1038.

[171] Moller, M., Weiss, J. and Wink, M. (2006) Reduction of Cytotoxicity of the Alkaloid Emetine through P-Glycoprotein (MDR1/ABCB1) in Human Caco-2 Cells and Leukemia Cell Lines. *Planta Medica*, **72**, 1121-1126. http://dx.doi.org/10.1055/s-2006-941546

[172] Belyaeva, T., Leontieva, E., Shpakov, A., Mozhenok, T. and Faddejeva, M. (2003) Sensitivity of Lysosomal Enzymes to the Plant Alkaloid Sanguinarine: Comparison with Other SH-Specific Agents. *Cell Biology International*, **27**, 887-895. http://dx.doi.org/10.1016/S1065-6995(03)00161-6

[173] Salminen, K.A., Meyer, A., Jerabkova, L., Korhonen, L.E., Rahnasto, M., Juvonen, R.O., *et al.* (2010) Inhibition of Human Drug Metabolizing Cytochrome P450 Enzymes by Plant Isoquinoline Alkaloids. *Phytomedicine*, **18**, 533-538.

[174] Adhami, V.M., Aziz, M.H., Mukhtar, H. and Ahmad, N. (2003) Activation of Prodeath Bcl-2 Family Proteins and Mitochondrial Apoptosis Pathway by Sanguinarine in Immortalized Human HaCaT Keratinocytes. *Clinical Cancer Research*, **9**, 3176-3182.

[175] Adhami, V.M., Aziz, M.H., Reagan-Shaw, S.R., Nihal, M., Mukhtar, H. and Ahmad, N. (2004) Sanguinarine Causes Cell Cycle Blockade and Apoptosis of Human Prostate Carcinoma Cells via Modulation of Cyclin Kinase Inhibitor-

Cyclin-Cyclin-Dependent Kinase Machinery. *Molecular Cancer Therapeutics*, **3**, 933-940.

[176] Malikova, J., Zdarilova, A. and Hlobilkova, A. (2006) Effects of Sanguinarine and Chelerythrine on the Cell Cycle and Apoptosis. *Biomedical Papers of the Medical Faculty of Palacký University*, **150**, 5-12. http://dx.doi.org/10.5507/bp.2006.001

[177] Ding, Z.H., Tang, S.C., Weerasinghe, P., Yang, X., Pater, A. and Liepins, A. (2002) The Alkaloid Sanguinarine Is Effective against Multidrug Resistance in Human Cervical Cells via Bimodal Cell Death. *Biochemical Pharmacology*, **63**, 1415-1421. http://dx.doi.org/10.1016/S0006-2952(02)00902-4

[178] Moller, M., Herzer, K., Wenger, T., Herr, I. and Wink, M. (2007) The Alkaloid Emetine as a Promising Agent for the Induction and Enhancement of Drug-Induced Apoptosis in Leukemia Cells. *Oncology Reports*, **18**, 737-744.

[179] Moller, M. and Wink, M. (2007) Characteristics of Apoptosis Induction by the Alkaloid Emetine in Human Tumour Cell Lines. *Planta Medica*, **73**, 1389-1396. http://dx.doi.org/10.1055/s-2007-990229

[180] Rosenkranz, V. and Wink, M. (2008) Alkaloids Induce Programmed Cell Death in Bloodstream Forms of Trypanosomes (*Trypanosoma b. brucei*). *Molecules*, **13**, 2462-2473. http://dx.doi.org/10.3390/molecules13102462

[181] Van Wyk, B.E. and Wink, M. (2004) Medicinal Plants of the World: An Illustrated Scientific Guide to Important Medicinal Plants and Their Uses. 1st Edition, Timber Press, Portland, 480 p.

[182] Bartak, P., Simanek, V., Vlckova, M., Ulrichová, J. and Vespalec, R. (2003) Interactions of Sanguinarine and Chelerythrine with Molecules Containing a Mercapto Group. *Journal of Physical Organic Chemistry*, **16**, 803-810. http://dx.doi.org/10.1002/poc.659

[183] Ulrichova, J., Dvorak, Z., Vicar, J., Lata, J., Smržová, J., Šedo, A. and Šimánek, V. (2001) Cytotoxicity of Natural Compounds in Hepatocyte Cell Culture Models: The Case of Quaternary Benzo[C]phenanthridine Alkaloids. *Toxicology Letters*, **125**, 125-132. http://dx.doi.org/10.1016/S0378-4274(01)00430-1

[184] Slaninova, I., Taborska, E., Bochorakova, H. and Slanina, J. (2001) Interaction of Benzo[C]phenanthridine and Protoberberine Alkaloids with Animal and Yeast Cells. *Cell Biology and Toxicology*, **17**, 51-63. http://dx.doi.org/10.1023/A:1010907231602

[185] Walterova, D., Ulrichova, J., Preininger, V., Simanek, V., Lenfeld, J. and Lasovsky, J. (1981) Inhibition of Liver Alanine Aminotransferase Activity by Some Benzophenanthridine Alkaloids. *Journal of Medicinal Chemistry*, **24**, 1100-1103. http://dx.doi.org/10.1021/jm00141a019

[186] Stiborova, M., Simanek, V., Frei, E., Hobza, P. and Ulrichová, J. (2002) DNA Adduct Formation from Quaternary Benzo[C]phenanthridine Alkaloids Sanguinarine and Chelerythrine as Revealed by the P-32-Postlabeling Technique. *Chemico-Biological Interactions*, **140**, 231-242. http://dx.doi.org/10.1016/S0009-2797(02)00038-8

[187] Das, M., Ansari, K.M., Dhawan, A., Shukla, Y. and Khanna, S.K. (2005) Correlation of DNA Damage in Epidemic Dropsy Patients to Carcinogenic Potential of Argemone Oil and Isolated Sanguinarine Alkaloid in Mice. *International Journal of Cancer*, **117**, 709-717. http://dx.doi.org/10.1002/ijc.21234

[188] Wink, M. (2006) Chapter 11 Importance of Plant Secondary Metabolites for Protection against Insects and Microbial Infections. In: Mahendra, R. and María Cecilia, C., Eds., *Advances in Phytomedicine*, Vol. 3, Elsevier, Amsterdam, 251-268.

12

Shengmai Suppressed Vascular Tension in Umbilical Arteries and Veins of Human and Sheep

Xiaohui Yin[1#], Xiuxia Gu[1#], Yun He[1], Di Zhu[1], Jie Chen[1], Jue Wu[1], Xueqin Feng[1], Jinhao Li[1], Caiping Mao[1], Zhice Xu[1,2*]

[1]Institute for Fetology & Reproductive Medicine Center, First Hospital of Soochow University, Suzhou, China
[2]Center for Prenatal Biology, Loma Linda University, Loma Linda, CA, USA
Email: [*]xuzhice@suda.edu.cn, zxu@llu.edu

Abstract

Objective—The umbilical cord is a critical pathway between mothers and fetuses, and regulations of umbilical vessel tension are important for fetal growth. Shengmai is an herbal medicine being used in treatments of cardiovascular diseases. However, effects of Shengmai on human blood vessels and related pharmacological mechanisms are unclear. Methods—This study investigated the effects of related mechanisms of Shengmai and its key compounds on human and sheep umbilical arteries and veins using organ bath systems. Key Findings—Shengmai significantly suppressed phenylephrine-stimulated vasoconstriction in umbilical arteries and veins. NG-Nitro-L-arginine Methyl Estercould not change the Shengmai-suppressed vasoconstriction in human and sheep umbilical vessels. Among four key compounds of Shengmai, Ginsenoside Re, Ginsenoside Rb1, Ginsenoside Rg1, and Schisandrin, only Ginsenoside Re showed the significant effect similar to Shengmai's in the umbilical vessels. In Ca^{2+}-free solution, Ginsenoside Re did not affect vasoconstriction. In addition, caffeine- or phenylephrine-stimulated vasoconstriction were not changed by Ginsenoside Re. Either charybdotoxin or glibenclamide could inhibit Ginsenoside Re-caused inhibition of the stimulated vasoconstriction in both human and sheep umbilical vessels, where 4-aminopyridine did not show the similar inhibitory effect. Conclusion—The results provide new information on Shengmai's effects and underlying mechanisms in umbilical vessels. Importantly, the information gained offers interesting potential for developing new drugs acting on umbilical cords for fetal medicine.

Keywords

Shengmai, Umbilical Arteries and Veins, Ginsenoside Re, α-Adrenergic Receptor

---

[*]Corresponding author.
[#]X. H. Yin and X. X. Gu contributed equally to this work.

1. Introduction

The umbilical cord with its blood vessels is a major or only pathway between mothers and fetuses, and critical functions of umbilical vessels are to supply and maintain blood flow as well as oxygen and nutrition for fetuses, which is necessary for life *in utero* [1] [2]. Any condition that can influence blood vessels of umbilical cord, may affect the supply blood and nutrition for fetuses, and may cause *in utero* hypoxia or fetal growth restriction [3]. Although *in utero* hypoxia is a common condition in clinic due to multiple factors [4]-[7], there have been limited approaches in dealing with that medical problem. Therefore, finding new drugs or methods against *in utero* hypoxia related to poor supply of blood flow is a consistent effort in both basic science and clinical work.

Shengmai is one of traditional herbal medicines being used frequently in clinical practice in treatments of various of cardiovascular diseases, including ischemic heart diseases, and stroke [8] [9]. In spite of that, there exist many experimental and clinical studies in demonstration of effects and mechanisms of Shengmai in cardiovascular systems or central blood vessel systems [8], it is unknown if Shengmai has any special vascular influence or effect on blood vessels of umbilical cords. The present study is focused on this topic.

Previous work showed that Shengmai consists of at least three major components, *Panax Ginseng, Ophiopogon Japonicus, and Schisandra Chinensis* [9]-[11]. Several antioxidant ingredients have been discovered in *Panax Ginseng* and *Schisandra*, including Ginseoside Rb1, Ginseoside Rg1, and Ginseoside Re(GRe) from *Panax Ginseng* and schizandrin from *Schisandra* [12]. They have been shown in preventing the oxidative damage in heart, brain, and other tissues, and being routinely used in treatment of coronary heart disease [9]. Shengmai also was demonstrated its effects in preventing circulatory shock and brain oxidative and ischemic damage during heatstroke [8]. Moreover, administration of Shengmai right after the onset of heat stroke is still considerably effective way for improving circulatory shock and inhibiting oxidative damage in the brain [8]. As mentioned above, since there has been no data on Shengmai's effects on the umbilical vessels, no information is available on possible influence as well as mechanisms of Shengmai on umbilical vessels. Obviously, addressing such questions is important.

In the present study, we investigated Shengmai's effects on both arteries and veins from human umbilical cords first. Considering inevitable variations among different human subjects, we also used umbilical cords from experimental healthy sheep in testing Shengmai's effects on sheep umbilical vessels. Subsequent experiments determined several key compounds of Shengmai and their vascular effects on umbilical vessels. In addition, we performed preliminary study on possible mechanisms that may be involved in vascular actions of Shengmai or its ingredients on umbilical vessels. Information gained is not only contribution to vascular pharmacology, but also to perinatal medicine and clinical work related to pregnancy.

2. Materials and Methods

2.1. Preparation of the Umbilical Cord Vessels

Human umbilical cord samples were obtained from 105 women after delivery at term at local hospitals. All deliveries were either vaginal deliveries or elective cesarean deliveries without complications. The median gestation at delivery was 39 weeks ± 8 days. The reasons for cesarean delivery included previous cesarean section and presumed cephalopelvic disproportion. The median parity value of the women at the time of delivery was 1 (range 0 - 3). There was no evidence of hypertensive disease, gestational diabetes mellitus (GDM) and other diseases for any of the subjects. The mean body mass index (BMI) of those cases was 22.32 kg/m^2 [13]. All procedures were approved by the Institute Committee.

All procedures were approved by the Institute Animal Care Committee and were incompliance with the Guidelines for NIHC are and Use of Laboratory Animals. The animal experiments were performed in chronically instrumented conscious sheep at 128 - 134 days of gestation (term 145 days). Animals were housed in individual study cage and in a light controlled room (12 h light/dark cycles) with food and water provided libitum. All sheep deliveries were elective cesarean deliveries, and umbilical cord samples were obtained immediately. All procedures were approved by the Institute Committee and in compliance with the Guidelines for national institute of health (NIH) Care and Use of Laboratory Animals.

Approximately 10 ± 5 cm segments were excised from middle part of umbilical cords between the placenta and fetus [13]. Then samples were immediately placed in the modified Krebs-Henseleit solution (K-H solution) at 4°C with composition (mmol/L): NaCl, 119 mmol/L, KCl, 4.7 mmol/L, NaHCO$_3$, 25 mmol/L, KH$_2$PO$_4$, 1.2 mmol/L, CaCl$_2$, 2.5 mmol/L, MgSO$_4$, 1.0 mmol/L, EDTA, 0.004 mmol/L, and D-glucose, 11 mmol/L, at 37°C at pH 7.4 with constant bubbling with 95% O$_2$/5% CO$_2$ [14]. Samples were used immediately following the preparation.

2.2. Vascular Experiments

Umbilical veins and arteries were carefully dissected from umbilical cords by removal of surrounding tissue using micro-dissecting instruments. Vessels were cut in rings with 3 - 5 mm length [13] [15]. Rings were then suspended individually on stainless steel hooks inserted into their lumens and stretched with an initial isometric tension of 2 g, in glass-jacketed organ baths as previously reported [16] [17]. Each bath contained 5 ml of K-H solution, pH 7.35 - 7.45, at 37°C, and constant bubbling with a mixture of 95% oxygen/5% carbon dioxide [18]. The upper hook was connected to a force transducer and changes in isometric force were recorded using Power-Lab system with Chart 7.0 software (AD Instruments, Australia). Rings were allowed to equilibrate for 120 minutes. During that period bath solution was replaced every 15 minutes with fresh K-H solution.

After 120 min of equilibration, each ring was contracted using KCl (60 mM) for reaching a maximum response, and then washed out. The KCl challenge was performed three times to test functional state of the vascular tissue. Optimal tension was adjusted throughout the equilibration period. After the last KCl challenge, a 30 - 40 minutes recovery period was allowed [14]. Following drugs were tested in the experiments.

The effect of Shengmai on human umbilical vein/artery (HUV/HUA) or sheep umbilical vein/artery (SUV/SUA) rings: When the rings were equilibrated, phenylephrine (PE, 10^{-4} mol/L) was added to produce steady contraction, and then Shengmai (10^{-4} mol/L) was applied. Vascular reactions were monitored for 120 min.

When the rings were equilibrated, NG-Nitro-L-arginine Methyl Ester (L-NAME, the nitric oxide synthase (eNOS) inhibitor, 10^{-5} mol/L) for 30 minutes and PE (10^{-4} mol/L) was added to produce steady contraction,and then 10^{-4} mol/L Shengmai was applied. Vascular reactions were monitored for at least 120 minutes.

When the sheep umbilical rings were equilibrated, following PE (10^{-4} mol/L) to produce steady contraction, Following key elements of Shengmaiwere used in testing: GRe (10^{-4} mol/L), Ginsenoside Rb1 (10^{-4} mol/L), Ginsenoside Rg1 (10^{-4} mol/L), or Schisandrin (10^{-4} mol/L) was added separately. Vessel tone was monitored and recorded for at least 120 minutes after adding the drug.

CaCl$_2$ dose-effect curve: SUV/SUA rings were washed 2 - 3 times with Ca^{2+}-free K-H solution (containing 1 μM EGTA). The vessel rings were preincubated with GRe (10^{-4} mol/L) for 30 minutes before application of KCl (60 mM). CaCl$_2$ was then added cumulatively (0.25 - 5 × 10^{-5} mol/L). The vehicle, instead of GRe, was used for the control group before add KCl (60 mM).

The effect of GRe on PE- or caffeine-induced contractions in SUV/SUA rings was tested in Ca^{2+}-free K-H solution. The SUV/SUA rings were washed 2 - 3 times with Ca^{2+}-free K-H solution. The rings were exposed to GRe (10^{-4} mol/L) for 30 minutes, and then add 10^{-5} mol/L PE or 20 mmol/L caffeine.

The effect of potassium channel antagonists on SUV/SUA rings was tested. Different potassium channel antagonists were applied 30 minutes before the addition of PE (10^{-4} mol/L). 4-aminopyridine (4-AP, 10^{-3} mol/L [19], Voltage-dependent K$^+$ (Kv) channels antagonist [19] [20], charybdotoxin (CTX, 10^{-7} mol/L [20], Ca^{2+}-activated K$^+$ (BKCa) channels antagonist [20]), Glibenclamide (10^{-6} mol/L [19], ATP-sensitive K$^+$ (KATP) channels antagonist [19] [20], or vehicle were used. Following steady vasoconstriction by PE (10^{-4} mol/L), GRe (10^{-4} mol/L) was added into the bath, and vascular responses were monitored and recorded for at least 120 minutes.

2.3. Drugs and Solutions

The modified K-H solution: NaCl, 119 mmol/L, KCl, 4.7 mmol/L, NaHCO$_3$, 25 mmol/L, KH$_2$PO$_4$, 1.2 mmol/L, CaCl$_2$, 2.5 mmol/L, MgSO$_4$, 1.0 mmol/L, EDTA, 0.004 mmol/L, and glucose, 11 mmol/L.

Shengmai was purchased from Suzhong Pharnaceutical Group (Jiangsu, China). GRe, Ginsenoside Rb1, Ginsenoside Rg1, and Schisandrol were purchased from Shanghai Sunny Biotech Co., Ltd. (Shanghai, China). Phenylephrine, NG-Nitro-L-arginine Methyl Ester (L-NAME), 4-AP, CTX, and Gli were purchased from Sigma-

Aldrich (USA).

2.4. Statistical Analysis

All data were expressed as means ± SEMs, the date was calculated from the concentration-response curve resulting performed by Graph Pad Prism (Version 5.01, Graph Pad Software Inc., La Jolla, CA, USA). All analog signals were recorded continuously throughout the study, and then digitized on a computer with Med-Lab acquisition software. And differences were evaluated for statistically significance ($P < 0.05$) by two-way ANOVA or t-test.

3. Results

3.1. The Effect of Shanghai on HUV/HUA and SUV/SUA

PE (10^{-4} mol/L) produced a concentration-related vasoconstriction in the HUV/HUA rings, where Shengmai (10^{-4} mol/L) could suppress PE-mediated vasoconstrictions significantly in the HUV/HUA rings (**Figure 1**).

After 120 min of equilibration, PE (10^{-4} mol/L) produced a dose-dependent vasoconstriction in the SUV/SUA rings, where Shengmai (10^{-4} mol/L) produced significant suppressed PE-mediated vasoconstriction in the SUV/SUA rings (**Figure 2**).

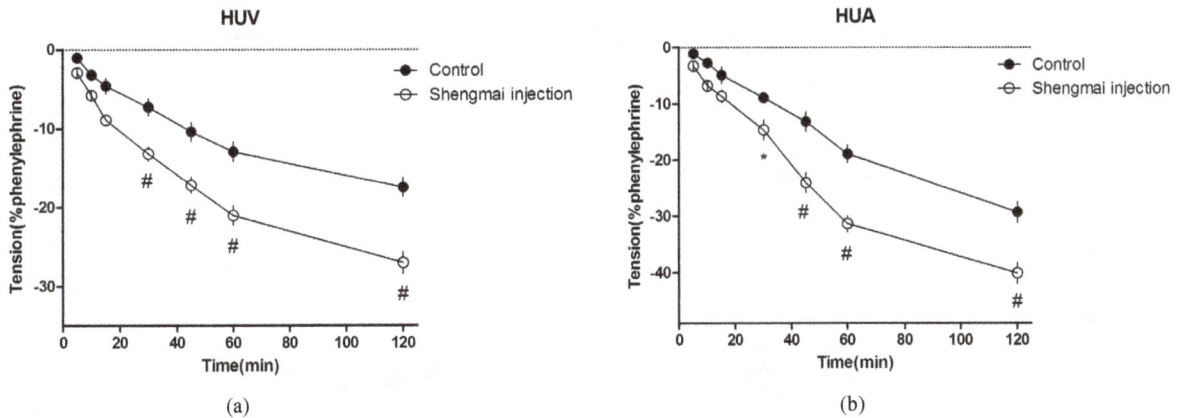

Figure 1. Shengmai suppressed phenylephrine-stimulated vasoconstrictions in human umbilical vein/artery (HUV/HUA). ((a): HUV n = 105 rings from 94 umbilical cords; (b): HUA n = 110 rings from 94 umbilical cords). Control vs Shengmai, #P < 0.01, *P < 0.05.

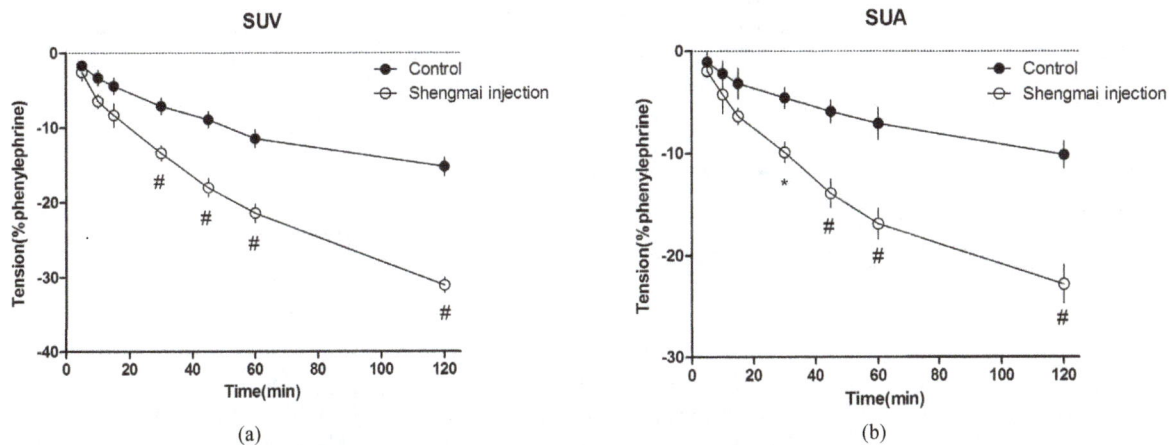

Figure 2. Shengmai suppressed phenylephrine-stimulated vasoconstrictions in sheep umbilical vein/artery (SUV/SUA) ((a): SUV n = 48 rings from 6 umbilical cords; (b): SUA n = 44 rings from 6 umbilical cords). Control vs Shengmai, #P < 0.01, *P < 0.05.

3.2. The effect of L-NAME on HUV/HUA and SUV/SUA

After 120 min of equilibration, PE (10^{-4} mol/L) produced dose-dependent contractions in HUV/HUA and SUV/SUA rings. There was no significant difference in the Shengmai-suppressed vascular tension between the groups with or without L-NAME (**Figure 3(A)**, **Figure 3(B)**).

3.3. The effect of Key Compounds of Shengmai on SUV/SUA

Following PE (10^{-4} mol/L)-produced steady vasoconstriction, Ginsenoside Re, Ginsenoside Rb1, Ginsenoside Rg1, or Schisandrin was added. GRe (10^{-4} mol/L) suppressed PE-stimulated vasoconstrictions in SUV/SUA rings, where Ginsenoside Rb1 (10^{-4} mol/L), Ginsenoside Rg1 (10^{-4} mol/L), and Schisandrin (10^{-4} mol/L) did not cause significant changes (**Figure 4**).

3.4. CaCl₂ Dose-Effect Curve

Following the rings were equilibrated in Ca^{2+}-free K-H solution, Ginsenoside Re (10^{-4} mol/L) was added 30 min before application of KCl to produce steady contraction. $CaCl_2$ was then added cumulatively. There was no statistical significance in vascular responses between the control and GRe groups (**Figure 5**).

3.5. The Effect of GRe on PE- or Caffeine-Induced Contractions in SUV/SUA

Following the rings were equilibrated in Ca^{2+}-free K-H solution and pre-treatment with GRe for 30 min, PE or

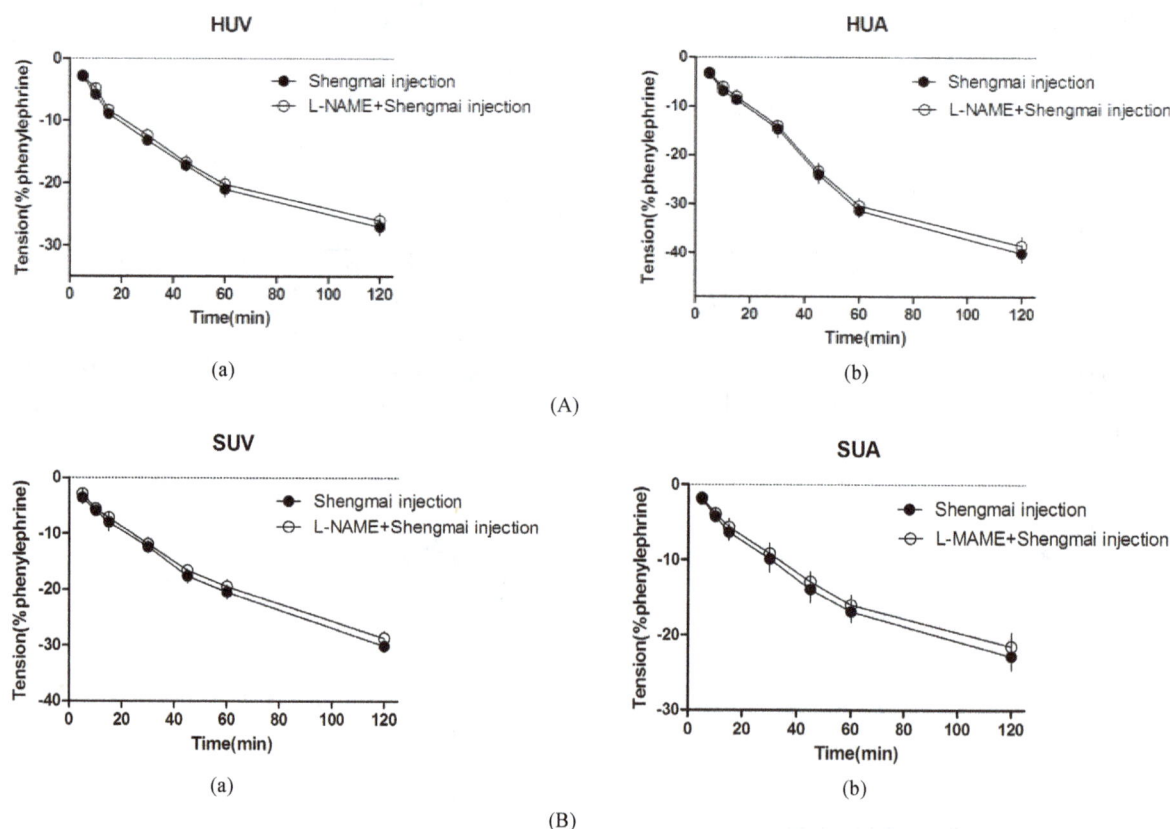

Figure 3. (A) Pre-treatment with NG-Nitro-L-arginine Methyl Ester (L-NAME) had no influence on Shengmai-suppressed vasoconstriction by phenylephrine in human umbilical vein/artery (HUV/HUA) ((a): HUV n = 105 rings from 90 umbilical cords; (b): HUA n = 110 rings from 94 umbilical cords); (B) Pre-treatment with NG-Nitro-L-arginine Methyl Ester (L-NAME) had no influence on Shanghai-suppressed phenylephrine-stimulated vasoconstrictions in sheep umbilical vein/artery ((a): SUV n = 48 rings from 6 umbilical cords; (b): SUA n = 44 rings from 6 umbilical cords). L-NAME + Shangmai: Following pre-treatment with L-NAME, Shanghai was added into the organ bath.

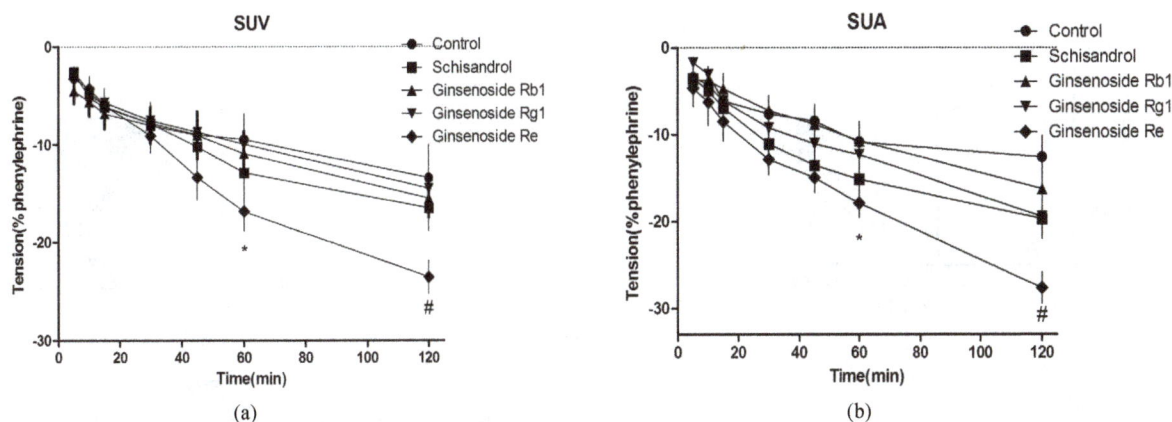

Figure 4. The effect of Ginsenoside Re, Ginsenoside Rb1, Ginsenoside Rg1, or Schisandrin on sheep umbilical vein/artery (SUV/SUA) stimulated by phenylephrine ((a): SUV n = 43 rings from 10 umbilical cords; (b): SUA n = 45 rings from 10 umbilical cords). Control vs Ginsenoside Re, #P < 0.01, *P < 0.05.

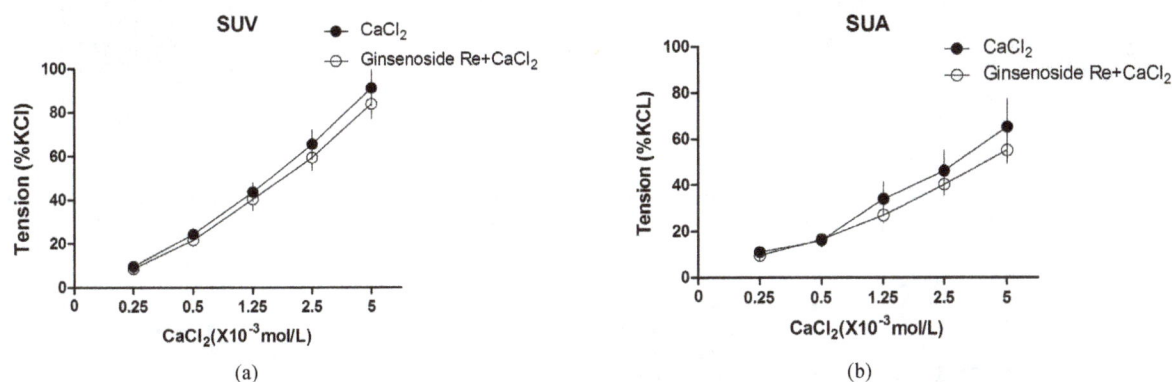

Figure 5. The effect of $CaCl_2$ on sheep umbilical vein/artery (SUV/SUA) ((a): SUV n = 24 rings from 6 umbilical cords; (b): SUA n = 20 rings from 6 umbilical cords).

caffeine was then applied. There was no significant difference in vascular responses between the control and GRe group (P > 0.05) in both SUV and SUA (**Figure 6**).

3.6. The Effect of Potassium Channel Antagonists on Ginsenoside Re-Induced Relaxation in SUV/SUA

Either CTX (10^{-7} mol/L) or Glibenclamide (10^{-6} mol/L) significantly reduced the GRe-suppressed vascular tension in SUV/SUA. However, the pre-treatment with 4-AP (10^{-3} mol/L) did not change the vascular response-caused by GRe (**Figure 7**).

4. Discussion

A number of clinical and experimental investigations have demonstrated the cardiovascular effects of Shengmai, and Shengmai has been often used in clinical treatments against stroke and cardiovascular diseases, including coronary heart disease, atherosclerosis, and hypertension [8] [9]. It is recently confirmed that blood vessels in umbilical cords can act differently from other vascular systems to chemical stimulation. However, there was no information regarding effects of Shengmai on either arteries and veins of umbilical cords as background of this study. Importantly, the umbilical cord serves as only important pathway between pregnant mothers and fetuses for supply of blood, oxygen, and nutrition. Thus, understanding influence of various chemicals or drugs on umbilical vessels is very important to perinatal medicine.

In the present study, Shengmai induced a significant decrease of vascular tone-stimulated by phenylephrine in both human and sheep umbilical arteries and veins, demonstrating that Shengmai could cause vasodilation or

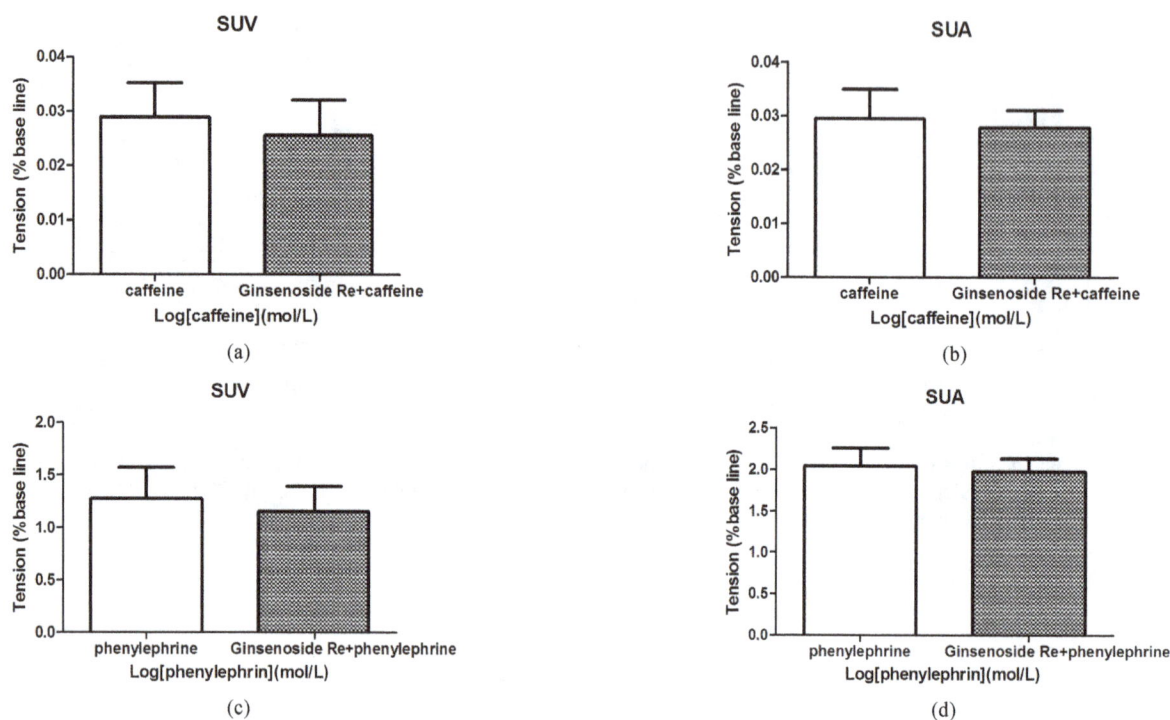

Figure 6. The effect of Ginsenoside Reon sheep umbilical vein/artery (SUV/SUA) stimulated by phenylephrine or caffeine ((a): SUV n = 24 rings from 6 umbilical cords; (b): SUA n = 20 rings from 6 umbilical cords).

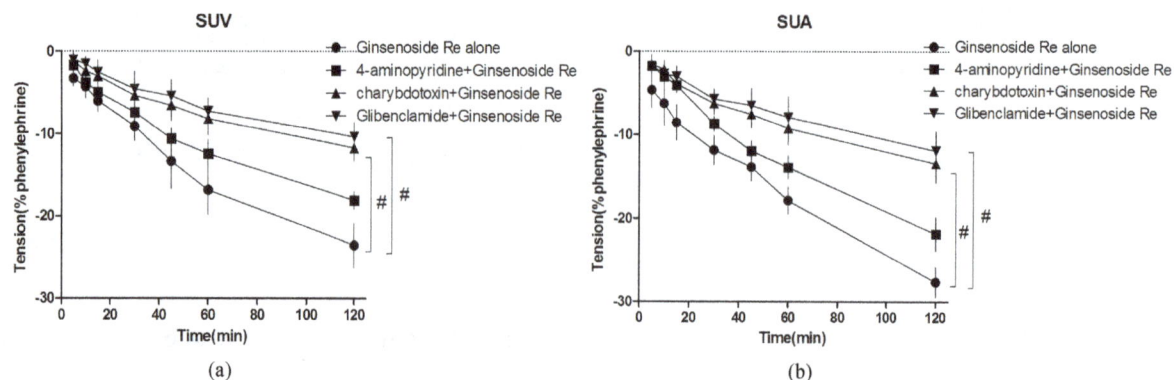

Figure 7. The effect of potassiumchannels antagonists on Ginsenoside Re-suppressed vascular tension in sheep umbilical vein/artery (SUV/SUA) ((a): SUV n = 36 rings from 8 umbilical cords; (b): SUA n = 34 rings from 8 umbilical cords). Ginsenoside Re alone vs charybdotoxin; Ginsenoside Re vs Glibenclamide, #P < 0.01.

suppress phenylephrine-produced vascular tension. Notably, this was the first study to show the effects of Shengmai on umbilical cords. Significance of the findings includes that may offer new opportunities for developing novel drugs or approaches targeting at regulations of umbilical cord blood vessels. For example, many clinical conditions may lead to *in utero* hypoxia as well as fetal growth restriction [4]. Increasing of umbilical blood flow could be helpful for those conditions. Thus, the Shengmai's effects on umbilical vessels may have great potentials in the field.

In the present study, possible mechanisms of Shengmai-suppress vasoconstriction by PE in the umbilical cord vessels were determined. The first possibility we considered was contribution from nitric oxide (NO) signaling pathway. It is well known that NO mainly from the endothelium in vascular systems, and plays critical roles in vascular relaxation [21] [22]. Damage of vascular endothelium or NO pathways may cause disability of vascular functions, particularly vasodilation [23]-[26]. In our experiments, following the pre-treatment with L-NAME in both human and sheep vessels, no significant changes was observed in Shengmai-mediated vascular responses, suggesting that Shengmai-produced vascular relaxation may not rely on NO.

Shengmai is a traditional herb medicine with many ingredients. Major biological compounds in Shengmai include Ginsenoside Re, Ginsenoside Rb1, Ginsenoside Rg1, and Schisandrin [12]. Previous study using those key compounds of Shengmai showed vascular effects on other vessel systems [27]-[30], including anti-oxidative influence [31] and inhibition of P-glycoprotein [32] [33]. It was unknown whether any of those four elements play major roles in Shengmai-mediated vascular dilation in umbilical cords. In the present study, we found Shengmai-produced vasodilation mainly depend on GRe, not other three compounds tested. Again, this is a new finding in demonstration of that GRe in Shengmai is critical for the suppression of PE-induced vasoconstriction effect in umbilical cord vessels.

After excluding possibility of NO involved, other mechanisms, including calcium and potassium signaling pathways, were considered in smooth muscle of umbilical vessels. Vascular smooth muscle requires Ca^{2+} for constrictions either from intracellular stores or the influx of extra-cellular Ca^{2+}. The major routes of Ca^{2+} influx include receptor-operated Ca^{2+} channel (ROCC) [34] and voltage-gated Ca^{2+} channel (VGCC) [35] [36]. PE is a α-adrenergic receptor agonist [37] that produces vasoconstriction mainly via VGCC. Extra-cellular high potassium makes VGCCs to open in response to membrane depolarization and allow Ca^{2+} ions to enter cells [38] and induce vasoconstriction. $CaCl_2$ could cause dose-dependent vasoconstriction linked to Ca^{2+} influx [36] [39]. Our study demonstrated that Shengmai and Ginsenoside Re could suppress PE-induced vasoconstriction in umbilical vessel rings. When the vessel rings were equilibrated in Ca^{2+}-free K-H solution with GRe, $CaCl_2$ was then added into the bath cumulatively. This treatment could not change the Ca^{2+} influx induced vasoconstriction in both umbilical arteries and veins, indicating that GRe-suppressed vascular tension may not be related to VGCC-mediated intracellular Ca^{2+} influx.

The sarcoplasmic reticulum (SR) can release stored Ca^{2+} in cells [40]. Caffeine could induce transient vasoconstriction mainly by Ca^{2+} release from the SR, where the SR Ca^{2+} flux is mediated by ryanodine receptors that can be opened in response to small trigger Ca^{2+} stimulation [41]. In Ca^{2+}-free K-H solution, PE-induced vasoconstriction was induced by activating IP3 (1, 4, 5-trisphosphate)-sensitivity calcium channels [42]. In the present study, GRe could not affect caffeine- or PE-induced vasoconstriction in Ca^{2+}-free K-H solution, suggesting that GRe-induced vascular tension may not be related to the Ca^{2+} release via the SR or IP3-sensitivity calcium pool [43].

Potassium channels integrate a variety of vasoactive signals to dilate or constrict blood vesselsvia regulations of the membrane potential (depolarization or hyper-polarization) in smooth muscle cells [20] [44]. In order to test the relationship between Shengmai- or GRe-induced vasodilation and K^+ channels, we determined the effects of the different antagonists on K^+ channels, including 4-AP, Glibenclamide, and CTX. The pre-treatment of vessel rings with 4-AP had no effects on the GRe-suppressed vascular tension. However, either CTX or Glibenclamide significantly reduced GRe-suppressed vessel tension inumbilical vessels. The results demonstrated that the Shengmai-mediate umbilical vascular response was related to potassium channel pathways. Since 4-AP had no influence on GRe-produced vascular changes, while CTX and Glibenclamide inhibited the effect of GRe, the data indicated that Ca^{2+}-activated K^+ channels and ATP-sensitive channels, not voltage-dependent K^+ channels, might play a role in the GRe- and Shengmai-suppressed vascular tension.

5. Conclusion

This was the first study to show that Shengmai and its compound GRe could suppress vascular tension-generated by PE in the umbilical cord. Since Shengmai could be used during pregnancy, the data increased understanding the effects of this herb drug on umbilical vessels. The possible mechanisms for Shengmai-reduced vascular tonemay not be related to NO pathways in the umbilical cords, and may not be linked to release of intracellular Ca^{2+} orentry of extra-cellular Ca^{2+}. However, potassium channels, particularly BKCa channels and ATP-sensitive channels, may play an important role in the GRe-suppressed vascular tension. Although further studies are required for detailed mechanisms of Shengmai on umbilical vessels, the new information gained in this study offers insight for understanding Shengmai's effects on umbilical cords.

Acknowledgements

Thanks to all the pregnant mothers and their families who participated in this study. This work was supported by Grant 2012CB947604; 2013BAI04B05; NSFC (81030006, 81320108006, 81370719, and 81370714); N3126908;

Jiangsu Key Discipline/Laboratory and "Chuang XinTuan Dui" funds; and Jiangsu Key Discipline of Human Assisted Reproduction Medicine funds.

Conflict of Interest

The authors declare that they have no conflict of interest.

References

[1]   Antoniou, E.E., Derom, C., Thiery, E., Fowler, T., Southwood, T.R. and Zeegers, M.P. (2011) The Influence of Genetic and Environmental Factors on the Etiology of the Human Umbilical Cord: The East Flanders Prospective Twin Survey. *Biology of Reproduction*, **85**, 137-143. http://dx.doi.org/10.1095/biolreprod.110.088807

[2]   Imamura, T., Potempa, J. and Travis, J. (2004) Activation of the Kallikrein-Kinin System and Release of New Kinins through Alternative Cleavage of Kininogens by Microbial and Human Cell Proteinases. *Biological Chemistry*, **385**, 989-996. http://dx.doi.org/10.1515/BC.2004.129

[3]   Ferguson, V.L. and Dodson, R.B. (2009) Bioengineering Aspects of the Umbilical Cord. *European Journal of Obstetrics & Gynecology*, **144**, S108-S113. http://dx.doi.org/10.1016/j.ejogrb.2009.02.024

[4]   Whitehead, C.L., Teh, W.T., Walker, S.P., Leung, C., Larmour, L. and Tong, S. (2013) Circulating MicroRNAs in Maternal Blood as Potential Biomarkers for Fetal Hypoxia *in-Utero*. *PLoS ONE*, **8**, e78487. http://dx.doi.org/10.1371/journal.pone.0078487

[5]   Smith, G.C. and Fretts, R.C. (2007) Stillbirth. *The Lancet*, **370**, 1715-1725. http://dx.doi.org/10.1016/S0140-6736(07)61723-1

[6]   Froen, J.F., Gardosi, J.O., Thurmann, A., Francis, A. and Stray-Pedersen, B. (2004) Restricted Fetal Growth in Sudden Intrauterine Unexplained Death. *Acta Obstetricia et Gynecologica Scandinavica*, **83**, 801-807. http://dx.doi.org/10.1080/j.0001-6349.2004.00602.x

[7]   Lawn, J.E., Cousens, S. and Zupan, J. (2005) 4 Million Neonatal Deaths: When? Where? Why? *The Lancet*, **365**, 891-900. http://dx.doi.org/10.1016/S0140-6736(05)71048-5

[8]   Nishida, H., Kushida, M., Nakajima, Y., Ogawa, Y., Tatewaki, N., Sato, S., *et al.* (2007) Amyloid-Beta-Induced Cytotoxicity of PC-12 Cell Was Attenuated by Shengmai-San through Redox Regulation and Outgrowth Induction. *Journal of Pharmacological Sciences*, **104**, 73-81. http://dx.doi.org/10.1254/jphs.FP0070100

[9]   Wang, N.L., Liou, Y.L., Lin, M.T., Lin, C.L. and Chang, C.K. (2005) Chinese Herbal Medicine, Shengmai San, Is Effective for Improving Circulatory Shock and Oxidative Damage in the Brain during Heatstroke. *Journal of Pharmacological Sciences*, **97**, 253-265. http://dx.doi.org/10.1254/jphs.FP0040793

[10]   Zhao, M.H., Rong, Y.Z. and Lu, B.J. (1996) [Effect of Shengmaisan on Serum Lipid Peroxidation in Acute Viral Myocarditis]. *Chinese Journal of Integrated Traditional and Western*, **16**, 142-145.

[11]   Fang, J., Jiang, J. and Luo, D.C. (1987) [Effect of Sheng Mai Decoction on Left Ventricular Function in Patients with Coronary Heart Disease. A Randomized, Double-Blind, Placebo-Controlled, Cross-Over Trial]. *Chinese Journal of Internal Medicine*, **26**, 403-406.

[12]   Zhan, S., Guo, W., Shao, Q., Fan, X., Li, Z. and Cheng, Y. (2014) A Pharmacokinetic and Pharmacodynamic Study of Drug-Drug Interaction between Ginsenoside Rg1, Ginsenoside Rb1 and Schizandrin after Intravenous Administration to Rats. *Journal of Ethnopharmacology*, **152**, 333-339. http://dx.doi.org/10.1016/j.jep.2014.01.014

[13]   Hehir, M.P., Moynihan, A.T., Glavey, S.V. and Morrison, J.J. (2009) Umbilical Artery Tone in Maternal Obesity. *Reproductive Biology and Endocrinology*, **7**, 6. http://dx.doi.org/10.1186/1477-7827-7-6

[14]   Pujol Lereis, V.A., Hita, F.J., Gobbi, M.D., Verdi, M.G. and Rodriguez, M.C. (2006) Rothlin RP. Pharmacological Characterization of Muscarinic Receptor Subtypes Mediating Vasoconstriction of Human Umbilical Vein. *British Journal of Pharmacology*, **147**, 516-523. http://dx.doi.org/10.1038/sj.bjp.0706654

[15]   Errasti, A.E., Velo, M.P., Torres, R.M., Sardi, S.P. and Rothlin, R.P. (1999) Characterization of Alpha1-Adrenoceptor Subtypes Mediating Vasoconstriction in Human Umbilical Vein. *British Journal of Pharmacology*, **126**, 437-442. http://dx.doi.org/10.1038/sj.bjp.0702320

[16]   Dennedy, M.C., Houlihan, D.D., McMillan, H. and Morrison, J.J. (2002) β_2- and β_3-Adrenoreceptor Agonists: Human Myometrial Selectivity and Effects on Umbilical Artery Tone. *American Journal of Obstetrics and Gynecology*, **187**, 641-647. http://dx.doi.org/10.1067/mob.2002.125277

[17]   Potter, S.M., Dennedy, M.C. and Morrison, J.J. (2002) Corticosteroids and Fetal Vasculature: Effects of Hydrocortisone, Dexamethasone and Betamethasone on Human Umbilical Artery. *BJOG: An International Journal of Obstetrics & Gynaecology*, **109**, 1126-1131. http://dx.doi.org/10.1111/j.1471-0528.2002.01540.x

[18] Topal, G., Foudi, N., Uydes-Dogan, B.S., Cachina, T., Kucur, M., Gezer, A., *et al.* (2010) Involvement of Prostaglandin F2alpha in Preeclamptic Human Umbilical Vein Vasospasm: A Role of Prostaglandin F and Thromboxane A2 Receptors. *Journal of Hypertension*, **28**, 2438-2445.

[19] Lam, F.F., Deng, S.Y., Ng, E.S., Yeung, J.H., Kwan, Y.W., Lau, C.B., *et al.* (2010) Mechanisms of the Relaxant Effect of a Danshen and Gegen Formulation on Rat Isolated Cerebral Basilar Artery. *Journal of Ethnopharmacology*, **132**, 186-192. http://dx.doi.org/10.1016/j.jep.2010.08.015

[20] Nelson, M.T. and Quayle, J.M. (1995) Physiological Roles and Properties of Potassium Channels in Arterial Smooth Muscle. *American Journal of Physiology*, **268**, C799-C822.

[21] Gao, W., Dong, X., Xie, N., Zhou, C., Fan, Y., Chen, G., *et al.* (2014) Dehydroabietic Acid Isolated from *Commiphora opobalsamum* Causes Endothelium-Dependent Relaxation of Pulmonary Artery via PI3K/Akt-eNOS Signaling Pathway. *Molecules*, **19**, 8503-8517. http://dx.doi.org/10.3390/molecules19068503

[22] Gauthier, K.M., Campbell, W.B. and McNeish, A.J. (2014) Regulation of $K_{Ca}2.3$ and Endothelium-Dependent Hyperpolarization (EDH) in the Rat Middle Cerebral Artery: The Role of Lipoxygenase Metabolites and Isoprostanes. *PeerJ*, **2**, e414. http://dx.doi.org/10.7717/peerj.414

[23] Shamsuzzaman, A.S., Gersh, B.J. and Somers, V.K. (2003) Obstructive Sleep Apnea: Implications for Cardiac and Vascular Disease. *The Journal of the American Medical Association*, **290**, 1906-1914. http://dx.doi.org/10.1001/jama.290.14.1906

[24] Phillips, B.G., Narkiewicz, K., Pesek, C.A., Haynes, W.G., Dyken, M.E. and Somers, V.K. (1999) Effects of obstructive Sleep Apnea on Endothelin-1 and Blood Pressure. *Journal of Hypertension*, **17**, 61-66. http://dx.doi.org/10.1097/00004872-199917010-00010

[25] Allahdadi, K.J., Walker, B.R. and Kanagy, N.L. (2005) Augmented Endothelin Vasoconstriction in Intermittent Hypoxia-Induced Hypertension. *Hypertension*, **45**, 705-709. http://dx.doi.org/10.1161/01.HYP.0000153794.52852.04

[26] Sumpio, B.E., Riley, J.T. and Dardik, A. (2002) Cells in Focus: Endothelial Cell. *The International Journal of Biochemistry & Cell Biology*, **34**, 1508-1512. http://dx.doi.org/10.1016/S1357-2725(02)00075-4

[27] Wang, L., Zhang, Y., Wang, Z., Li, S., Min, G., Chen, J., *et al.* (2012) Inhibitory Effect of Ginsenoside-Rd on Carrageenan-Induced Inflammation in Rats. *Canadian Journal of Physiology and Pharmacology*, **90**, 229-236. http://dx.doi.org/10.1139/y11-127

[28] Kou, J., Tian, Y., Tang, Y., Yan, J. and Yu, B. (2006) Antithrombotic Activities of Aqueous Extract from Radix Ophiopogon Japonicus and Its Two Constituents. *Biological and Pharmaceutical Bulletin*, **29**, 1267-1270. http://dx.doi.org/10.1248/bpb.29.1267

[29] Chiu, P.Y., Luk, K.F., Leung, H.Y., Ng, K.M. and Ko, K.M. (2008) Schisandrin B Stereoisomers Protect against Hypoxia/Reoxygenation-Induced Apoptosis and Inhibit Associated Changes in Ca^{2+}-Induced Mitochondrial Permeability Transition and Mitochondrial Membrane Potential in H9c2 Cardiomyocytes. *Life Sciences*, **82**, 1092-1101. http://dx.doi.org/10.1016/j.lfs.2008.03.006

[30] Chai, H., Wang, Q., Huang, L., Xie, T. and Fu, Y. (2008) Ginsenoside Rb1 Inhibits Tumor Necrosis Factor-Alpha-Induced Vascular Cell Adhesion Molecule-1 Expression in Human Endothelial Cells. *Biological and Pharmaceutical Bulletin*, **31**, 2050-2056. http://dx.doi.org/10.1248/bpb.31.2050

[31] Yim, T.K. and Ko, K.M. (1999) Methylenedioxy Group and Cyclooctadiene Ring as Structural Determinants of Schisandrin in Protecting against Myocardial Ischemia-Reperfusion Injury in Rats. *Biochemical Pharmacology*, **57**, 77-81. http://dx.doi.org/10.1016/S0006-2952(98)00297-4

[32] Fong, W.F., Wan, C.K., Zhu, G.Y., Chattopadhyay, A., Dey, S., Zhao, Z., *et al.* (2007) Schisandrol A from Schisandra Chinensis Reverses P-Glycoprotein-Mediated Multidrug Resistance by Affecting Pgp-Substrate Complexes. *Planta Medica*, **73**, 212-220. http://dx.doi.org/10.1055/s-2007-967120

[33] Pan, Q., Lu, Q., Zhang, K. and Hu, X. (2006) Dibenzocyclooctadiene Lingnans: A Class of Novel Inhibitors of P-Glycoprotein. *Cancer Chemotherapy and Pharmacology*, **58**, 99-106. http://dx.doi.org/10.1007/s00280-005-0133-1

[34] Ito, S., Suki, B., Kume, H., Numaguchi, Y., Ishii, M., Iwaki, M., *et al.* (2010) Actin Cytoskeleton Regulates Stretch-Activated Ca^{2+} Influx in Human Pulmonary Microvascular Endothelial Cells. *American Journal of Respiratory Cell and Molecular Biology*, **43**, 26-34. http://dx.doi.org/10.1165/rcmb.2009-0073OC

[35] van Kesteren, R.E. and Geraerts, W.P. (1998) Molecular Evolution of Ligand-Binding Specificity in the Vasopressin/Oxytocin Receptor Family. *Annals of the New York Academy of Sciences*, **839**, 25-34. http://dx.doi.org/10.1111/j.1749-6632.1998.tb10728.x

[36] Rembold, C.M. (1992) Regulation of Contraction and Relaxation in Arterial Smooth Muscle. *Hypertension*, **20**, 129-137. http://dx.doi.org/10.1161/01.HYP.20.2.129

[37] Ives, S.J., Andtbacka, R.H., Kwon, S.H., Shiu, Y.T., Ruan, T., Noyes, R.D., *et al.* (2012) Heat and Alpha1-Adrenergic Responsiveness in Human Skeletal Muscle Feed Arteries: The Role of Nitric Oxide. *Journal of Applied Physiology*,

113, 1690-1698.

[38] Striessnig, J., Pinggera, A., Kaur, G., Bock, G. and Tuluc, P. (2014) L-type Ca Channels in Heart and Brain. *Wiley Interdisciplinary Reviews: Membrane Transport and Signaling*, **3**, 15-38. http://dx.doi.org/10.1002/wmts.102

[39] Hermsmeyer, K., Sturek, M. and Rusch, N.J. (1988) Calcium Channel Modulation by Dihydropyridines in Vascular Smooth Muscle. *Annals of the New York Academy of Sciences*, **522**, 25-31. http://dx.doi.org/10.1111/j.1749-6632.1988.tb33339.x

[40] Connolly, M.J., Prieto-Lloret, J., Becker, S., Ward, J.P. and Aaronson, P.I. (2013) Hypoxic Pulmonary Vasoconstriction in the Absence of Pretone: Essential Role for Intracellular Ca^{2+} Release. *The Journal of Physiology*, **591**, 4473-4498. http://dx.doi.org/10.1113/jphysiol.2013.253682

[41] Perez, C.G., Copello, J.A., Li, Y., Karko, K.L., Gomez, L., Ramos-Franco, J., *et al.* (2005) Ryanodine Receptor Function in Newborn Rat Heart. *American Journal of Physiology-Heart and Circulatory Physiology*, **288**, H2527-H2540. http://dx.doi.org/10.1152/ajpheart.00188.2004

[42] Navarro-Dorado, J., Garcia-Alonso, M., van Breemen, C., Tejerina, T. and Fameli, N. (2014) Calcium Oscillations in Human Mesenteric Vascular Smooth Muscle. *Biochemical and Biophysical Research Communications*, **445**, 84-88. http://dx.doi.org/10.1016/j.bbrc.2014.01.150

[43] Cribbs, L.L. (2006) T-Type Ca^{2+} Channels in Vascular Smooth Muscle: Multiple Functions. *Cell Calcium*, **40**, 221-230. http://dx.doi.org/10.1016/j.ceca.2006.04.026

[44] Jackson, W.F. (2000) Ion Channels and Vascular Tone. *Hypertension*, **35**, 173-178. http://dx.doi.org/10.1161/01.HYP.35.1.173

13

Co-Localization of Alpha1-Adrenoceptors and GPR55: A Novel Prostate Cancer Paradigm?

Kalyani Chimajirao Patil, Laura McPherson, Craig James Daly

College of Medical, Veterinary & Life Sciences, School of Life Sciences, University of Glasgow, Glasgow, UK
Email: Craig.Daly@Glasgow.ac.uk

Abstract

α_1-adrenoceptors (α_1-ARs) and "cannabinoid-like" G Protein Coupled Receptor 55 (GPR55) belong to the G-protein coupled receptor (GPCR) family and play a crucial role in regulating prostate function. Although physical and functional interactions between the cannabinoid and adrenergic systems have been reported, analysis of functional interactions between α_1-AR and GPR55 in normal and neoplastic prostate has not been reported. Since GPR55 levels are high in rodent adrenal gland, we propose a function link between the adrenergic system and GPR55 receptor. Confocal Laser Scanning Microscopy (CLSM) was employed to examine the endogenous α_1-AR and GPR55 expression and their co-localization, expressed as fluorescence, *in vitro* in human androgen-insensitive PC-3 and androgen-sensitive LNCaP prostatic carcinoma cell lines, using the fluorescent ligands—Syto 62 (nuclear stain), BODIPY FL-Prazosin (QAPB; fluorescent quinazoline α_1-AR ligand) and Tocriflour (T1117; a novel fluorescent diarylpyrazole cannabinoid/GPR55 ligand). Fluorescent ligand binding in untreated PC-3 cells and LNCaP cells and spheroids showed heterogeneous expression of both α_1-ARs and GPR55. A small proportion of cells had both α_1-ARs and GPR55 in relatively equal numbers indicating a degree of co-localization. Co-localization of fluorescent ligand binding exhibited a stronger correlation in LNCaP (0.87) as compared to PC-3 (0.63) cells. Upregulation of α_1-AR was observed in PC-3 cells following chronic doxazosin incubation. Robust T1117 binding, suggestive of GPR55 upregulation, was also observed in these cells. The presence of subtype-rich cells with a degree of co-localization between α_1-ARs and GPR55 indicates a possibility for dimerisation or functional interaction and a new paradigm for functional synergism in which interactions may be either between cells or involve converging intracellular signaling processes.

Keywords

Prostate, α_1-Adrenoceptor, GPR55, Doxazosin

1. Introduction

Prostate cancer (PCa) is the most common non-cutaneous male cancer and the second highest cause of cancer-related deaths in Western society [1]. PCa mortality results from bone and lymph node metastasis and the progression from androgen-dependent to androgen-independent PCa cell growth [2]. The disease is heterogeneous in terms of grade, oncogene/tumor suppressor gene expression, genetics, and its molecular, cellular and hormonal profile is complex [1]. These alterations and heterogeneity result in the failure of androgen ablation therapy and chemotherapy, which are major therapeutic modalities for advanced PCa [3]. Therefore, considerable efforts are directed towards developing treatment strategies targeting receptors that are a part of the molecular circuitry controlling tumor growth.

1.1. Adrenoceptor

In PCa, the involvement of a wide range of G-protein coupled receptors (GPCRs) has been described [4]. The α_1-adrenoceptors (α_1-ARs) are of particular interest given their role in prostate function, and use as a therapeutic target. A recent comprehensive review of prostatic α_1-ARs outlines the complex signaling pathways and additional GPCRs that this receptor can interact with [5]. Currently, the recognized subtypes of α_1-ARs are α_{1A}, α_{1B}, α_{1D} [6]. α_{1A}-AR subtypes are the main prostate receptors and predominate in prostate stroma. α_{1D}-AR subtype is also found in the stroma whereas α_{1B}-AR is mainly found in the epithelium [7]. Functional studies suggest a predominance of α_1-ARs which have low affinity for the quinazoline drug, Prazosin, and these have been classed as α_{1L}-AR, a functional phenotype of α_{1A}-adrenoceptor, in mouse prostate [8].

The role of α_1-ARs in human prostate is undisputed and therefore, is the most commonly targeted GPCR in the prostate. The α_1-AR antagonists belonging to quinazoline family of drugs have therapeutic benefit in PCa as they induce apoptosis in the epithelial and smooth muscle cells of the prostate without affecting their proliferative capacity [9] [10]. Therapeutically, quinazolines decrease the incidence of PCa by 31.7% [11]. Evidence highlights the emerging therapeutic significance of two quinazoline drugs, Terazosin and Doxazosin as anti-tumor agents in PCa therapy. Doxazosin mesylate (brand name: Cardura), a subtype non-selective α_1-adrenoceptor antagonist, promotes smooth muscle relaxation. Doxazosin has also been documented to induce apoptosis and anoikis in PCa cells, both *in vitro* and *in vivo* [12]. The apoptotic activity of this quinazoline antagonist is independent of: 1) ability to antagonize α_1-AR; and 2) the hormone sensitivity of cells (*i.e.* androgen dependency) but dependent upon number and distribution of smooth muscle cells in the tissue [9]. It induces apoptosis by a) increasing caspase-3 activity in a concentration and time dependent manner which activate intracellular cascade promoting anoikis and subsequently, apoptosis; b) cleavage of focal adhesion kinases (FAK), a non-receptor tyrosine kinase mediating cell proliferation and migration, by caspases and c) decreasing Akt phosphorylation which has been shown to interfere with the apoptotic action of doxazosin [13] [14].

1.2. Endocannabinoids

Several studies have evaluated the role of the endocannabinoid system, consisting of classic cannabinoid receptors, CB1 and CB2, two endogenous ligands (anandamide and 2-arachidonoylglycerol) and several enzymes required in their production and degradation, in different PCa tissue/cell lines [15]. High CB1 receptor immunoreactivity score in PCa tissue was found to be associated with PCa severity and outcome [16]. Also, CB2 receptor expression was demonstrated in multiple PCacell lines (PC-3, DU-145, LNCaP, CWR22Rv1 and CA-HPV-10) [17]-[21]. However, role of a putative cannabinoid receptor GPR55, a 319-amino acid multi-pass membrane protein phylogenetically distinct from CB1 and CB2, in tumor progression suggests its importance as a possible cancer biomarker. High levels of GPR55 have been associated with aggressive cancers [22] and tumor angiogenesis [23].

We have previously shown co-localization between T1117, a fluorescent form of the cannabinoid CB1 receptor antagonist AM251, which showed binding affinity for GPR55 [24] and BODIPY FL-Prazosin (QAPB), a fluorescent ligand for all α_1-AR subtypes [25] in vascular tissue indicating their possible interaction in the cardiovascular system. Since tissue distribution of GPR55 overlaps significantly with α_1-AR in prostate, and GPR55 shares similar pharmacology with the classical cannabinoid (CB1) receptors [26], we investigated the degree of heterogeneity and possibility of interaction between α_1-AR and GPR55 by examining their distribution and co-localization *in vitro* using two commonly used prostate carcinoma cell lines; LNCaP and PC-3. The

LNCaP and PC-3 cell lines were selected as they display appropriate cellular characteristics and are widely used to model androgen-dependent early stage PCa and androgen-independent later refractory stage disease, respectively. Importantly, our findings provide preliminary evidence of co-localization and possible interaction between α_1-AR and GPR55 and its physiological importance in neoplastic prostatic cell *in vitro* which has never been studied prior to this study.

2. Materials and Methods

2.1. Materials

Stock concentrations of fluorescent ligands were dissolved in dimethyl sulphoxide (DMSO), and diluted in distilled water as required. Ligands were obtained from the following sources: BODIPY FL-Prazosin (QAPB) and Syto 62 from Invitrogen (Invitrogen Ltd., Paisley, UK); Tocrifluor T1117 (N-(piperidin-1-yl)-5-(4-(4-(3-(5-carboxamidotetramethylrhodaminyl) propyl)) phenyl)-1-(2,4-dicholrophenyl)-4-methyl-1H pyrazole-3-carboxamide) from Tocris (Bristol, UK) and Doxazosin from Pfizer (Sandwich, UK).

2.2. Cell Culture

The human androgen-insensitive, PC-3 (ATCC: CRL-1435) and androgen-sensitive, LNCaP (ATCC: CRL-1740) prostatic carcinoma cell lines were obtained from American Type Culture Collection repository. Cells were cultured in the appropriate media recommended by the supplier supplemented with 10% Fetal Bovine Serum (FBS), Penicillin-Streptomycin (Pen-Strep) and L-Glutamine in a humidified incubator at 37°C, 95% O_2 and 5% CO_2 until confluent. Upon attaining confluence, the cells were trypsinized and rinsed in media and PBS. Subsequently, cells were re-suspended and plated to glass coverslips 24 hours before use.

2.3. Confocal Analysis

BODIPY FL-Prazosin (QAPB, 0.1 µM) and Tocriflour (T1117, 0.1 µM) were applied in combination to determine the receptor expression and co-localization in a) control untreated PC-3 and LNCaP cells and LNCaP-derived spheroids (24 hours) and b) PC-3 cells under chronic doxazosin treatment (6 weeks; 1 µM) allowed to regrow in drug-free media (2 weeks). Incubation media also included a fluorescent nuclear stain Syto 62 (1 µg/ml). Cell images are representative of at least three independent experiments in all cases.

2.4. Microscopic Examination

Cells were imaged using a Bio-Rad Radiance 2100 Confocal Laser Scanning Microscope (CLSM) using either an oil immersion lens 20× (NA 0.75) or 40× objective (NA 1.0). The CLSM was fitted with an argon ion, Green Helium Neon (HeNe) and red diode laser. In all comparative studies, laser intensity and photomultiplier tube (PMT) settings were identical. Fluorescent ligands were imaged as follows: QAPB (ex 488 nm, em 515 nm); T1117 (ex 543 nm, em 590 nm) and Syto 62 (ex 637 nm, em 660 nm). Multi-channel images are displayed as merged channels. Detailed analysis methods have previously been published [27].

2.5. Data Analysis

Data was collected, recorded and quantified using ImageJ 1.44p. Co-localization was quantified using the JA-CoP plugin for ImageJ and expressed as a Pearsons Correlation between two fluorophores generated from n = 4 for PC-3 cells and n = 5 for LNCaP cells. Graphs were drawn using GraphPad PRISM 5.0. Data was expressed as mean ± SEM (Standard Error Mean) of at least 3 independent experiments. Statistical tests such as students T-tests were carried out and significance was defined as P < 0.05.

3. Results

3.1. Co-Localization of Adrenergic and Cannabinoid Binding Sites in Prostate Cancer Cells

Figure 1 shows the binding pattern of QAPB and T1117 in PC-3 and LNCaP cells (control). In control cell population, heterogeneity extended to the expression of both α_1-ARs and GPR55. A spectrum of phenotypes was observed within the cell population, from those expressing predominantly α_1-AR to those harboring predomi-

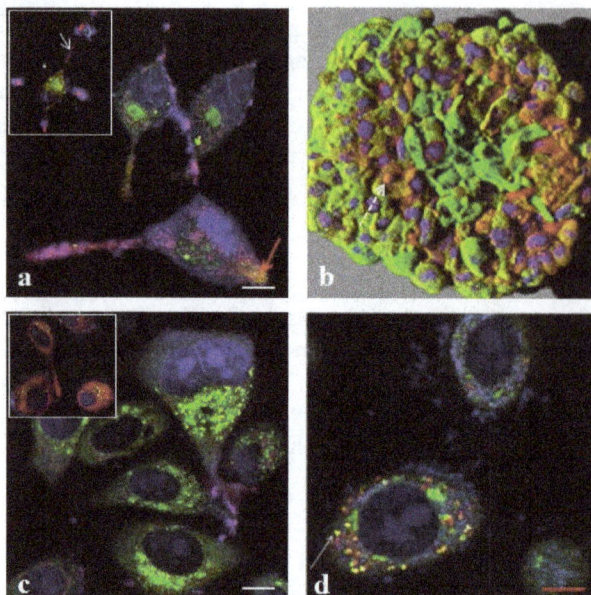

Figure 1. Fluorescent ligand binding and co-localization in PC-3 and LNCaP cells and LNCaP-derived spheroids. (a) Confocal scan of LNCaP cells after incubation with QAPB and fluorescent cannabinoid ligand T1117 (both 0.1 μM) showing a combination of cells expressing α_1-AR (green), GPR55 (red) or both in relatively equal amounts (yellow; red arrow). Inset: LNCaP cells showing high GPR55 concentration (red fluorescence; white arrow) within the cell processes; (b) LNCaP-derived spheroids showing similar heterogeneity in receptor expression with certain areas showing co-localization of α_1-AR and GPR55 (dotted arrow); (c) Confocal images of PC-3 cells showing α_1-AR positive cells (QAPB binding-induced green fluorescence) and GPR55 positive cells (T1117 binding-induced red fluorescence) (inset); (d) Arrow indicates overlapping regions (yellow) of receptor location suggesting a degree of co-localization of α_1-ARs and GPR55. Nuclei stained with Syto 62 (1 μg/ml). Calibration bar ((a) and (c)) indicates 20 microns and for (d) indicates 15 microns.

nantly GPR55 (**Figure 1(c)**). Importantly, it was apparent that PC-3 cells do not simply express α_1-ARs and GPR55 in equal proportions. A small proportion of cells had both α_1-ARs and GPR55 in relatively equal numbers reflected by the yellow fluorescence indicating a degree of co-localization of QAPB and T1117 (**Figure 1(d)**). LNCaP cells (in some but not all) (**Figure 1(a)**) and spheroids (**Figure 1(b)**) also demonstrated clear degree of co-localization between α_1-AR and GPR55. Co-localization (correlation analysis) of QAPB and T1117 binding revealed a stronger correlation in LNCaP (0.87 ± 0.03) cells *vs* PC-3 (0.63 ± 0.02) cells. Interestingly, T1117 binding was always associated with the long processes and cell tips of LNCaP cells (**Figure 1(a)**).

3.2. Chronic Doxazosin Treatment Elicits Upregulation of Intracellular α_1-AR and GPR55 Expression, Accompanied by Stimulated Growth of PC-3 Cells

The even distribution of binding sites, in certain areas and apparent co-localization of QAPB and T1117 in control PC-3 cells suggested co-expression and possibility of strong physical/functional association between the two receptors. To determine whether the functional antagonism of α_1-AR might result in altered GPR55 expression, ligand binding studies were performed in cells that received 1 μM doxazosin treatment for 6 weeks and returned to drug-free media for 2 weeks. The QAPB and T1117-binding induced fluorescence were determined in doxazosin-treated PC-3 cells normalized against fluorescence seen in untreated cells. Chronic administration of doxazosin resulted in significant ($P < 0.05$) increase in the fluorescence induced by QAPB binding suggesting upregulation in α_1-AR (**Figure 2(a)**). T1117-binding induced fluorescence was significantly higher ($P < 0.01$) following chronic treatment with the α_1-antagonist (**Figure 2(b)**). Sample cells are shown for comparison (**Figure 2(c)**, **Figure 2(d)**).

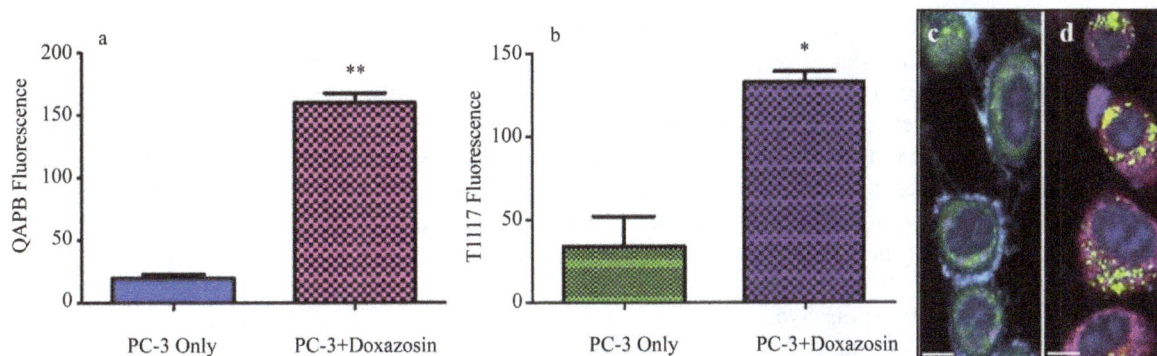

Figure 2. Chronic doxazosin treatment causes upregulation of α_1-AR and GPR55 expression. (a) Quantitative fluorescence measurement of QAPB binding in the presence and absence of doxazosin; (b) Analysis of GPR55 expression determined by T1117 fluorescence in PC-3 cells showing upregulation after chronic doxazosin treatment. As a positive control, PC-3 cells showing normal growth mechanisms were used. Results are expressed as mean ± SEM. $^*P < 0.05$, $^{**}P < 0.01$. (c)-(d) Confocal images of PC-3 cells before (c) and after (d) chronic doxazosin treatment (1 µM, 6 weeks). A predominance of intracellular GPR55 was observed in response to chronic administration of doxazosin. Each image is a representative of those generated from three independent experiments. (Scale bar 20 microns).

4. Discussion

In recent years, a wealth of information describing the molecular mechanics of GPCR cycle involving agonist activation, internalization, downregulation and sequestration have been obtained. In addition, significant amount of evidence has highlighted the importance of GPCR dimerisation and co-localization that may alter receptor function, pharmacology or regulatory properties [28]. However, heterodimerisation dynamics and its generality in controlling receptor expression are not widely explored. Fluorescent ligand binding *in vitro* in PC-3 and LNCaP cells and LNCaP-derived spheroids demonstrated clear degree of co-localization (in some but not all cells) between α_1-AR and GPR55. Homodimerisation and more selective heterodimerisation between individual α_1-AR subtypes have been reported [29]. Assays showing functional interactions between cannabinoid and adrenoceptor ligands have, in fact, confirmed that adrenoceptor heterodimerisation may extend beyond $\alpha\alpha$ and $\alpha\beta$ interactions [24]. Although the resolution of current fluorescence-based study was insufficient to confirm the existence of α_1-AR and GPR55 heterodimer, it does indicate their co-localization which is a pre-requisite of dimerization. In addition, evidence from recent molecular pharmacological studies has shown that co-expressed receptors can interact [26] [30] [31]. It can be hypothesized that co-localized α_1-ARs and cannabinoid together potentiate the action of neurotransmitters in the prostate since the autonomic nervous system plays an important role in prostatic functions [32]. The co-localization of α_1-ARs and GPR55 suggest a new paradigm for synergism in which interactions may be either between cells or involve converging intracellular signaling processes.

In PCa cells, fluorescent ligand binding studies showed binding sites for both T1117 and QAPB in different cellular locations (**Figure 1**). The binding of QAPB appeared to be more punctuate, both on the cell surface and intracellularly whereas binding sites for T1117 were more diffuse as seen earlier from the studies on vascular endothelium [24]. This pattern of binding allowed the classification of "subtype-rich" cells which could be classed as either expressing predominantly α_1-AR or predominantly GPR55. The presence of 'subtype-rich' cells was also observed in PC-3 cells. The significance of this is currently unknown, but it suggests that a subpopulation of cells have a preferred receptor expression profile in respect of GPCR's.

Upregulation of intracellular α_1-AR observed in PC-3 cells following removal of chronic α_1-AR antagonism can be considered an adaptive response to chronic administration of doxazosin. This adaptive change may manifest as withdrawal response after long-term α_1-AR antagonist use and can explain "α_1-AR blocker withdrawal syndrome" as an aftermath of chronic stimulation of α_1-AR. Aarons *et al.* (1980) have already reported this common outcome of an adaptive response to long-term β-AR antagonist use *via* upregulation of tissue β-ARs [33]. Although chronic doxazosin treatment has shown to alter α_1-AR properties in rat prostate [34] [35], to our knowledge, there is no report of withdrawal response, *via* α_1-AR upregulation, due to chronic administration of doxazosin in PCa cells.

In the present study, novel interaction between α_1-AR and GPR55 was identified *in vitro* in control untreated and doxazosin-treated PC-3 cells. The apparently high expression of intracellular α_1-AR in PC-3 cells showed that chronic doxazosin-induced response had an α_1-AR component. This was expected; intriguingly, robust intracellular T1117 binding-fluorescence suggestive of GPR55 upregulation was also observed in these cells. This suggests that co-expression of α_1-AR tempered the activity of GPR55 resulting in a dramatic increase in its intracellular expression in heterologous cells. It is possible that functional and perhaps physical association with α_1-AR leads to changes in the localization of GPR55 to "active" areas in the intracellular compartment of a cell enriched with signaling molecules. The pre-requisite of this event is that the two receptors should be in close proximity, influencing their ability to transduce signals. Our co-localization study supports such a notion. In addition, our observation that PC-3 cells, high in GPR55, grow at a furious rate when returned to drug-free media (data not shown) supports our hypothesis that in a clinical setting, removal of α_1-antagonism and the resultant stimulation of α_1-AR may allow lysophosphotidylinositol (LPI), an endogenous natural ligand for GPR55 synthesized intracellularly from membrane phosphoinositols by phospholipase A2 (PLA2), formation *via* activation of PLA(2) to stimulate GPR55-mediated accelerated proliferation. A link between α_1-AR stimulation and activation of PLA(2) has been reported [36] and if this could be demonstrated in prostatic smooth muscle then we would have a direct link between α_1-AR stimulation and LPI production. The growth aspect is further substantiated by our observation of high levels of T1117 binding sites in the long processes of LNCaP cells.

It therefore is plausible that complex functional interaction between α_1-AR and GPR55 exist whereby α_1-AR antagonism directly affects GPR55 functionality by overexpression after chronic doxazosin treatment to support tumorigenesis by promoting cell growth and drug resistance. Therefore, the α_1-ARs\GPR55 ratio could identify the metastatic prognosis of PCa cells and may serve as a useful biomarker or predictor of metastatic PCa. If our hypothesis is correct, then using carefully constructed, stable, non-toxic fluorescent ligands for the receptors, the number of 'hot' cells can be determined in a biopsy by clinicians/uropathologists to monitor the efficacy of anti-cancer therapy which the individual is undergoing and gauge the potential/progression to aggressive PCa. These results present both α_1-ARs and GPR55 and catecholamines as potentially significant targets for specific therapeutic modalities for treating PCa.

5. Conclusion

The present study suggested an interaction between α_1-AR and GPR55 *via* co-localization/dimerization providing rationale for further studies on mechanisms of cross talk between different subfamilies of GPCRs. These results open a new avenue of research oriented on delineating direct physical and functional interactions between the cannabinoid and adrenergic systems that were primarily attributed to only CB1 receptor mediated presynaptic inhibition of noradrenergic transmission [37]-[40]. We suggest, therefore, in the light of our findings and the wide, overlapping distribution of α_1-AR and GPR55, re-evaluation of interactions between adrenergic and GPR55 systems in cells and tissues that co-express both using higher resolution techniques with fluorescent ligands. In addition, our finding that the α_1-AR antagonist doxazosin alters GPR55 receptor number in cells endogenously expressing both α_1-AR and GPR55 needs to be studied *in vivo* due to the potential clinical significance of doxazosin in suppressing prostate tumourigenicity [6]. The recent observation that GPR55 is expressed in PCa cell line [41], suggests that some of the anti-tumor effects of α_1-AR antagonist [6] may be the result of indirect action on GPR55 in addition to the blockade of α_1-AR. However, the unexpected, novel "GPR55" phenomenon finding, possibly conferring the properties of tumor growth and drug resistance, demonstrates the significant impact of α_1-AR antagonists, particularly, doxazosin, in prostate carcinogenesis. To our knowledge, the current study in PC-3 cells is the first demonstration that chronic doxazosin treatment affects GPR55 expression. Since GPR55 has emerged as a lipid-sensitive modulator of oncogenesis, undoubtedly, pharmacology of LPI-GPR55 autocrine signaling system warrants focused research to develop novel therapeutics targeting the protein or its ligand for the purposes of inhibiting cancer growth and limit the risk of metastases. Moreover, studies need to be designed to investigate any association between GPR55 expression and other membrane receptors as well as with cancer remission, relapse or resistance following treatment with various chemotherapeutic inhibitory agents.

References

[1]   Russell, P.J. and Kingsley, E.A. (2003) Human Prostate Cancer Cell Lines. *Methods in Molecular Medicine Prostate Cancer Methods and Protocols*, **81**, 21-39. http://dx.doi.org/10.1385/1-59259-372-0:21

[2]   Isaacs, J.T. (1994) The Role of Androgens in Prostatic Cancer. *Vitamins & Hormones*, **49**, 433-502.
        http://dx.doi.org/10.1016/S0083-6729(08)61152-8

[3]   Crawford, E.D., Eisenberger, M.A., McLeod, D.C., Spaulding, J., Benson, R., Dorr, F.A., Blumenstein, B.A., Davis,
        M.A. and Goodman, P.J. (1989) A Controlled Randomized Trial of Leuprolide with and without Flutamide in Prostatic
        Cancer. *New England Journal of Medicine*, **321**, 419-424. http://dx.doi.org/10.1056/NEJM198908173210702

[4]   Daaka, Y.G. (2004) Proteins in Cancer: The Prostate Cancer Paradigm. *Sci STKE*, **216**, 1-10.

[5]   Hennenberg, M., Stief, C.G. and Gratzke, C. (2014) Prostatic α1-adrenoceptors: New Concepts of Function, Regulation,
        and Intracellular Signaling. *Neurology & Urodynamics*, **33**, 1074-1085. http://dx.doi.org/10.1002/nau.22467

[6]   Kyprianou, N., Chon, J. and Benning, C.M. (2000) Effects of Alpha1-Adrenoceptor (α_1-AR) Antagonists on Cell Pro-
        liferation and Apoptosis in the Prostate: Therapeutic Implications in Prostatic Disease. *The Prostate Supplement*, **9**,
        42-46. http://dx.doi.org/10.1002/1097-0045(2000)45:9+<42::AID-PROS9>3.0.CO;2-U

[7]   Desiniotis, A. and Kyprianou, N. (2011) Advances in the Design and Synthesis of Prazosin Derivatives over the Last
        Ten Years. *Expert Opinion on Therapeutic Targets*, **15**, 1405-1418. http://dx.doi.org/10.1517/14728222.2011.641534

[8]   Gray, K., Short, J. and Ventura, S. (2008) The α1A-Adrenoceptor Gene Is Required for the α1L-Adrenoceptor-Medi-
        ated Response in Isolated Preparations of the Mouse Prostate. *British Journal of Pharmacology*, **155**, 103-109.
        http://dx.doi.org/10.1038/bjp.2008.245

[9]   Kyprianou, N., Litvak, J., Alexander, R.B., Borkowski, A. and Jacobs, S.C. (1998) Induction of Prostate Apoptosis by
        Doxazosin. *Journal of Urology*, **159**, 1810-1815. http://dx.doi.org/10.1016/S0022-5347(01)63162-8

[10]   Chon, J., Isaacs, J.T., Borkowski, A., Partin, A.W., Jacobs, S.C. and Kyprianou, N. (1999) α-1 Adrenoceptor Antagon-
        ists Terazosin and Doxazosin Induce Prostate Apoptosis without Affecting Cell Proliferation in Patients with Benign
        Prostatic Hyperplasia. *Journal of Urology*, **161**, 2002-2008. http://dx.doi.org/10.1016/S0022-5347(05)68873-8

[11]   Harris, A.M., Warner, B.W., Wilson, J.M., Becker, A., Rowland, R.G., Conner, W., Lane, M., Kimbler, K., Durbin,
        E.B., Baron, A.T. and Kyprianou, N. (2007) Effect of α_1-Adrenoceptor Antagonist Exposure on Prostate Cancer Inci-
        dence: An Observational Cohort Study. *The Journal of Urology*, **178**, 2176-2180.
        http://dx.doi.org/10.1016/j.juro.2007.06.043

[12]   Kyprianou, N. (2003) Doxazosin and Terazosin Suppress Prostate Growth by Inducing Apoptosis: Clinical Signific-
        ance. *The Journal of Urology*, **169**, 1520-1525. http://dx.doi.org/10.1097/01.ju.0000033280.29453.72

[13]   Walden, P.D., Globina, Y. and Nieder, A. (2004) Induction of Anoikis by Doxazosin in Prostate Cancer Cells Is Asso-
        ciated with Activation of Caspase-3 and a Reduction of Focal Adhesion Kinase. *Urological Research*, **32**, 261-265.
        http://dx.doi.org/10.1007/s00240-003-0365-7

[14]   Garrison, J. and Kyprianou, N. (2006) Doxazosin Induces Apoptosis of Benign and Malignant Prostate Cells via a
        Death Receptor-Mediated Pathway. *Cancer Research*, **66**, 464-472.
        http://dx.doi.org/10.1158/0008-5472.CAN-05-2039

[15]   Henstridge, C.M. (2012) Off-Target Cannabinoid Effects Mediated by GPR55. *Pharmacology*, **89**, 179-187.
        http://dx.doi.org/10.1159/000336872

[16]   Chung, S.C., Hammarsten, P., Josefsson, A., Stattin, P., Granfors, T. and Egevad, L. (2009) A High Cannabinoid CB_1
        Receptor Immune-Reactivity Is Associated with Disease Severity and Outcome in Prostate Cancer. *European Journal
        of Cancer*, **45**, 174-182. http://dx.doi.org/10.1016/j.ejca.2008.10.010

[17]   Melck, D., Rueda, D., Galve-Roperh, I., De Petrocellis, L., Guzmán, M. and Di Marzo, V. (1999) Involvement of the
        cAMP/Protein Kinase A Pathway and of Mitogen-Activated Protein Kinase in the Anti-Proliferative Effects of Anan-
        damide in Human Breast Cancer Cells. *FEBS Letters*, **463**, 235-240. http://dx.doi.org/10.1016/S0014-5793(99)01639-7

[18]   Sánchez, M.G., Ruiz-Llorente, L., Sánchez, A.M. and Díaz-Laviada, I. (2003) Activation of Phosphoinositide
        3-Kinase/PKB Pathway by CB_1 and CB_2 Cannabinoid Receptors Expressed in Prostate PC-3 Cells: Involvement in
        Raf-1 Stimulation and NGF Induction. *Cellular Signalling*, **15**, 851-859.
        http://dx.doi.org/10.1016/S0898-6568(03)00036-6

[19]   Nithipatikom, K., Endsley, M.P., Isbell, M.A., Falck, J.R., Iwamoto, Y., Hillard, C.J. and Campbell, W. (2004)
        2-Arachidonoylglycerol: A Novel Inhibitor of Androgen-Independent Prostate Cancer Cell Invasion. *Cancer Research*,
        64, 8826-8830. http://dx.doi.org/10.1158/0008-5472.CAN-04-3136

[20]   Sarfaraz, S., Afaq, F., Adhami, V.M. and Mukhtar, H. (2005) Cannabinoid Receptor as a Novel Target for the Treat-
        ment of Prostate Cancer. *Cancer Research*, **65**, 1635-1641. http://dx.doi.org/10.1158/0008-5472.CAN-04-3410

[21]   Brown, I., Cascio, M.G., Wahle, K.W., Smoum, R., Mechoulam, R. and Ross, R.A. (2010) Cannabinoid Recep-
        tor-Dependent and -Independent Anti-Proliferative Effects of Omega-3 Ethanolamides in Androgen Receptor-Positive
        and -Negative Prostate Cancer Cell Lines. *Carcinogenesis*, **31**, 1584-1591. http://dx.doi.org/10.1093/carcin/bgq151

[22]   Andradas, C., Caffarel, M.M., Perez-Gomez, E., Salazar, M., Lorente, M., Velasco, G., Guzman, M. and Sanchez, M.

(2011) The Orphan G Protein-Coupled Receptor GPR55 Promotes Cancer Cell Proliferation via ERK. *Oncogene*, **30**, 245-252. http://dx.doi.org/10.1038/onc.2010.402

[23] Bondarenko, A., Waldeck-Weiermair, M., Naghdi, S., Poteser, M., Malli, R. and Graier, W. (2010) GPR55-Dependent and -Independent Ion Signaling in Response to Lysophosphatidylinositol in Endothelial Cells. *British Journal of Pharmacology*, **161**, 308-320. http://dx.doi.org/10.1111/j.1476-5381.2010.00744.x

[24] Daly, C.J., Ross, R.A., Whyte, J., Henstridge, C.M., Irving, A.J. and McGrath, J.C. (2010) Fluorescent Ligand Binding Reveals Heterogeneous Distribution of Adrenoceptors and "Cannabinoid-Like" Receptors in Small Arteries. *British Journal of Pharmacology*, **159**, 787-796. http://dx.doi.org/10.1111/j.1476-5381.2009.00608.x

[25] Daly, C.J., Milligan, C.M., Milligan, G., Mackenzie, J.F. and Mcgrath, J.C. (1998) Cellular Localization and Pharmacological Characterization of Functioning Alpha-1 Adrenoceptors by Fluorescent Ligand Binding and Image Analysis Reveals Identical Binding Properties of Clustered and Diffuse Populations of Receptors. *The Journal of Pharmacology and Experimental Therapeutics*, **286**, 984-990.

[26] Hudson, B.D., Hébert, T.E. and Kelly, M. (2010) Physical and Functional Interactions between CB_1 Cannabinoid Receptors and $\beta2$-Adrenocepors. *British Journal of Pharmacology*, **160**, 627-642. http://dx.doi.org/10.1111/j.1476-5381.2010.00681.x

[27] Daly, C.J. and McGrath, J.C. (2011) Previously Unsuspected Widespread Cellular and Tissue Distribution of Beta-Adrenoceptors and Its Relevance to Drug Action. *Trends in Pharmacological Sciences*, **32**, 219-226. http://dx.doi.org/10.1016/j.tips.2011.02.008

[28] Angers, S., Salapour, A. and Bouvier, M. (2002) Dimerization: An Emerging Concept for G Protein—Coupled Receptor Ontogeny and Function. *Annual Review of Pharmacology and Toxicology*, **42**, 409-435. http://dx.doi.org/10.1146/annurev.pharmtox.42.091701.082314

[29] Milligan, G., Pediani, J., Fidock, M. and López-Giménez, J.F. (2004) Dimerization of Alpha1-Adrenoceptors. *Biochemical Society Transactions*, **32**, 847-850.

[30] Uberti, M., Hague, C., Oller, H., Minneman, K. and Hall, R. (2005) Heterodimerisation with β_2-Adrenergic Receptors Promotes Surface Expression and Functional Activity of α_{1D}-Adrenergic Receptors. *Journal of Pharmacology and Experimental Therapeutics*, **313**, 16-23. http://dx.doi.org/10.1124/jpet.104.079541

[31] Copik, A.J., Ma, C., Kosaka, A., Sahdeo, S., Trane, A., Ho, H., Dietrich, P.S., Yu, H., Ford, A.P., Button, D. and Milla, M.E. (2009) Facilitatory Interplay in α_{1a} and β_2 Adrenoceptor Function Reveals a Non-Gq Signaling Mode: Implications for Diversification of Intracellular Signal Transduction. *Molecular Pharmacology*, **75**, 713-728. http://dx.doi.org/10.1124/mol.108.050765

[32] Pennefather, J.N., Lau, W.A., Mitchelson, F. and Ventura, S. (2000) The Autonomic and Sensory Innervation of the Smooth Muscle of the Prostate Gland: A Review of Pharmacological and Histological Studies. *Journal of Autonomic Pharmacology*, **20**, 193-206. http://dx.doi.org/10.1046/j.1365-2680.2000.00195.x

[33] Aarons, R.D., Nies, A.S., Gal, J., Hegstrand, L.R. and Molinoff, P.B. (1980) Elevation of Beta-Adrenergic Receptor Density in Human Lymphocytes after Propranolol Administration. *Journal of Clinical Investigation*, **65**, 949-957. http://dx.doi.org/10.1172/JCI109781

[34] Foster Jr., H.E., Yono, M., Shin, D., Takahashi, W., Pouresmail, M., Afiatpour, P. and Latifpour, J. (2004) Effects of Chronic Administration of Doxazosin on α_1-Adrenoceptors in the Rat Prostate. *The Journal of Urology*, **172**, 2465-2470. http://dx.doi.org/10.1097/01.ju.0000138475.89790.88

[35] Yono, M., Poster Jr., H.E., Shin, D., Takahashi, W., Pouresmail, M. and Latifpour, J. (2004) Doxazosin Treatment Causes Differential Alterations of α_1-Adrenoceptor Subtypes in the Rat Kidney, Heart and Aorta. *Life Sciences*, **75**, 2605-2614. http://dx.doi.org/10.1016/j.lfs.2004.08.001

[36] Kreda, S.M., Sumner, M., Fillo, S., Ribeiro, C.M., Luo, G.X., Xie, W., Daniel, K.W., Shears, S., Collins, S. and Wetsel, W.C. (2001) α_1-Adrenergic Receptors Mediate LH-Releasing Hormone Secretion through Phospholipases C and A_2 in Immortalized Hypothalamic Neurons. *Endocrinology*, **142**, 4839-4851.

[37] Schlicker, E., Timm, J., Zentner, J. and Gothert, M. (1997) Cannabinoid CB_1 Receptor-Mediated Inhibition of Noradrenaline Release in the Human and Guinea-Pig Hippocampus. *Naunyn-Schmiedeberg's Archives of Pharmacology*, **356**, 583-589. http://dx.doi.org/10.1007/PL00005093

[38] Schultheiss, T., Flau, K., Kathmann, M., Gothert, M. and Schlicker, E. (2005) Cannabinoid CB_1 Receptor-Mediated Inhibition of Noradrenaline Release in Guinea-Pig Vessels, but Not in Rat and Mouse Aorta. *Naunyn-Schmiedeberg's Archives of Pharmacology*, **372**, 139-146. http://dx.doi.org/10.1007/s00210-005-0007-4

[39] Pakdeechote, P., Dunn, W.R. and Ralevic, V. (2007) Cannabinoids Inhibit Noradrenergic and Purinergic Sympathetic Cotransmission in the Rat Isolated Mesenteric Arterial Bed. *British Journal of Pharmacology*, **152**, 725-733. http://dx.doi.org/10.1038/sj.bjp.0707397

[40] Tam, J., Trembovler, V., Di Marzo, V., Petrosino, S., Leo, G., Alexandrovich, A., Regev, E., Casap, N., Shteyer, A.,

Ledent, C., Karsak, M., Zimmer, A., Mechoulam, R., Yirmiya, R., Shohami, E. and Bab, I. (2008) The Cannabinoid CB$_1$ Receptor Regulates Bone Formation by Modulating Adrenergic Signaling. *The FASEB Journal*, **22**, 285-294. http://dx.doi.org/10.1096/fj.06-7957com

[41] Pineiro, R., Maffucci, T. and Falasca, M. (2011) The Putative Cannabinoid Receptor GPR55 Defines a Novel Autocrine Loop in Cancer Cell Proliferation. *Oncogene*, **30**, 142-152. http://dx.doi.org/10.1038/onc.2010.417

14

Acute Toxicity (Lethal Dose 50 Calculation) of Herbal Drug Somina in Rats and Mice

Muhammad Ahmed

Department of Pharmacology and Toxicology, Faculty of Pharmacy, Umm Al-Qura University, Makkah, Kingdom of Saudi Arabia
Email: hma00ahmed@hotmail.com

Abstract

Somina (herbal preparation) prepared by Hamdard Laboratories (Waqf) Pakistan is a mixture of five different medicinal plants, widely prescribed for the treatment of mental illness. For acute toxicity, the Karber arithmetic method for the calculation of LD50 and Hodge and Sterner toxicity scale was used. In this study, different doses (10, 100, 285, 500, 1000, 5000 and 10,000 mg/kg) of the extract was administered orally to the different groups of rats and mice. Signs of toxicity and possible death of animals were monitored for 24 hrs to calculate the median lethal dose (LD50) of somina. At the end of the study, all the animals in all the dose groups were sacrificed and the internal organ-body was compared with values from the control group. The LD50 was found to be >10,000 mg/kg body weight upon oral administration in mice and rats as no mortality was observed after single dose administration. According to Hodge and Sterner toxicity scale, the obtained value of LD 50 > 10,000 mg/kg classified the Somina as Practically non-toxic herbal medicine.

Keywords

Acute Toxicity, Somina, Median Lethal Dose (LD50), Karber Arithmetic Method for the Calculation of LD50, Hodge and Sterner Toxicity Scale

1. Introduction

Somina (Herbal drug) prepared by Hamdard Laboratories (Waqf) Pakistan in powdered form is widely used in Unani system of medicine for the treatment of mental illness. It is claimed that somina possesses sedative, hypnotic and anxiolytic activities [1]. Somina is composed of five different medicinal plants.

Sesamum indicum, Prunus amygdalus, Papaver somniferum, Lactuca serriola (seed extracts), *Lagenaria vulgaris.*

In the literature, different properties of these medicinal plants have been reported. *Sesamum indicum* was reported to have antioxidant [2] and anti-inflammatory activities [3]. *Prunus amygdalus* keeps medicinal properties such as anti-inflammatory, sedative, anti-hyperlipidemia, antitumor and antioxidant and Antimicrobial [4]. Anticonvulsant [5] and analgesic activity [6] of *Papaver somniferum* were cited in the literature. *Lactuca serriola* was found to possess spasmogenic, spasmolytic, bronchodilator, and vasorelaxant activities [7]. Since ancient times *Lagenaria vulgaris* has been utilized for treatment of jaundice, diabetes, ulcer, piles, colitis, hypertension and skin diseases [8]. Despite the popular use of these plants, some toxicological studies have previously performed and the results showed that at different doses *Lagenaria vulgaris* (2 g/kg: [9]), *Lactuca serriola* (6 g/kg; [10]), *Prunus amygdalus* (2 g/kg: [11]), *Sesamum indicum* (500 mg/kg: [12]) were found to be well tolerated. However, toxicity or safety of Individual constituents has reported in the literature but screening has not yet done on somina as whole to confirm its safety for the use in folkloric medicine. This study was conducted to investigate the toxicity of somina having all ingredients together.

2. Materials and Methods

2.1. Formation of Different Doses of Somina

Somina is available in powder form. Recommended dose of somina for human is 10 g/70kg. In the present study, different doses of somina were used as shown in **Table 1**.

All doses were prepared by dissolving its powder in distilled water at the time of administration for the determination of LD50.

2.2. Animals

40 Adult NMRI mice (20 - 25 g) and 40 adult Sprague-Dawley Rats (200 - 250 g) of either sex were obtained from Dr. Hafiz Muhammad Ilyas Institute of Pharmacology and Herbal Sciences (Dr. HMIIPHS) and were housed in groups of 5 per cage for seven days prior to experimentation in an ideal laboratory environment as per OCED [13]. Each experimental group consisted of five animals. University and Departmental committee for Research and Ethics had approved all the experimental protocols. Each animal was used only once. For ethical reason, all animals were sacrificed at the end of the study [14].

2.3. Toxicological/Safety Evaluation Studies in Mice

Eight groups containing five NMR-I mice (25 - 30 g) in each and eight groups containing five rats (200 - 250 g) were used in this study. All animals were treated orally once and different doses (control, 10, 100, 285, 500, 1000, 5000, 10,000 mg/kg) were administered as shown in **Table 1**.

Animals were weighed before the dose administration. All the animals were kept under continuous observation for 6 hours after the administration of the dose, for any change in behavior or physical activities. After 24 hrs, all survived mice were anesthetized with pentothal sodium (40 mg/kg) and autopsied.

Table 1. Different doses of somina (herbal drug).

S. No.	Dose	Ratio
1	10 mg/kg	Less than human dose
2	100 mg/kg	Approximately similar to human dose
3	285 mg/kg	2 times greater than human dose
4	500 mg/kg	4 time greater than human dose
5	1000 mg/kg	7 time greater than human dose
6	5000 mg/kg	35 time greater than human dose
7	10,000 mg/kg	70 time greater than human dose
8	Saline (10 ml/kg)	Control group

2.4. Calculation of Median Lethal Dose (LD50)

For each mouse, the observation was made for 24 hr and symptoms of toxicity and rate of mortality in each group were noted. At the end of study period, expired animals were counted for the calculation of LD50. The arithmetic method of Karber [15] was used for the determination of LD50.

$$LD50 = LD100 - \sum (a \times b)/n$$

n = total number of animal in a group.
a = the difference between two successive doses of administered extract/substance.
b = the average number of dead animals in two successive doses.
LD100 = Lethal dose causing the 100% death of all test animals.
Hodge and Sterner scale (**Table 2**) was used for the evaluation of toxicity with the help of LD50 [16].

3. Results

From the experiment, the results reveal that the somina has not been found to be toxic even at 10,000 mg/kg or 10 mg/kg that is 70 times higher than the human dose in experimental animals (rats and mice) as shown in **Table 3**. The animals received 10,000 mg/kg orally was not found to cause any mortality and non-significant changes were observed in wellness parameters used for evaluation of toxicity. Behavioral pattern like salivation, sleep cycle and corner sitting of the treated animals were found to enhance (**Table 3**). However, the low doses did not produce any pronounced effect. Autopsy revealed that no changes were observed in organ structure and weight.

Table 2. Hodge and sterner toxicity scale.

S. No.	Term	LD50 (Rat, Oral)
1	Extremely Toxic	Less than 1 mg/kg
2	Highly Toxic	1 - 50 mg/kg
3	Moderately Toxic	50 - 500 mg/kg
4	Slightly Toxic	500 - 5000 mg/kg
5	Practically Non-Toxic	5000 - 15,000 mg/kg

Table 3. Toxicological study of different doses of somina administered orally in mice and rats.

S. No.	Groups	Dose/Day	Mortality (x/N)	Symptoms (2 hr)
\multicolumn{5}{Toxicity in Mice}				
1	Group I	Saline (10 ml/kg)	0/5	Nil
2	Group II	10 mg/kg	0/5	Nil
3	Group III	100 mg/kg	0/5	Nil
4	Group IV	285 mg/kg	0/5	Nil
5	Group V	500 mg/kg	0/5	Nil
6	Group VI	1000 mg/kg	0/5	Nil
7	Group VII	5000 mg/kg	0/5	Corner Sitting,
8	Group VIII	10,000 mg/kg	0/5	Corner Sitting, Salivation, Drowsy
\multicolumn{5}{Toxicity in Rats}				
1	Group I	Saline (10 ml/kg)	0/5	Nil
2	Group II	10 mg/kg	0/5	Nil
3	Group III	100 mg/kg	0/5	Nil
4	Group IV	285 mg/kg	0/5	Nil
5	Group V	500 mg/kg	0/5	Nil
6	Group VI	1000 mg/kg	0/5	Nil
7	Group VII	5000 mg/kg	0/5	Corner Sitting, Palpeberalptosis
8	Group VIII	10,000 mg/kg	0/5	Corner Sitting, Salivation, Palpeberalptosis, Drowsy

LD50 Value: As per observations and calculations (Karber, 1931), the LD50 value of somina after oral administration was found to be more than 10,000 mg/kg body weight.

According to Hodge and Sterner (2005) toxicity scale, somina is said to be in non-toxic herbal drug category (**Table 2**).

4. Discussion

Although, the somina is used in folkloric medicine for the treatment of mental illness and research had been done to investigate its said effect [1] [17] but the present study was conducted to reveals the safety evaluation of somina, because it contain different constituent and it is a mixture of five medicinal plants. However, each plant contains different active compounds have medicinal and toxic effects. That's why it is mandatory to evaluate the toxicity of herbal drugs (somina) whose adverse effects and toxic doses are mostly unknown [18]. Previously reported data revealed the toxic effect of different herbs at different doses such as Kava, germander (*Teucrium-chamaedrys*). Chaparral (*Larrea tridentate*) causes severe liver injury [19]. Licorice can induce hypokalemic myopathy [20] and Kelp (seaweed) can cause hyperthyroidism [21]. In the present study, the somina was found to be safe up to 10,000 mg/kg orally.

This present study is in agreement with other previous studies in which different doses of constituent of somina is reported to be safe like *Lagenaria vulgaris* at the dose of 2 g/kg [9], *Lactuca serriola* at the dose of 6 g/kg [10], *Prunus amygdalus* at the dose of 2 g/kg [11], while *Sesamum indicum* did not produce any toxicity up to the dose of 500 mg/kg [12]. In the present study, a maximum dose of somina was used in all above of reported literature doses were less than the present study. Although the present study confirms that somina is practically non-toxic [16]. In the present study, other organs like kidney, heart and spleen did not show any significant change.

5. Conclusion

In conclusion, the results of the present study conclude that somina is safe or practically non-toxic when administered orally. This study is the preliminary study; in the future, this research is offering an outset to continue the research by administering the somina through different routes in different animals' species and in human.

Acknowledgements

Author is grateful to Prof. S. I Ahmed (Late) Former Dean Faculty of Pharmacy, University of Karachi, Hamdard University Karachi and Director of HMIIPHS, Hamdard University Karachi for his support, encouragement at every step of this study and Hamdard Foundation Pakistan for financial support.

Ethical Approval

Author hereby declared that the experimental protocol was approved by the University and Departmental committee for Research and Ethics. Each animal was used only once. For ethical reason, all animals were sacrificed at the end of the study (AVMA Guideline, 2013). Experimental protocol was followed according to Guidelines for Care and Use of Laboratory Animals in Biomedical Research (2010). All rules were followed as well as specific national laws where applicable.

Competing Interests

The author has no conflict of interest to report.

References

[1]   Azmat, A., Ahmed, M., Zafar, N. and Ahmad, S.I. (2008) Neuropharmacological Profile of Somina (Herbal Drug) in Mice and Rats. *Pakistan Journal of Pharmacology*, **25**, 53-58.

[2]   Hu, Q., Xu, J., Chen, S. and Yang, F. (2004) Antioxidant Activity of Extracts of Black Sesame Seed (*Sesamum indicum* L.) by Supercritical Carbon Dioxide Extraction. *Journal of Agricultural and Food Chemistry*, **25**, 943-947.

[3]   Hsu, D., Chu, P.Y. and Liu, M.Y. (2012) Emerging Trends in Dietary Components for Preventing and Combating Disease. Sesame Seed (*Sesamum indicum* L.) Extracts and Their Anti-Inflammatory Effect. *American Chemical Society ACS Symposium Series*, **1093**, 335-341. http://dx.doi.org/10.1021/bk-2012-1093.ch019

[4]   Thebo, N., Sheikh, W., Bhangar, M.I., Iqbal, P. and Nizamani, M.H. (2012) Therapeutic and Antioxidant Potential in the Shell Extract of *Prunus amygdalus* against Dermal Mycosis. *Medicinal & Aromatic Plants*, **1**, 108. http://dx.doi.org/10.4172/2167-0412.1000108

[5]   Heidari, M.R. and Bayat, M. (2003) Effect of Methanol Extract of *Papaver somniferum* L. on Seizure Induced by Picrotoxin in Male Mice. *Journal of Rafsanjan University of Medical Sciences and Health Services*, **2**, 187-194.

[6]   Calixto, J.B., Scheidt, C., Otuki, M. and Santos, A.R. (2001) Biological Activity of Plant Extracts: Novel Analgesic Drugs. *Expert Opinion on Emerging Drugs*, **6**, 261-279. http://dx.doi.org/10.1517/14728214.6.2.261

[7]   Janbaz, K.H., Latif, M.F., Saqib, F., Imran, I., Zia-Ul-Haq, M. and De Feo, V. (2013) Pharmacological Effects of *Lactuca serriola* L. in Experimental Model of Gastrointestinal, Respiratory, and Vascular Ailments. *Evidence-Based Complementary and Alternative Medicine*, **2013**, Article ID: 304394, 9 p. http://dx.doi.org/10.1155/2013/304394

[8]   Prajapati, R.P., Kalariya, M., Parmar, S.K. and Sheth, N.R. (2010) Phytochemical and Pharmacological Review of *Lagenaria sicereria*. *Journal of Ayurveda and Integrative Medicine*, **1**, 266-272. http://dx.doi.org/10.4103/0975-9476.74431

[9]   Saha, P., Mazumder, U.K., Haldar, P.K., Islam, A. and Kumar, S.R.B. (2011) Evaluation of Acute and Sub Chronic Toxicity of *Lageneria seceraria* Aerial Parts. *International Journal of Pharmaceutical Sciences and Research*, **2**.

[10] Sayyah, M., Hadidi, N. and Kamalinejad, M. (2004) Analgesic and Anti-Inflammatory Activity of *Lactuca sativa* Extract in Rats. *Journal of Ethnopharmacology*, **92**, 325-329. http://dx.doi.org/10.1016/j.jep.2004.03.016

[11] Shah, K.H., Patel, J.B., Shrma, V.J., Shrma, R.M., Patel, R.P. and Chaunhan, U.M. (2011) Evaluation of Antidiabetic Activity of *Prunus amygdalus* Batsch in Streptozotocin Induced Diabetic Mice. *The Research Journal of Pharmaceutical, Biological and Chemical Sciences*, **2**, 429-434.

[12] Palanisamy, B. and Shanmugasundaram, K. (2012) Acute and Subacute Oral Toxicity Studies of Ethanolic Extract of *Sesamum indicum* Seeds (Linn.) in Winstar Albino Rats. *Journal of Global Pharma Technology*, **4**, 17-23.

[13] OECD (2001) Guidelines for Testing of Chemicals. Acute Oral Toxicities up and down Procedure. 425, 1-26. www.oecd.org/dataoecd/17/51/1948378.pdf

[14] AVMA Guidelines for the Euthanasia of Animals: 2013 Edition.

[15] Karber, G. (1931) Beitrag zur kollecktiven Behandlung pharmakologischer Reihenversuche. *Arch. Exptl. Pathol. Pharmakol*, **162**, 480-483.

[16] Hodge, A. and Sterner, B. (2005) Toxicity Classes. In: Canadian Center for Occupational Health and Safety. http://www.ccohs.ca/oshanswers/chemicals/id50.htm

[17] Azmat, A., Ahmed, M., Haider, S., Haleem, D.J., Zafar, N. and Ahmad, S.I. (2012) Enhanced Memory Processes under the Influence of Herbal Drug Somina and Its Effect on Brain Serotonin. *African Journal of Pharmacy and Pharmacology*, **6**, 2458-2463. http://dx.doi.org/10.5897/AJPP11.612

[18] Elvin-Lewis, M. (2001) Should We Be Concerned about Herbal Remedies. *Journal of Ethnopharmacology*, **75**, 141-164. http://dx.doi.org/10.1016/S0378-8741(00)00394-9

[19] Stickel, F., Egerer, G. and Seitz, H.K. (2000) Hepatotoxicity of Botonicals. *Public Health Nutrition*, **3**, 113-124. http://dx.doi.org/10.1017/S1368980000000161

[20] Shintani, S., Murase, H., Tsukagoshi, H. and Shiigai, T. (1992) Glycyrrhizin (Licorice)-Induced Hypokalemic Myopathy: Report of 2 Cases and Review of the Literature. *European Neurology*, **32**, 44-51. http://dx.doi.org/10.1159/000116786

[21] Clark, C.D., Bassett, B. and Burge, M.R. (2003) Effect of Kelp Supplementation on Thyroid Function in Euthyroid Subjects. *Endocrine Practice*, **9**, 363-369. http://dx.doi.org/10.4158/EP.9.5.363

15

Cyclodextrin-Modified Film Dosage Forms for Oral Candidiasis Treatment

Yoshifumi Murata[1]*, Kyoko Kofuji[1], Shushin Nakano[2], Ryosei Kamaguchi[2]

[1]Faculty of Pharmaceutical Science, Hokuriku University, Kanazawa, Japan
[2]Morishita Jintan Co. Osaka Technocenter, Hirakata, Japan
Email: *y-murata@hokuriku-u.ac.jp

Abstract

Oral candidiasis is a common disease in patients with dry mouth. In this study, film dosage forms (FD) incorporating miconazole nitrate, an antifungal agent, were prepared with water-soluble polysaccharide and cyclodextrin (CD). The dissolution profiles of the drug from the FDs were investigated in limited dissolution medium. Soft films were obtained from sodium alginate containing 0.5% α-CD, β-CD, or γ-CD. Most FDs were easy to handle, though the film tearing resistance was lower than that of CD-free FDs. Addition of CD to the FD accelerated the drug dissolution rate. Interestingly, this phenomenon was also observed in FDs prepared with pullulan. In contrast, acceleration of the drug dissolution rate was not observed when CD polymer was added to the base solution. The initial drug dissolution rate was controllable by the amount of CD added to the FD. Therefore, FDs prepared with these materials are useful to treat oral candidiasis in patients with dry mouth syndrome.

Keywords

Film Dosage Form, Natural Polysaccharide, Cyclodextrins, Miconazole, Oral Candidiasis

1. Introduction

Dry mouth syndrome is a risk factor for oral diseases, including microbial infections, such as dental caries, periodontitis, and candidiasis [1]. Decreased saliva secretion occurs as a symptom of disease, such as diabetes, or as an adverse effect of drug administration [2]. Aging also decreases salivation [3] and can cause difficulty swallowing in the elderly. Saliva plays an important role in cleaning the oral cavity, and has an antimicrobial activity. Oral candidiasis is a fungal infection caused by *Candida* strains, including *Candida albicans. Candida*

---

*Corresponding author.

strains are not harmful to healthy individuals, but can cause infections in immunocompromised patients. Oral candidiasis is common in patients with dry mouth [4]. Miconazole nitrate (MCZ) is an antifungal agent widely used to treat *Candida* infections. It is well known that systemic MCZ administration can cause drug interaction-sowing to cytochrome P450 inhibition [5]. Therefore, MCZ is directly applied to the tongue to avoid side effects that occur following gastrointestinal absorption [6]. MCZ gel preparations are commonly used to topically treat oral candidiasis. The patient has to apply the gel evenly in the oral cavity with their tongue. However, this procedure is tedious for patients, and is difficult for elderly patients.

Film is an excellent dosage form for oral care. When film dosage forms (FD) are placed in a small amount of liquid, they swell quickly and release the incorporated drug. FDs prepared with natural polysaccharides, including sodium alginate (ALG) and pullulan (PUL), which are safe for ingestion were previously characterized [7]. These polysaccharides can form films using simple methods that do not require dissolution in organic solvents. For FDs incorporating MCZ, the drug dissolution rate is enhanced by the addition of a surfactant to the base solution [8]. The surfactant used to prepare FDs is selected considering safety, formability, and patient comfort.

Cyclodextrins (CDs) are cyclic oligosaccharides with cone-shaped cavities, which affect the physicochemical properties of organic compounds by forming inclusion complexes. CDs have been studied to enhance the solubility of poorly water-soluble drugs, to improve the stability of unstable compounds, and as a masking agent for medicines and foods [9]-[11]. Some natural CDs are safe for oral administration, particularly α-CD, β-CD, and γ-CD, which are widely used as food additives [12]. In the present study, FDs were modified by the addition of CD to control the MCZ dissolution rate in limited dissolution medium. Additionally, FDs modified using the adsorbent, cyclodextrin polymer (CDP), were also investigated [13] [14].

2. Experimental

2.1. Materials

ALG was obtained from NacalaiTesque Inc. (300 cps, Kyoto, Japan), and 1.5% (w/w) ALG was prepared in deionized water as thefilm base solution. Guluronicacid-rich ALG (IL-6G) was supplied by Kimica Co. (Tokyo, Japan). PUL was supplied by Hayashibara Biochemical Laboratories (Okayama, Japan), and polysaccharides produced by *Bifidobacteriumlongum* JBL05 (BPS) were supplied by Morishita Jintan (Osaka, Japan). MCZ ($C_{18}H_{14}C_{14}N_2O$ HNO_3, M.W. 479.14), the three CDs (α-CD, β-CD, γ-CD), and the three CDPs (α-CDP, β-CDP, γ-CDP) were obtained fromWako Pure Chemicals (Osaka, Japan). All other chemicals were of reagent grade.

2.2. FD Preparation

A CD or CDP was added with agitationto 10 g of the film base solution.The mixture was thoroughly mixed with sonication, and 3.0 g of each solution was poured into individual plastic Petri dishes (diameter: 54 mm). After 24 h at 37°C, the circular films formed on each dish were transferred to a desiccator. Film formation was considered to have failed if a circular film was not obtained, the film had cracks, or the film could not be removed from the bottom of the dish. In the present method, 3 mg of MCZ was theoretically incorporated into each FD.

2.3. Film Thickness and Rheological Properties

Film thickness was measured at 10 points on each film using a micrometer (CLM1-15QM; Mitutoyo, Kawasaki, Japan) with a set pressure of 0.5 N. Measurements were made on 3 films, and the mean thickness was calculated for each type. The rheological properties of each film were determined using a rheometer (SUN RHEO TEX SD-700#; Sun Scientific Co., Tokyo, Japan) at room temperature. The film was fixed on a vial (inner diameter: 1.4 mm; outer diameter: 18.8 mm) using a rubber band (Kyowa Co., Osaka, Japan), and was probed with a cylindrical adapter (diameter: 5.0 mm). Stress and strain were measured at the point at which the adapter broke through the film. The tests were performed in triplicate.

2.4. Solubility of MCZ

The solubility of MCZ was measured in physiological saline containing CD or CDP. MCZ was added to the test solution and shaken at 37°C for 24 h. The suspension was removed using a pre-heated plastic syringe (Terumo Co., Tokyo, Japan) at 37°C and filtered using asyringe driven filter unit (Millex-HV, pore size: 0.45 μm, Millipore Co., Danvers, MA, USA). The solution was diluted with physiological saline and injected onto a high performance liquid chromatography (HPLC) column.

2.5. Determination of MCZ Content

The HPLC system (Hitachi Co., Tokyo, Japan) consisted of a pump (L-2130), UV-detector (L-2400), auto-sampler (L-2200), and chromate-integrator (D-2500) connected to a packed column (150 mm × 4.6 mm, Cosmosil 5C_{18}-MS-II, NacalaiTesque, Kyoto, Japan). To determine the concentration of MCZ, HPLC was conducted at ambient temperature using an eluent consisting of 10 mM KH_2PO_4 and acetonitrile (1:4) at a flow rate of 0.8 ml/min [15]. The detector wavelength was set at 230 nm.

2.6. MCZ Dissolution Test

The FD was placed in a plastic dish, and 10 ml dissolution medium (physiological saline preheated to 37°C) was added. The dish was shaken at 300 rpm in a shaker incubator (SI-300; As One Co., Osaka, Japan) at 37°C. After 1, 3, 5, 10, 15, 20, 30, 45, or 60 minutes, 0.3 ml of the medium was removed using a plastic syringe and filtered through a syringe driven filter unit (pore size: 0.45 μm). Aliquots of the filtered solution (80 μl) were placed into micro-test tubes (1.5 ml), and 720 μl of methanol was added to precipitate the polysaccharide dissolved from the FD. Samples were mixed and centrifuged (7700 × g, 5 min; H-1300; Kokusan Co., Saitama, Japan), and the supernatants were injected onto the HPLC column. All tests were performed in triplicate.

3. Results and Discussion

The polysaccharides used in this study can form thin films, termed FDs, using a casting method. FDs were formed by pouring 1.5% ALG, 1.2% BPS, or 4% PUL containing MCZ (1 mg/g) into a Petri dish and evaporating the solvent. Addition of CDs to the film base solution affected FD formation. As shown in **Figure 1**, a circular, soft film was obtained from 1.5% ALG solutions containing 0.5% α-CD, with a thickness of 43 μm. FDs were also obtained using ALG containing 0.5% β-CD and 0.5% γ-CD, as shown in **Table 1**, although the film

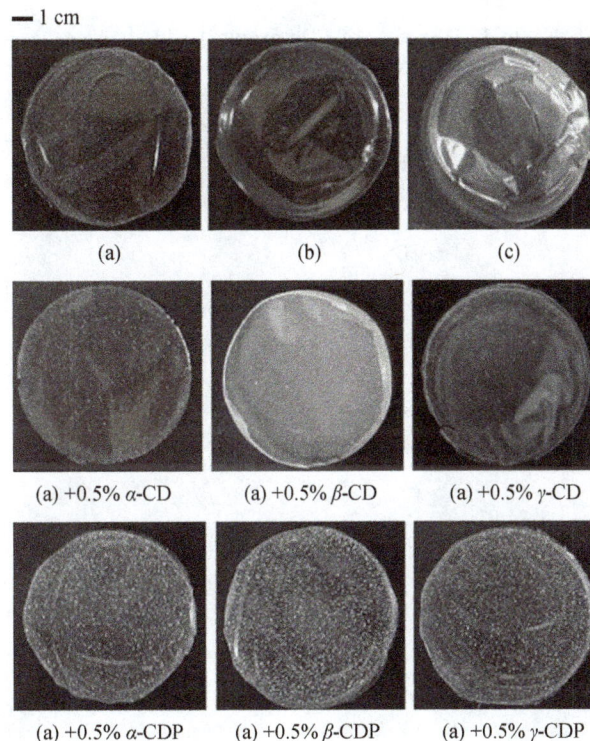

Figure 1. Pictures of FDs prepared with polysaccharides containing MCZ. (a) 1.5% ALG (b) 4% PUL (c) 1.2% BPS.

prepared with solution containing 0.8% γ-CD was cracked. In the case of 1.5% ALG containing CDP, the FD thickness was approximately 200 µm. MCZ and other additives were homogeneously dispersed in the FDs, as shown in **Figure 2**. FDs were also obtained when 4% PUL containing 0.5% γ-CD was used; however, 1.2% BPS containing 0.5% CD did not form FDs.

To use FDs incorporating MCZ in oral candidiasis therapy, they must be easy to handle, since the form is directly applied to the target region. **Figure 3** shows the additive effect of CD on the rheological properties of FDs prepared with ALG. Although γ-CD or γ-CDP lowered the resistance of FDs to tearing, each FD had sufficient strength to be treated by hand.

Since the FD film matrix consists of a water-soluble polysaccharide, it immediately swells in physiological saline at 37°C, leading to erosion and MCZ release. **Figure 4** shows the MCZ dissolution profiles from FDs prepared with 1.5% ALG. FDs prepared with ALG released 8.8% ± 0.7% of the incorporated MCZ into the test solution at 5 min. The initial dissolution rate increased following addition of CDs to the film base. For example, 24% ± 8% of the MCZ was released at 5 min from FDs prepared with ALG containing 0.5% α-CD. Addition of β-CD or γ-CD to the FDs also accelerated the drug dissolution rate. This phenomenon was also observed in FDs prepared with the other alginate, IL-6G. However, addition of 0.5% CDPs to the base solution did not affect the drug dissolution profile. The MCZ dissolution rate increased when CD was added to 4% PUL. For example, the amount of MCZ dissolved at 5 min increased from 36% ± 4% to 68% ± 9% following the addition of 0.5% α-CD to the film base. In addition, the initial MCZ dissolution rate increased when CD-free FD was dipped into the test solution containing 0.15% CD.

Table 2 shows the additive effect of CD or CDP on MCZ solubility in physiological saline at 37°C. When 0.15% α-CD was added to the test solution, the solubility increased 1.5-fold, as compared to α-CD free test solution. A similar effect was observed using β-CD and γ-CD. In contrast, MCZ solubility was not affected by the addition of α-CDP, β-CDP, or γ-CDP. CDs can form complexes with some water-insoluble compounds, thereby increasing their solubility. Therefore, the acceleration of MCZ dissolution from FD may be attributable to complex formation between the polysaccharide matrix and CDs in the base solution.

Figure 5 shows the additive effect of γ-CD on the MCZ dissolution rate from FDs. As the amount of γ-CD incorporated in the FDs increased, the MCZ dissolution rate increased. To treat oral candidiasis, FDs containing

Table 1. Thickness of FDs prepared with 1.5% ALG containing 0.5% additive.

Additive	Thickness (µm)
α-CD	43 ± 5
β-CD	45 ± 6
γ-CD	71 ± 4
α-CDP	217 ± 5
β-CDP	220 ± 3
γ-CDP	209 ± 22

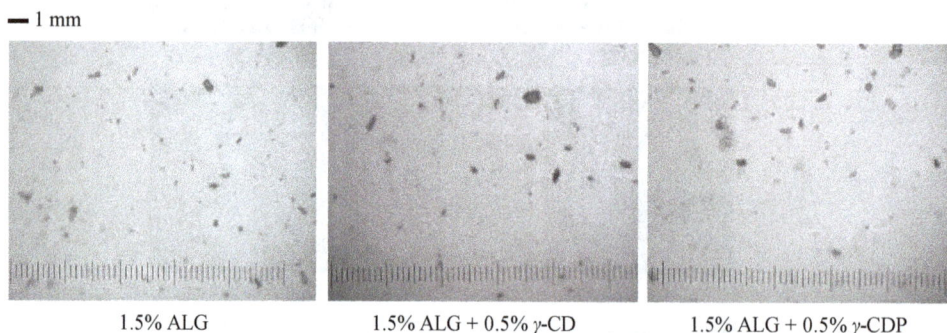

— 1 mm

| 1.5% ALG | 1.5% ALG + 0.5% γ-CD | 1.5% ALG + 0.5% γ-CDP |

Figure 2. Stereo-microphotographs of FD surfaces.

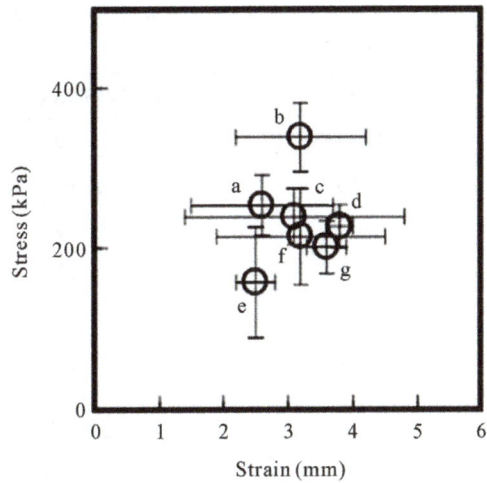

Figure 3. Rheological properties of FDs prepared with 1.5% ALG containing 0.5% CD or CDP. (a: additive free, b: α-CD, c: β-CD, d: γ-CD, e: α-CDP, f: β-CDP, g: γ-CDP).

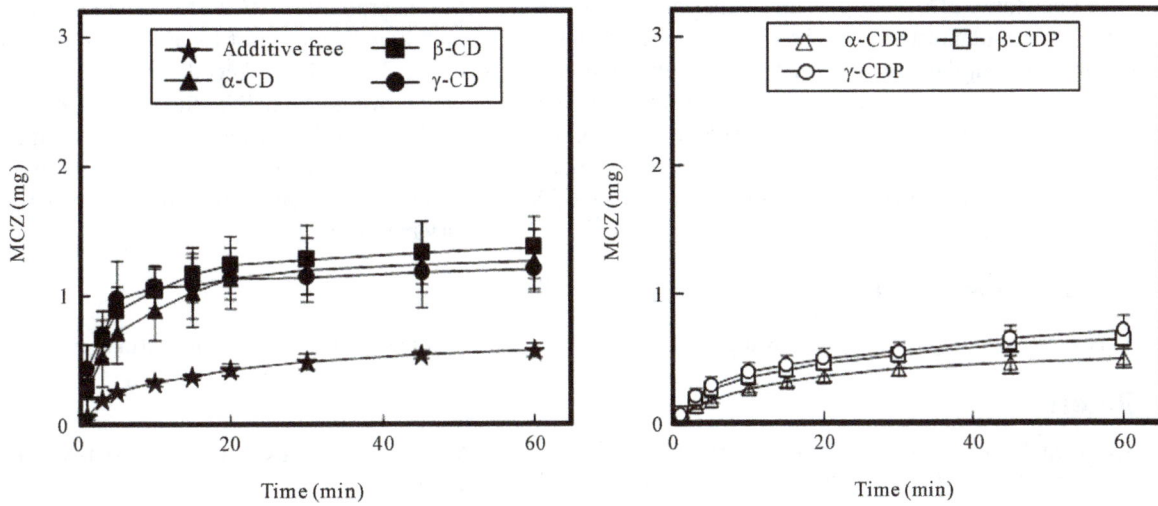

Figure 4. Release profiles of MCZ from FDs prepared with 1.5% ALG in physiological saline containing CD or CDP.

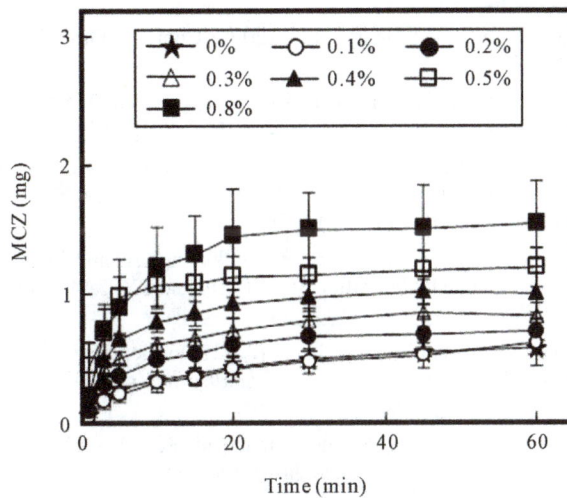

Figure 5. Effect of γ-CD concentration on MCZ release from FDs.

Table 2. Solubility of MCZ in physiological saline containing 0.15% additive at 37°C.

Additive	Solubility (mM)
additive free	1.2
α-CD	1.8
β-CD	1.8
γ-CD	1.9
α-CDP*	1.1
β-CDP*	1.2
γ-CDP*	1.1

*Suspension.

MCZ are administered in the oral cavity to act directly at the affected site. These data show that the amount of MCZ that reached the site per unit time could be controlled by the addition of CDs.

In this study, FDs were prepared with polysaccharides and CDs incorporating MCZ. All materials used are safe for oral administration. When treating oral candidiasis, the antifungal agent must be applied repeatedly to completely treat the disease [16]. Therefore, the dissolution rate of MCZ in saliva affects the antifungal activity. FD easily disintegrates upon contact with a small amount of saliva, allowing it to deliver the incorporated MCZ to the affected part of the oral cavity. The MCZ dissolution rate can be controlled by the amount of CD added to the base FD solution. Thus, FDs prepared with water-soluble polymers, such as polysaccharides, are useful for treating localized problems in the oral cavity and simplify the administration of drugs to patients. This preparation is a candidate for the treatment of oral candidiasis caused by dry mouth syndrome.

Acknowledgements

This work was supported in parts by a grant from The OTC Self-Medication Promotion Foundation (2014).

References

[1] Han, P., Suarez-Durall, P. and Mulligan, R. (2015) Dry Mouth: A Critical Topic for Older Adult Patients. *Journal of Prosthodontic Research*, **59**, 6-19. http://dx.doi.org/10.1016/j.jpor.2014.11.001

[2] NoboruKuroiwa, D., Ruiz Da Cunha Melo, M.A., Balducci, I., Bortolin Lodi, K., Ghislaine Oliveira Alves, M. and Dias Almeida, J. (2014) Evaluation of Salivary Flow and Drug Interactions in Patients with a Diagnosis of Diabetes Mellitus. *Minerva Stomatologica*, **63**, 421-426.

[3] Gonsalves, W.C., Wrightson, A.S. and Henry, R.G. (2008) Common Oral Conditions in Older Persons. *American Family Physician*, **78**, 845-852.

[4] Garcia-Cuesta, C., Sarrion-Pérez, M.G. and Bagán J.V. (2014) Current Treatment of Oral Candidiasis: A Literature Review. *Journal of Clinical and Experimental Dentistry*, **6**, 576-582. http://dx.doi.org/10.4317/jced.51798

[5] Niwa, T., Imagawa, Y. and Yamazaki, H. (2014) Drug Interactions between Nine Antifungal Agents and Drugs Metabolized by Human Cytochromes P450. *Current Drug Metabolism*, **15**, 651-679. http://dx.doi.org/10.2174/1389200215666141125121511

[6] Gronlund, J., Saari, T.I., Hagelberg, N., Neuvonen, P.J., Olkkola, K.T. and Laine, K. (2011) MiconazoleOral Gel Increases Exposure to Oral Oxycodone by Inhibition of CYP2D6 and CYP3A4. *Antimicrobial Agents and Chemotherapy*, **55**, 1063-1067. http://dx.doi.org/10.1128/AAC.01242-10

[7] Murata, Y., Kofuji, K., Nishida, N. and Kamaguchi, R. (2012) Development of Film Dosage Form Containing Allopurinol for Prevention of Oral Mucositis.*International Scholarly Research Network Pharmaceutics*, **2012**, Article ID: 764510. http://dx.doi.org/10.5402/2012/764510

[8] Murata, Y., Isobe, T., Kofuji, K., Nishida, N. and Kamaguchi, R. (2013) Development of Film Dosage Forms Containing Miconazole for the Treatment of Oral Candidiasis. *Pharmacology & Pharmacy*, **4**, 325-330. http://dx.doi.org/10.4236/pp.2013.43047

[9] Stella, V.J. and He, Q. (2008) Cyclodextrins. *Toxicologic Pathology*, **36**, 30-42.

http://dx.doi.org/10.1177/0192623307310945

[10] Tamamoto, L.C., Schmidt, S.J. and Lee, S.Y. (2010) Sensory Properties of Ginseng Solutions Modified by Masking Agents. *Journal of Food Science*, **75**, 341-347. http://dx.doi.org/10.1111/j.1750-3841.2010.01749.x

[11] Ogawa, N., Takahashi, C. and Yamamoto, H. (2015) Physicochemical Characterization of Cyclodextrin-Drug Interactions in the Solid State and the Effect of Water on these Interactions. *Journal of Pharmaceutical Science*, **104**, 942-954. http://dx.doi.org/10.1002/jps.24319

[12] Irie, T. and Uekama, K. (1997) Pharmaceutical Applications of Cyclodextrins. III. Toxicological Issues and Safety Evaluation. *Journal of Pharmaceutical Science*, **86**, 147-954. http://dx.doi.org/10.1021/js960213f

[13] García-Fernández, M.J., Tabary, N., Martel, B., Cazaux, F., Oliva, A., Taboada, P., Concheiro, A. and Alvarez-Lorenzo, C. (2013) Poly-Cyclodextrins as Ethoxzolamide Carriers in Ophthalmic Solutions and in Contact Lenses. *Carbohydrate Polymers*, **98**, 1343-1352. http://dx.doi.org/10.1016/j.carbpol.2013.08.003

[14] Simões, S.M., Veiga, F., Ribeiro, A.C., Figueiras, A.R., Taboada, P., Concheiro, A. and Alvarez-Lorenzo, C. (2014) Supramolecular Gels of Poly-α-Cyclodextrin and PEO-Based Copolymers for Controlled Drug Release. *European Journal of Pharmaceutics and Biopharmaceutics*, **87**, 579-588. http://dx.doi.org/10.1016/j.ejpb.2014.04.006

[15] Pershing, L.K., Corlett, J. and Jorgensen, C. (1994) *In Vivo* Pharmacokinetics and Pharmacodynamics of Topical Ketoconazole and Miconazole in Human Stratum Corneum. *Antimicrobial Agents and Chemotherapy*, **38**, 90-95. http://dx.doi.org/10.1128/AAC.38.1.90

[16] Garcia-Cuesta, C., Sarrion-Pérez, M.G. and Bagán, J.V. (2014) Current Treatment of Oral Candidiasis: A Literature Review. *Journal of Clinical and Experimental dentistry*, **6**, 576-582. http://dx.doi.org/10.4317/jced.51798

16

Antidiabetic Effects of Omega-3 Polyunsaturated Fatty Acids: From Mechanism to Therapeutic Possibilities

Yuko Iwase, Noriyasu Kamei, Mariko Takeda-Morishita*

Laboratory of Drug Delivery Systems, Faculty of Pharmaceutical Sciences, Kobe Gakuin University, Kobe, Japan
Email: *mmtakeda@pharm.kobegakuin.ac.jp

Abstract

Diabetes mellitus (DM) is chronic disease characterized by hyperglycemia and insulin resistance caused by dysfunction of pancreatic β cells. Over the past few decades, epidemiological studies have suggested that dietary long-chain polyunsaturated fatty acids such as docosahexaenoic acid and eicosapentaenoic acid decrease the risk of metabolic diseases including DM. The mechanisms underlying the therapeutic efficacy of dietary long-chain polyunsaturated fatty acids in treating DM have been partly revealed. In this review, the authors describe the antidiabetic effects of long-chain polyunsaturated fatty acids and also discuss their possibilities as therapeutics for DM in the light of recent findings.

Keywords

Omega-3 Polyunsaturated Fatty Acids, Diabetes, Insulin Secretion, Docosahexaenoic Acid

1. Introduction

Diabetes mellitus (DM) is a chronic disease in which the blood glucose level is too high because the body experiences insulin deficiency, decreased ability to use insulin, or both. The World Health Organization (WHO) has estimated that 347 million people worldwide have DM and projects that DM will be the seventh leading cause of death in 2030 [1]. According to the American Diabetes Association, most DM cases can be classified into two types: type 1 diabetes (T1DM) and type 2 diabetes (T2DM) [2]. T1DM is an immune-mediated disease characterized by an absolute deficiency of insulin secretion. T1DM patients have autoimmune destruction of pancreatic

---

*Corresponding author.

β cells, which leads to the absolute insulin deficiency. T2DM accounts for 90% - 95% of all DM cases. T2DM patients have both hyperglycemia and hyperinsulinemia. Recent reports have shown that insulin resistance in the brain correlates strongly with Alzheimer's disease (AD) and that AD and DM are risk factors for each other. Because AD causes brain insulin resistance, oxidative stress, and cognitive impairment, it is sometimes called "type 3 DM" [3]-[7].

Most T2DM patients are obese as a result excessive food intake, a high-fat diet, or lack of physical activity. Chronic inflammation caused by obesity has emerged as an important physiological mechanism linked to insulin resistance and T2DM. Obesity is associated with increased production of proinflammatory cytokines and activation of the inflammatory pathways in key metabolic tissues. Obesity itself causes insulin resistance. To cope with insulin resistance, pancreatic β cell mass increases to provide the required amount of insulin to maintain a normal blood glucose level in the early stages of DM [8]. However, hyperglycemia over a long period causes abnormal insulin secretion, which exhausts pancreatic β cells. Pancreatic β cell dysfunction leads to the accumulation of M1 macrophages in the pancreas and the secretion of inflammatory cytokines. Inflammatory cytokines cause inflammation and worsen insulin resistance.

Obesity also induces insulin resistance in adipose tissue [9]-[14]. Accumulated triacylglycerol in adipose tissue resulting from obesity increases both the size and number of adipocytes. Enlarged adipocytes secrete inflammatory cytokines such as tumor necrosis factor-alpha (TNF-α) and interleukin-6 (IL-6), and induce insulin resistance. Enlarged adipocytes also secrete the chemokine monocyte chemoattractant protein-1 (MCP-1) [13] [15]-[17]. M1 macrophages express MCP-1 receptors, and MCP-1 secretion causes M1 macrophage migration and accumulation in adipose tissue, leading to worsening of inflammation and insulin resistance. In addition, brain inflammation has been linked to obesity, and brain inflammation resulting from obesity inhibits leptin delivery into the brain (hypothalamus) [18]-[24]. Inflammation induces insulin resistance and aggravates DM. Therefore, suppressing inflammation is a promising approach to antidiabetic treatment. Administration of omega-3 polyunsaturated fatty acids (n-3 PUFAs) is one approach for suppressing inflammation. Some experiments have shown that n-3 PUFAs have anti-inflammatory effects in the hypothalamus [18]-[24].

Fatty acids are organic acids with an aliphatic chain and a carboxyl group. Aliphatic acids with one double bond are monounsaturated fatty acids, and those with more than one double bond are PUFAs. PUFAs can be divided into two categories: the n-6 family (n-6 PUFA), which is derived from linolenic acid, and the n-3 family (n-3 PUFA), which is derived from α-linolenic acid [25]. Over the past few decades, epidemiological studies have suggested that n-3 PUFAs such as docosahexaenoic acid (DHA) and eicosapentaenoic acid (EPA) decrease the risk of coronary heart disease, hypertension, and stroke, and improve mood disorders and cognitive function. Greenland Inuit who eat a diet rich in seafood containing a high level of n-3 PUFAs have low rates of coronary heart disease and DM compared with Danes who eat a typical Western diet [26] [27].

As shown in **Figure 1**, in this review, the authors focus on the mechanisms underlying the hypoglycemic action and antidiabetic effects of n-3 PUFAs in terms of the roles of the G protein-coupled receptor 120 (GPR120) as well as their possibilities as therapeutics for DM in Section 2 (Insulin-sensitizing effects of n-3 PUFAs *via* GPR120), peroxisome proliferator-activated receptors (PPARs), and sterol regulatory element-binding proteins (SREBPs) in Section 3 (Insulin-sensitizing effects of n-3 PUFAs *via* SREBP and PPARs). Improvements in endothelial dysfunction induced by n-3 PUFAs and the use of n-3 PUFAs as a DM biomarker that reflects blood n-3 PUFA concentration are also described in Section 4 (Improvement of vascular endothelial dysfunction by n-3 PUFAs).

2. Insulin-Sensitizing Effects of n-3 PUFAs *via* GPR120

The antidiabetic effect of n-3 PUFAs is based on the secretion of glucagon-like peptide-1 (GLP-1), which is mediated partly by GPR120 [28]. Incretins, peptide hormones secreted in response to food intake, increase endogenous insulin secretion. GLP-1, a 30-amino acid peptide hormone derived from proglucagon, is the most potent incretin hormone and is secreted from lower intestinal L cells. Secreted GLP-1 is rapidly degraded by dipeptidyl peptidase-4 (DPP-4), which causes the short half-life for GLP-1 of <2 min [29] [30]. In cultured cells, GLP-1 secretion by GLUTag, STC-1, and NCI-H716 cells has been reported [31]-[33]. Food intake stimulates GLP-1 secretion by L cells [34], and the direct administration of nutrients to the apical lumen of L cells also increases their secretion of GLP-1 [35] [36]. Elrick and co-workers reported in 1964 that insulin secretion induced by oral glucose administration was higher than that induced by intravenous administration [37]. It was proposed

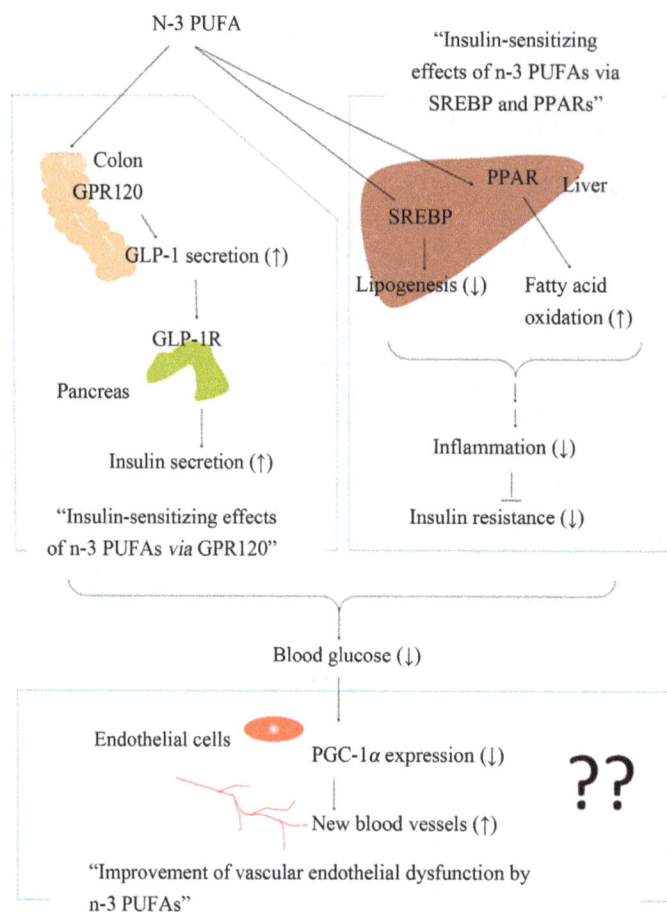

Figure 1. A schematic representation of the effects of n-3 PUFAs on the hypoglycemic action and antidiabetic effects in this review. The role of GPR120, and the role of SREBP and PPAR are described in Section 2 and Section 3, respectively. Improvements in endothelial dysfunction induced by n-3 PUFAs are described in Section 4.

that this phenomenon reflects the stimulation of insulin secretion by GLP-1 secreted by L cells in response to oral glucose administration.

Of note, GLP-1-induced insulin release requires hyperglycemia because GLP-1 causes only minimal stimulation of insulin secretion under normal circumstances. The insulinotropic effect of GLP-1 is linked to hyperglycemia, and GLP-1 does not cause hypoglycemia. Several studies have reported a significant reduction in GLP-1 secretion in response to food intake in T2DM patients [38]-[40]. However, the elimination rate of GLP-1 is similar in T2DM patients and in healthy individuals [41].

Green and co-workers reported that exposure to 5 mM glucose increases GLP-1 secretion, glucose transporter 4 (GLUT4) protein content, and subsequent glycogen synthesis in myocytes. GLP-1 secretion increases the GLUT4 protein level in skeletal muscle or fat, which increases glucose uptake and glycogen synthesis [42]. Thus, stimulation of GLP-1 secretion is one promising approach to inducing antidiabetic effects. Many antidiabetic agents that work by stimulating GLP-1 secretion, such as the GLP-1 agonists exenatide, and liraglutide, have been reported. Studies have shown that the increase in GLP-1 secretion stimulated by mastication leads to suppression of insulin resistance [43]-[45]. GLP-1 secretion by long-chain monounsaturated fatty acids also has been reported in murine, rat, and human L cells [33] [46] [47]. Hirasawa and co-workers showed that stimulation of GPR120 by α-linolenic acid, which was one of the n-3 PUFAs, promotes the secretion of GLP-1 *in vitro* and *in vivo*, and increases circulating insulin. GPR120, one of the G-protein coupled receptors, is highly expressed in mature adipose tissue, inflammatory macrophages, and lower intestinal L cells [48]-[51]. Hirasawa and co-workers suggested that n-3 PUFA intake might be useful in the treatment of DM [49]. In fact, Morishita and co-workers reported that direct administration of n-3 PUFAs such as DHA, EPA, and EPA-ethyl esters into the intestine stimulates GLP-1 release in rats [52]-[55]. In their proof of concept study for DHA as DM therapeutics, the strong effects of intracolonic administration of DHA on blood glucose, plasma GLP-1 concentration, and pancreatic islets were clearly demonstrated (**Figures 2(a)-(c)**) [53]. The blood glucose concentrations were decreased by DHA intracolonic administration, and plasma GLP-1 concentrations tended to be higher in DHA intracolonic administrated mice. In addition, DHA treatment stimulated pancreatic β cells apoptosis and suppressed cell growth in DM mice. Furthermore, insulin sensitivity was improved by a diet containing DHA and EPA for 8 weeks compared with a diet containing linolenic acid [56]. The study suggested the high possibility of DHA or EPA as DM therapeutics as well as importance of their targeting to the lower intestine.

In GPR120-knockdown mice, DHA treatment did not suppress the secretion of inflammatory cytokines such as TNF-α and IL-6, and did not attenuate the release of the chemokine, MCP-1. These changes led to anti-inflammatory effects and improved insulin sensitivity. These results show clearly that the anti-inflammatory effects and anti-insulin-resistance effects of DHA are GPR120 dependent [49].

Dysfunctional GPR120 has been reported in both obese rats and humans [57]. A GPR120-specific agonist improved insulin sensitivity in obese mice [58], indicating that the induction of GLP-1 secretion through GPR120 has antidiabetic effects. n-3 PUFA bound to GPR120 causes suppression of the toll-like receptor pathway and the TNF-α pathway, which leads to anti-inflammatory effects. β-Arrestin 2 plays an important role in these pathways. Luan and co-workers showed that β-arrestin 2 was strongly downregulated in diabetic mouse models and that knockdown of β-arrestin 2 exacerbated insulin resistance, whereas the administration of β-arrestin 2 restored insulin sensitivity in mice [59]. They also showed that insulin stimulated the formation of new β-arrestin 2 signal complexes, in which β-arrestin 2 scaffolds Akt and Src to the insulin receptor. Loss or dysfunction

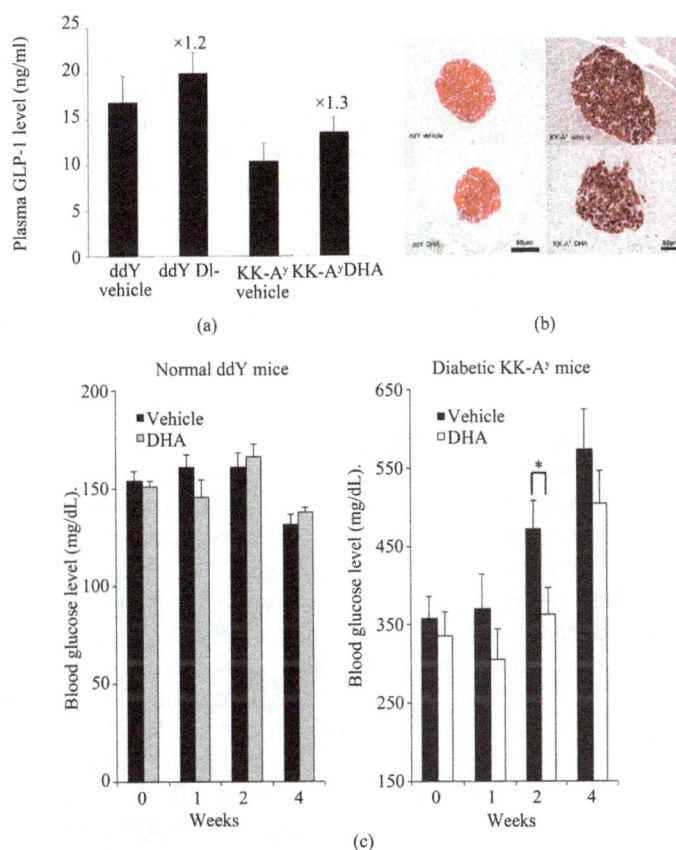

Figure 2. The effects of intracolonic administration of DHA on (a) blood glucose, (b) plasma GLP-1 secretion, and (c) pancreatic islets. Each data points represents the mean ± S.E.M. (n = 9 - 10). $^{*}p < 0.05$, significant difference between vehicle- and DHA-treatment group. Reproduced with permission from [53].

of β-arrestin 2 causes a deficiency in this signal complex and disturbance of insulin signaling *in vivo*, thereby contributing to the development of insulin resistance and progression of T2DM.

Whether insulin resistance is improved by n-3 PUFAs is controversial [60]-[62]. Some reports have shown that fish oil intake alleviates insulin resistance by suppressing inflammation caused by macrophages *in vitro* but not *in vivo*. Shida and co-workers reported that the improvement in insulin resistance by n-3 PUFAs correlated strongly with the intestinal GPR120 location [53]. To be most effective in controlling the blood glucose level with n-3 PUFAs (or fish intake), n-3 PUFAs must reach the colon or lower intestine. They suggested that n-3 PUFAs must be administrated directly to the colon because orally ingested fatty acids do not easily reach the colon [53]. In addition, Ichimura and co-workers reported a human GPR120 variant [57] and that the risk of obesity or insulin resistance relates to the GPR120 variant. In T2DM, patients with a mutation in the gene encoding GPR120, an n-3 PUFA-rich diet intake did not always improve insulin sensitivity or DM.

Other genetic risk factors may also be involved in the absence of improvement in insulin resistance in response to n-3 PUFA supplementation. For instance, because the brain uptake of DHA is strongly influenced by the apolipoprotein E ε4 allele (APOE4), DHA intake has no beneficial effects on cognition in people with APOE4, and this allele is a strong risk factor for AD [19]. Therefore, restoring insulin resistance by providing an n-3 PUFA-rich diet should be considered in future trials of genetic risk factors ideally before the first stage of DM.

3. Insulin-Sensitizing Effects of n-3 PUFAs *via* SREBP and PPARs

After a meal, the increased circulating levels of glucose and insulin promote *de novo* fatty acid synthesis and impair β-oxidation, leading to the development of hepatic steatosis. Lipid accumulation in the liver in the form of excess ectopic lipids is caused by elevated levels of circulating serum triacylglycerol and free fatty acids, and is preceded by inflammatory and endoplasmic reticulum stress, which leads to insulin resistance and impaired insulin secretion [63]. N-3 PUFAs suppress hepatic lipid synthesis through the suppression of hepatic SREBP-1 expression by accelerating its transcript decay [64]. For instance, dietary n-3 PUFAs decrease the transcription of the genes encoding hepatic lipogenic or glycolytic enzymes, such as fatty acid synthase, acetyl-CoA carboxylase, stearoyl-CoA desaturase, malic enzyme, l-pyruvate kinase, and glucokinase [65]. Mice fed a high-fat and high-glucose diet for 4 weeks gained weight and exhibited abnormal glucose tolerance, increased serum TNF-α and IL-6 concentrations, and increased expression of hepatic fatty acid synthetase [66]. However, mice fed the high-fat and high-glucose diet supplemented with 1% EPA exhibited normal body weight and levels of serum TNF-α and IL-6. Furthermore, hepatic mRNA of fatty acid synthetase, acetyl-CoA carboxylase, SREBP1c, and PPAR-γ were decreased to the control levels.

The expression of lipogenic enzymes or fatty acid synthesis-regulating proteins is suppressed by EPA, which prevents the development of hepatic steatosis and ameliorates insulin resistance. Additionally, n-3 PUFAs stimulate hepatic lipid metabolism through binding to PPARs, which regulates the expression of genes associated with lipid metabolism and adipocyte differentiation. Experiments with PPAR-α-null mice showed mitigation of high-fat diet-induced insulin resistance and improvement in the efficacy of n-3 PUFAs [67]. Wild-type mice fed a high-fat diet containing 27% safflower oil for 2 weeks exhibited a decreased glucose infusion rate (GIR) to half of that of mice fed a normal diet and the emergence of insulin resistance. However, only a limited decrease in GIR was seen in wild-type mice fed the high-fat diet containing 27% safflower oil supplemented with 1% fish oil. By contrast, the high-fat diet containing 27% safflower oil and 1% fish oil fed to PPAR-α-null mice caused hepatic accumulation of triacylglycerol and insulin resistance.

Increased visceral fat deposition alters serum adiponectin level. Serum adiponectin secretion is lower in T2DM patients than in healthy individuals, and this difference is implicated in insulin resistance. Therefore, an increase in serum adiponectin level may indicate an antidiabetic effect. In mice, a diet containing n-3 PUFAs decreased adipose mass, suppressed systemic inflammation, and increased adiponectin transcription in adipose tissue and serum adiponectin concentration [68]-[71]. However, in PPAR-α-null mice, increasing the serum adiponectin concentration did not ameliorate insulin resistance [67]. Taken together, these data suggest that n-3 PUFA intake may attenuate inflammation and endoplasmic reticulum stress, thereby reducing insulin resistance and impaired insulin secretion.

4. Improvement of Vascular Endothelial Dysfunction by n-3 PUFAs

In this section, the authors focus on DM complications. WHO classifies DM complications into two categories:

microvascular or damage to small blood vessels, and macrovascular or damage to larger blood vessels [72]. Microvascular complications include damage to the eyes, which can lead to blindness, damage to the kidneys, which can lead to renal failure, and neural damage, which can lead to diabetic foot disorders. Macrovascular complications include cardiovascular diseases such as heart attack, stroke, and insufficient blood flow to the legs. There is evidence from large randomized controlled trials that good metabolic control in people with T1DM or T2DM can delay the onset and progression of these complications. These diabetic complications are based on vascular endothelial dysfunction, which is caused by PPAR-γ coactivator 1α (PGC-1α), a member of the transcription coactivator family [73].

Vascular endothelial dysfunction occurs frequently in DM. PGC-1α protein expression is elevated in vascular endothelial cells from diabetic model mice and DM patients. Sawada and co-workers reported that vascular endothelial cells from diabetic model mice or DM patients, which expressed high levels of PGC-1α protein, exhibited significantly less migration compared with control cells, suggesting that PGC-1α contributes to the decrease in cell migration [73]. Vascular endothelial cells that overexpress PGC-1α display significant repression of migration, as measured in migration assays. PGC-1α activates Notch signaling, which is a powerful inhibitor of endothelial migration and sprouting angiogenesis, and inhibits endothelial cell migration, leading to vascular endothelial growth factor (VEGF) resistance. Sawada and co-workers also showed that endothelial cells that overexpress PGC-1α exhibited significantly blunted formation of new blood vessels and strong inhibition of the rate of recovery of blood flow and reendothelialization in *in vivo* experiments compared with control cells. Another report has indicated that Notch signaling inhibition can rescue VEGF resistance in diabetic endothelial cells and improve blood flow recovery in the murine hind limb ischemia model [74]. By contrast, lack of PGC-1α decreased blood flow recovery in the murine hind limb ischemia model.

In skeletal muscle, PGC-1α expression regulates mitochondrial biosynthesis, increases GLUT4 expression, and increases insulin secretion, all of which increase glucose uptake and insulin sensitivity. In other words, the increase in PGC-1α expression in skeletal muscle ameliorates insulin resistance. Conjugated linolenic acid and n-3 PUFAs increase mitochondrial biosynthesis and metabolic rate in skeletal muscle cells [12]. N-3 PUFAs increased PGC-1α expression in skeletal muscle cells by up to 165% of the level in control cells not exposed to n-3 PUFAs [75].

To date, there have been no reports on whether PGC-1α expression in endothelial cells is related to antidiabetic effects. In endothelial cells cultured in 25 mM glucose, the PGC-1α mRNA and protein expression levels were doubled compared with control levels, suggesting that a continuous high blood glucose level can increase PGC-1α protein expression in endothelial cells in DM. Because n-3 PUFAs have a hypoglycemic effect, the improvement in endothelial cell dysfunction based on the suppression of PGC-1α expression is expected upon normalization of blood glucose by n-3 PUFAs. The control of PGC-1α expression in endothelial cells by n-3 PUFAs might be a novel therapeutic target for preventing DM complications. In addition, the n-3 PUFA concentration might serve as a DM biomarker. For instance, studies have shown that higher serum n-3 PUFA concentration is associated with a long-term lower risk of T2DM [76], increased serum and cerebrospinal fluid n-3 PUFA concentrations correlate strongly with a decrease in the phosphorylation of tau protein in cerebrospinal fluid [7], and serum n-3 PUFA concentration is closely related to the antidiabetic effects of the DPP-4 inhibitors [77].

5. Conclusions

In this review, the authors have focused on the hypoglycemic and antidiabetic effects of n-3 PUFAs from two points of view. The first is the insulin-sensitizing effect caused by n-3 PUFAs, which is based on GLP-1 secretion mediated by GPR120. Because this effect correlates strongly with the intestinal GPR120 location, targeted delivery of n-3 PUFAs to the colon is essential for the most effective control of blood glucose level by n-3 PUFAs. The second is the insulin-sensitizing effect of n-3 PUFAs mediated by SREBP and PPAR, which alter lipid metabolism and suppress inflammation, and can thereby ameliorate insulin resistance.

Further, the DM complication of blood vessel damage caused by endothelial dysfunction is improved by repressing PGC-1α expression in endothelial cells. We propose that controlling of PGC-1α expression in endothelial cells with n-3 PUFAs might provide a novel therapeutic approach to preventing blood vessel damage as a DM complication. In addition, n-3 PUFA concentration may be useful as a DM biomarker because the n-3 PUFA concentration correlates strongly with DM risk.

Recent human clinical trials with n-3 PUFAs in DM patients are listed in **Table 1** as recent human clinical

Table 1. Recent human clinical trials with n-3 PUFAs in diabetes patients.

Study aim	Dose	Term	Case	Endpoints and major findings	Ref.
To assess the effects of n-3 PUFAs on insulin concentration and lipid profiles among pregnant women with DM.	120 mg DHA and 180 mg EPA	6 wks.	28 gestational diabetic patients and 28 placebo controls.	No effect on fasting blood glucose and triglyceride. Decrease insulin, insulin resistance.	[78]
To investigate the effects of n-3 PUFAs on the cardiovascular biomarker and lipid profile parameters.	1 g fish oil	3 mos.	36 T2DM with cardiac autonomic neuropathy patients: 21 receiving fish oil and 15 receiving placebo.	Decrease N-terminal pro-brain natriuretic peptide, triglyceride and HDL cholesterol. No effect on LDL cholesterol.	[79]
To investigate whether n-3 PUFAs would change the fatty acids profile of the cerebro spinal fluid.	430 mg DHA and 150 mg EPA	6 mos.	33 mild Alzheimer's disease patients: 18 receiving n-3 PUFA supplement and 15 receiving placebo.	Increase n-3 PUFAs concentration of the cerebrospinal fluid. Decrease total and phosphorylated tau protein of the cerebrospinal fluid.	[7]
To investigate whether n-3 PUFAs would ameliorate the adipose tissue inflammation.	4 g n-3 PUFA ethyl esters	3 mos.	33 patients: 19 receiving n-3 PUFA tablet and 14 receiving placebo.	Decrease MCP-1 and triglyceride. No effect on adiponectin, IL-6 TNF-α, HDL cholesterol and LDL cholesterol.	[60]
To investigate the effects of n-3 PUFAs on inflammatory gene expression in the duodenum.	3 g DHA and EPA	2 mos.	12 patients (mean age 54.1 y, BMI 33.7).	No effects on inflammatory gene expression such as IL-6, TNF-α, IL-18 and STAT3.	[62]
To investigate the effect of n-3 PUFAs on nerve structure and function in T1DM (Whether n-3 PUFAs prevents or limits nerve damage in T1DM).	375 mg EPA, 280 mg DPA and 510 mg DHA	12 mos.	T1DM patients. Both gender. Age 18 y and older.	On going. Phase II Estimated primary completion data: January 2015. Change in corneal nerve fibre length.	*
To test whether vitamin D3 and/or EPA + DHA supplementation reduces the risk of T2D and improves insulin sensitivity.	465 mg EPA, 375 mg DHA and/or vitamin D3		T2DM patients. Both gender. Age 50 y and older.	On going. Estimated primary completion data: October 2017. Measure insulin sensitivity, beta-cell function and HbA1c levels.	*
To investigate the effects of n-3 PUFAs on atherothrombotic biomarkers in T2DM and Cardiovascular Disease.	1000 mg EPA and 1000 mg DHA		T2DM patients (HbA1c > 6.5%) with cardiovascular disease.	On going. Estimated primary completion data: April 2015. Change insulin sensitivity, fasting glucose and HbA1c levels.	*
To examine the effects of n-3 PUFAs on fasting insulin, glucose, insulin sensitivity in Chinese T2DM patients.	4 g fish oil (1200 mg EPA and 800 mg DHA)	6 mos.	240 T2DM patients: fasting glucose between 7.0 - 14.0 mmol/L, HbA1c < 9%, male, age 40 - 80 y.	On going. Estimated primary completion data: December 2014.	*
To investigate whether aspirin versus placebo and/or supplementation with n-3 PUFAs or placebo prevents the serious vascular events.	1 g n-3 PUFAs ethyl esters and/or 100 mg aspirin		T1DM and T2DM patients, age > 40 y, without previous history of vascular disease.	On going. Phase IV Estimated primary completion data: December 2016.	*

*ClinicalTrials.gov: available from http://clinicaltrials.gov/ct2/home.

trials with n-3 PUFAs in diabetes patients. Some of them are ongoing. Outcome of these researches is highly expected, and it will clarify the antidiabetic effects of n-3 PUFAs and the role of n-3 PUFAs in the treatment of DM.

References

[1]   World Health Organization (2015) Diabetes. Fact Sheet No. 312. http://www.who.int/mediacentre/factsheets/fs312/en/

[2]   American Diabetes Association (2012) Diagnosis and Classification of Diabetes Mellitus. *Diabetes Care*, **35**, S64-S71.

[3]   de la Monte, S.M. and Wands, J.R. (2008) Alzheimer's Disease is Type 3 Diabetes-Evidenced Review. *Journal of Diabetes Science and Technology*, **2**, 1101-11138. http://dx.doi.org/10.1177/193229680800200619

[4]   Duarte, A.I., Candeias, E., Correia, S.C., *et al.* (2013) Crosstalk between Diabetes and Brain: Glucagon-Like Peptide-1 Mimetics as a Promising Therapy against Neurodegeneration. *Biochimica et Biophysica Acta*, **1832**, 527-541.

[5]   Janson, J., Laedtk, T., Parisi J.E., *et al.* (2004) Increases Risk of Type 2 Diabetes in Alzheimer's Disease. *Diabetes*, **53**, 474-481. http://dx.doi.org/10.2337/diabetes.53.2.474

[6]   Takalo, M., Haapasalo, A., Martiskainen, H., *et al.* (2014) High-Fat Diet Increases Tau Expression in the Brain of T2DM and AD Mice Independently of Peripheral Metabolic Status. *Journal of nutritional Biochemistry*, **25**, 634-641. http://dx.doi.org/10.1016/j.jnutbio.2014.02.003

[7]   Freund, L.Y., Vedin, I., Cederholm, T., *et al.* (2014) Transfer of Omega-3 Fatty Acids across the Blood-Brain Barrier after Dietary Supplementation with a Docosahexaenoic Acid-Rich Omega-3 Fatty Acid Preparation in Patients with Alzheimer's Disease: The OmegAD Study. *Journal of International Medicine*, **275**, 428-436. http://dx.doi.org/10.1111/joim.12166

[8]   Weir, G.C., Laybutt, D.R., Kaneto, H., *et al.* (2001) Beta-Cell Adaptation and Decompensation during the Progression of Diabetes. *Diabetes*, **50**, S154-S159. http://dx.doi.org/10.2337/diabetes.50.2007.S154

[9]   Kanda, H., Tateya, S., Tamori, Y., *et al.* (2006) MCP-1 Contributes to Macrophage Infiltration into Adipose Tissue, Insulin Resistance, and Hepatic Steatosis in Obesity. *Journal of Clinical Investigation*, **116**, 1494-1505. http://dx.doi.org/10.1172/JCI26498

[10]   Kamei, N., Tobe, K., Suzuki, R., *et al.* (2006) Overexpression of Macrophage Chemoattractant Protein-1 in Adipose Tissue Cause Macrophage Recruitment and Insulin Resistance. *The Journal of Biological Chemistry*, **281**, 26602-26614. http://dx.doi.org/10.1074/jbc.M601284200

[11]   Flachs, P., Horakova, O., Brauner P., *et al.* (2005) Polyunsaturated Fatty Acids of Marine Origin up Regulate Mitochondrial Biogenesis and Induce β-Oxidation in White Fat. *Diabetologia*, **48**, 2365-2375. http://dx.doi.org/10.1007/s00125-005-1944-7

[12]   Vaughan, R.A., Garcia-Smith, R., Bisoffiet M., *et al.* (2012) Conjugated Linoleic Acid or Omega 3 Fatty Acids Increase Mitochondrial Biosynthesis and Metabolism in Skeletal Muscle Cells. *Lipid in Health and Disease*, **11**, 142-152. http://dx.doi.org/10.1186/1476-511X-11-142

[13]   Weisberg, S.P., McCann, D., Desai, M., *et al.* (2003) Obesity Is Associated with Macrophage Accumulation in Adipose Tissue. *Journal of Clinical Investigation*, **112**, 1796-1808. http://dx.doi.org/10.1172/JCI200319246

[14]   Xu, H., Barnes, G.T., Yang, Q., *et al.* (2003) Chronic Inflammation in Fat Plays a Crucial Role in the Development of Obesity-Related Insulin Resistance. *Journal of Clinical Investigation*, **112**, 1821-1830. http://dx.doi.org/10.1172/JCI200319451

[15]   Lazar, M.A. (2006) The Humoral Side of Insulin Resistance. *Nature Medicine*, **12**, 43-44. http://dx.doi.org/10.1038/nm0106-43

[16]   Sell, H. and Eckel, J. (2007) Monocyte Chemotactic Protein-1 and Its Role in Insulin Resistance. *Current Opinion in Lipidology*, **18**, 258-262. http://dx.doi.org/10.1097/MOL.0b013e3281338546

[17]   Sell, H. and Eckel, J. (2009) Chemotactic Cytokines, Obesity and Type 2 Diabetes: *In Vivo* and *in Vitro* Evidence for a Possible Causal Correlation? *Proceedings of the Nutrition Society*, **68**, 378-384. http://dx.doi.org/10.1017/S0029665109990218

[18]   Pimentel, G.D., Lira, F.S., Rosa, J.C., *et al.* (2013) High-Fat Fish Oil Diet Prevents Hypothalamic Inflammatory Profile in Rats. *ISRN Inflammation*, **2013**, Article ID: 419823.

[19]   Vandal, M., Alata, W., Tremblay, C., *et al.* (2014) Reduction in DHA Transport to the Brain of Mice Expressing Human APOE4 Compared to APOE2. *Journal of Neurochemistry*, **129**, 516-526. http://dx.doi.org/10.1111/jnc.12640

[20]   Afshordel, S., Hagl, S., Werner, D., *et al.* (2015) Omega-3 Polyunsaturated Fatty Acids Improve Mitochondrial Dysfunction in Brain Aging—Impact of Bcl-2 and NPD-1 Like Metabolites. *Prostaglandins, Leukotrienes, and Essential Fatty Acids*, 92, 23-31.

[21]   Eckert, G.P., Chang, S., Eckmann, J., *et al.* (2011) Liposome-Incorporated DHA Increases Neuronal Survival by Enhancing Non-Amyloidogenic APP Processing. *Biochimica et Biophysica Acta*, **1808**, 234-243.

[22]   Wellhauser, L. and Belsham, D.D. (2014) Activation of the Omega-3 Fatty Acid Receptor GPR120 Mediates Anti-Inflammatory Actions in Immortalized Hypothalamic Neurons. *Journal of Neuroinflammation*, **27**, 60. http://dx.doi.org/10.1186/1742-2094-11-60

[23]   Cintra, D.E., Ropelle, E.R., Moraes, J.C., *et al.* (2012) Unsaturated Fatty Acids Revert Diet-Induced Hypothalamic Inflammation in Obesity. *PLoS ONE*, **7**, e30571. http://dx.doi.org/10.1371/journal.pone.0030571

[24]   Zhao, Y., Calon, F., Julien, C., *et al.* (2011) Docosahexaenoic Acid-Derived Neuroprotectin D1 Induces Neuronal Survival via Secretase- and PPARγ-Mediated Mechanisms in Alzheimer's Disease Models. *PLoS ONE*, **6**, e15816. http://dx.doi.org/10.1371/journal.pone.0015816

[25] Wall, R., Ross, R.P., Fitzgerald, G.F. and Stanton, C. (2010) Fatty Acids from Fish: The Anti-Inflammatory Potential of Long-Chain Omega-3 Fatty Acids. *Nutrition Reviews*, **68**, 280-289. http://dx.doi.org/10.1111/j.1753-4887.2010.00287.x

[26] Bang, H.O. and Dyerberg, J. (1972) Plasma Lipids and Lipoproteins in Greenlandic West Coast Eskimos. *Acta Medica Scandinavica*, **192**, 85-94. http://dx.doi.org/10.1111/j.0954-6820.1972.tb04782.x

[27] Kromann, N. and Green, A. (1980) Epidemiological Studies in the Upernavik District, Greenland. Incidence of Some Chronic Diseases 1950-1974. *Acta Medica Scandinavica*, **208**, 401-406. http://dx.doi.org/10.1111/j.0954-6820.1980.tb01221.x

[28] Lim, G.E. and Brubaker, P.L. (2006) Glucagon-Like Peptide 1 Secretion by the L-Cell. The View from Within. *Diabetes*, **55**, S70-S77. http://dx.doi.org/10.2337/db06-S020

[29] Kieffer, T.J., McIntosh, C.H. and Pederson, R.A. (1995) Degradation of Glucose-Dependent Insulinotropic Polypeptide and Truncated Glucagon-Like Peptide 1 *in Vitro* and *in Vivo* by Dipeptidyl Peptidase IV. *Endocrinology*, **136**, 3585-3596.

[30] Holst, J.J. (2006) Glucagon-Like Peptide-1: From Extract to Agent: The Claude Bernard Lecture, 2005. *Diabetologia*, **49**, 253-260. http://dx.doi.org/10.1007/s00125-005-0107-1

[31] Drucker, D.J., Jin, T., Asa, S.L., *et al.* (2006) Activation of Proglucagon Gene Transcription by Protein Kinase-A in a Novel Mouse Enteroendocrine Cell Line. *Molecular Endocrinology*, **8**, 1646-1655.

[32] Abello, J., Ye, F., Bosshard, A., *et al.* (1994) Stimulation of Glucagon-Like Peptide-1 Secretion by Muscarinic Agonist in a Murine Intestinal Endocrine Cell Line. *Endocrinology*, **134**, 2011-2017.

[33] Reimer, R.A., Darimont, C., Gremlich, S., *et al.* (2001) A Human Cellular Model for Studying the Regulation of Glucagon-Like Peptide-1 Secretion. *Endocrinology*, **142**, 4522-4528. http://dx.doi.org/10.1210/endo.142.10.8415

[34] Drucker, D.J. (2006) The Biology of Incretin Hormones. *Cell Metabolism*, **3**, 153-165. http://dx.doi.org/10.1016/j.cmet.2006.01.004

[35] Rocca, A.S. and Brubaker, P.L. (1999) Role of the Vagus Nerve in Mediating Proximal Nutrient-Induced Glucagon-Like Peptide-1 Secretion. *Endocrinology*, **140**, 1687-1694.

[36] Roberge, J.N. and Brubaker, P.L. (1993) Regulation of Intestinal Proglucagon-Derived Peptide Secretion by Glucose-Dependent Insulinotropic Peptide in a Novel Enteroendocrine Loop. *Endcrinology*, **133**, 233-240.

[37] Elrick, H., Stimmler, L., Hlad Jr., C.J. and Rai, Y. (1964) Plasma Insulin Responses to Oral and Intravenous Glucose Administration. *Journal of Clinical Endocrinology Metabolism*, **24**, 1076-1082. http://dx.doi.org/10.1210/jcem-24-10-1076

[38] Toft-Nielsen, M.B., Damholt, M.B., Madsbad, S., *et al.* (2001) Determinants of the Impaired Secretion of Glucagon-Like Peptide-1 in Type 2 Diabetic Patients. *Journal of Clinical Endocrinology Metabolism*, **86**, 3717-3723. http://dx.doi.org/10.1210/jcem.86.8.7750

[39] Vilsbøll, T., Krarup, T., Deacon, C.F., *et al.* (2001) Reduced Postprandial Concentrations of Intact Biologically Active Glucagon-Like Peptide 1 in Type 2 Diabetic Patients. *Diabetes*, **50**, 609-613. http://dx.doi.org/10.2337/diabetes.50.3.609

[40] Muscelli, E., Mari, A., Casolaro, A., *et al.* (2008) Separate Impact of Obesity and Glucose Tolerance on the Incretin Effect in Normal Subjects and Type 2 Diabetic Patients. *Diabetes*, **57**, 1340-1348. http://dx.doi.org/10.2337/db07-1315

[41] Vilsbøll, T., Agersø, H., Krarup, T. and Holst, J.J. (2003) Similar Elimination Rates of Glucagon-Like Peptide-1 in Obese Type 2 Diabetic Patients and Healthy Subjects. *Journal of Clinical Endocrinology and Metabolism*, **88**, 220-224. http://dx.doi.org/10.1210/jc.2002-021053

[42] Green, C.J., Henriksen, T.I., Pedersen, B.K. and Solomon, T.P. (2012) Glucagon Like Peptide-1-Induced Glucose Metabolism in Differentiated Human Muscle Satellite Cells Is Attenuated by Hyperglycemia. *PLoS ONE*, **7**, e44284. http://dx.doi.org/10.1371/journal.pone.0044284

[43] Sonoki, K., Iwase, M. Takata, Y., *et al.* (2013) Effect of Thirty-Times Chewing per Bite on Secretion of Glucagon-Like Peptide-11 in Health Volunteers and Type 2 Diabetic Patients. *Endocrine Journal*, **60**, 311-319. http://dx.doi.org/10.1507/endocrj.EJ12-0310

[44] Tsuchiya, M., Niijima-Yaoita, F., Yoneda, H., *et al.* (2014) Long-Term Feeding on Powdered Food Causes Hyperglycemia and Signs of Systemic Illness in Mice. *Life Science*, **103**, 8-14. http://dx.doi.org/10.1016/j.lfs.2014.03.022

[45] Yamazaki, T., Yamori, M., Asai, K., *et al.* (2013) Mastication and Risk for Diabetes in Japanese Population: A Cross-Sectional Study. *PLoS ONE*, **8**, e4113. http://dx.doi.org/10.1371/journal.pone.0064113

[46] Rocca, A.S. and Brubaker, P.L. (1995) Stereospecific Effects of Fatty Acids on Proglucagon-Derived Peptide Secretion in Fetal Rat Intestinal Cultures. *Endocrinology*, **136**, 5593-5599.

[47] Brubaker, P.L., Schloos, J. and Drucker, D.J. (1998) Regulation of Glucagon-Like Peptide-1 Synthesis and Secretion in

the GLUTag Enteroendocrine Cell Line. *Endocrinology*, **139**, 4108-4114.

[48] Oh, D.Y., Talukdar, S., Bae, E.J., *et al.* (2010) GPR120 Is an Omega-3 Fatty Acid Receptor Mediating Potent Anti-Inflammatory and Insulin-Sensitizing Effects. *Cell*, **142**, 687-698. http://dx.doi.org/10.1016/j.cell.2010.07.041

[49] Hirasawa, A., Tsumaya, K., Awaji, T., *et al.* (2005) Free Fatty Acids Regulate Gut Incretin Glucagon-Like Peptide-1 Secretion through GPR120. *Nature Medicine*, **11**, 90-94. http://dx.doi.org/10.1038/nm1168

[50] Katsuma, S., Hatae, N., Yano, T., *et al.* (2005) Free Fatty Acids Inhibit Serum Deprivation-Induced Apoptosis through GPR120 in a Murine Enteroendocrine Cell Line STC-1. *Journal of Biological Chemistry*, **280**, 19507-19515. http://dx.doi.org/10.1074/jbc.M412385200

[51] Adachi, T., Tanaka, T., Takemoto, K., *et al.* (2006) Free Fatty Acids Administrated into the Colon Promote the Secretion of Glucagon-Like Peptide-1 and Insulin. *Biochemical and Biophysical Research Communications*, **340**, 332-357. http://dx.doi.org/10.1016/j.bbrc.2005.11.162

[52] Morishita, M., Tanaka, T., Shida, T. and Takayama, K. (2008) Usefulness of Colon Targeted DHA and EPA as Novel Diabetes Medications That Promote Intrinsic GLP-1 Secretion. *Journal of Controlled Release*, **132**, 99-104. http://dx.doi.org/10.1016/j.jconrel.2008.09.001

[53] Shida, T., Kamei, N. and Takeda-Morishita, M. (2013) Colonic Delivery of Docosahexaenoic Acid Improves Impaired Glucose Tolerance via GLP-1 Secretion and Suppresses Pancreatic Islet Hyperplasia in Diabetic KK-A^y Mice. *International Journal of Pharmacology*, **450**, 63-69. http://dx.doi.org/10.1016/j.ijpharm.2013.04.029

[54] Morishita, M., Kajita, M., Suzuki, A., *et al.* (2000) The Dose-Related Hypoglycemic Effects of Insulin Emulsions Incorporating Highly Purified EPA and DHA. *International Journal of Pharmacology*, **201**, 175-185. http://dx.doi.org/10.1016/S0378-5173(00)00411-7

[55] Suzuki, A., Morishita, M., Kajita, M., *et al.* (1998) Enhanced Colonic and Rectal Absorption of Insulin Using a Multiple Emulsion Containing Eicosapentaenoic Acid and Docosahexaenoic Acid. *Journal of Pharmaceutical Sciences*, **87**, 1196-1202. http://dx.doi.org/10.1021/js980125q

[56] Andersen, G., Harnack, K., Erbersdobler, H.F. and Somoza, V. (2008) Dietary Eicosapentaenoic Acid and Docosahexaenoic Acid Are More Effective than Alpha-Linolenic Acid in Improving Insulin Sensitivity in Rats. *Annals of Nutrition and Metabolism*, **52**, 250-256. http://dx.doi.org/10.1159/000140518

[57] Ichimura, A., Hirasawa, A., Poulain-Godefroy, O., *et al.* (2012) Dysfunction of Lipid Sensor GPR120 Leads to Obesity in Both Mouse and Human. *Nature*, **483**, 350-354. http://dx.doi.org/10.1038/nature10798

[58] Oh, D.Y., Walenta, E., Akiyama, T.E., *et al.* (2014) A GPR120-Selective Agonist Improves Insulin Resistance and Chronic Inflammation in Obese Mice. *Nature Medicine*, **20**, 942-947. http://dx.doi.org/10.1038/nm.3614

[59] Luan, B., Zhao, J., Wu, H., *et al.* (2009) Deficiency of A Beta-Arrestin-2 Signal Complex Contributes to Insulin Resistance. *Nature*, **457**, 1146-1149. http://dx.doi.org/10.1038/nature07617

[60] Spencer, M., Finlin, B.S., Unal, R., *et al.* (2013) Omega-3 Fatty Acids Reduce Adipose Tissue Macrophages in Human Subjects with Insulin Resistance. *Diabetes*, **62**, 1709-17171. http://dx.doi.org/10.2337/db12-1042

[61] de Caterina, R., Madonna, R., Bertolotto, A. and Schmidt, E.B. (2007) N-3 Fatty Acids in the Treatment of Diabetic Patients. *Diabetes Care*, **30**, 1012-1026. http://dx.doi.org/10.2337/dc06-1332

[62] Labonté, M.È., Couture, P., Tremblay, A.J., Hogue, J.C., Lemelin, V. and Lamarche, B. (2013) Eicosapentaenoic and Docosahexaenoic Acid Supplementation and Inflammatory Gene Expression in the Duodenum of Obese Patients with Type 2 Diabetes. *Nutrition Journal*, **12**, 98. http://dx.doi.org/10.1186/1475-2891-12-98

[63] Brookheart, R.T., Michel, C.T. and Schaffer, J.F. (2009) As a Matter of Fat. *Cell Metabolism*, **10**, 9-12. http://dx.doi.org/10.1016/j.cmet.2009.03.011

[64] Xu, J., Teran-Garcia, M., Park, J.H., *et al.* (2001) Polyunsaturated Fatty Acids Suppress Hepatic Sterol Regulatory Element-Binding Protein-1 Expression by Accelerating Transcript Decay. *Journal of Biological Chemistry*, **276**, 9800-9807. http://dx.doi.org/10.1074/jbc.M008973200

[65] Xu, J., Nakamura, M.T., Cho, H.P. and Clarke, S.D. (2007) Sterol Regulatory Element Binding Protein-1 Expression Is Suppressed by Dietary Polyunsaturated Fatty Acids. *Journal of Biological Chemistry*, **274**, 23577-23583. http://dx.doi.org/10.1074/jbc.274.33.23577

[66] Liu, X., Xue, Y., Liu, C., *et al.* (2013) Eiocasapentaenoic Acid-Enriched Phospholipid Ameliorates Insulin Resistance and Lipid Metabolism in Diet-Induced-Obese Mice. *Lipid in Health and Disease*, **12**, 109. http://dx.doi.org/10.1186/1476-511X-12-109

[67] Neschen, S., Morino, K., Dong, J., *et al.* (2007) N-3 Fatty Acids Preserve Insulin Sensitivity *in Vivo* in a Peroxisome Proliferator-Activated Receptor-α-Dependent Manner. *Diabetes*, **56**, 1034-1041. http://dx.doi.org/10.2337/db06-1206

[68] Wu, J.H., Cahill, L.E. and Mozaffarian, D. (2013) Effects of Fish Oil on Circulating Adiponectin: A Systematic Review and Meta-Analysis of Randomized Controlled Trials. *Journal of Endocrinology and Metabolism*, **98**, 2451-2459.

http://dx.doi.org/10.1210/jc.2012-3899

[69] Flachs, P., Mohamed-Ali, V. and Horakova, O. (2006) Polyunsaturated Fatty Acids of Marine Origin Induce Adiponectin in Mice Fed a High-Fat Diet. *Diabetologia*, **49**, 394-397. http://dx.doi.org/10.1007/s00125-005-0053-y

[70] Banga, A., Unal, R., Tripathi, P., *et al.* (2009) Adiponectin Translation Is Increased by the PPARgamma Agonist Pioglitazone and Omega-3 Fatty Acids. *American Journal of Physiology, Endocrinology and Metabolism*, **296**, E480-E489. http://dx.doi.org/10.1152/ajpendo.90892.2008

[71] Tishinsky, J.M., Ma, D.W. and Robinson, L.F. (2011) Eicosapentaenoic Acid and Rosiglitazone Increase Adiponectin in an Additive and PPARγ-Dependent Manner in Human Adipocytes. *Obesity*, **19**, 262-268. http://dx.doi.org/10.1038/oby.2010.186

[72] World Health Organization. Diabetes Programme [Article Online]. http://www.who.int/diabetes/action_online/basics/en/index3.html

[73] Sawada, N., Jiang, A., Takizawa, F., *et al.* (2014) Endothelial PGC-1α Mediates Vascular Dysfunction in Diabetes. *Cell Metabolism*, **19**, 246-258. http://dx.doi.org/10.1016/j.cmet.2013.12.014

[74] Cao, L., Aran, P.R., Kim, J., *et al.* (2010) Modulating Notch Signaling to Enhance Neovascularization and Reperfusion in Diabetic Mice. *Biomaterials*, **31**, 9048-9056. http://dx.doi.org/10.1016/j.biomaterials.2010.08.002

[75] Bryner, R.W., Woodworth-Hobbs, M.E., Williamson, D.L. and Always, S.E. (2012) Docosahexaenoic Acid Protects Muscle Cells from Palmitate-Induced Atrophy. *ISRN Obesity*, **2012**, Article ID: 647348.

[76] Virtanen, J.K., Mursu, J., Voutilainen, S., Uusitupa, M. and Tuomainen, T.P. (2014) Serum Omega-3 Polyunsaturated Fatty Acids and Risk of Incident Type 2 Diabetes in Men: The Kuopio Ischemic Heart Disease Risk Factor Study. *Diabetes Care*, **37**, 1189-1196. http://dx.doi.org/10.2337/dc13-1504

[77] Iwasaki, M., Hoshian, F., Tsuji, T., *et al.* (2012) Predicting Efficacy of Dipeptidyl Peptidase-4 Inhibitors in Patients with Type 2 Diabetes: Association of Glycated Hemoglobin Reduction with Serum Eicosapentaenoic Acid and Docosahexaenoic Acid Levels. *Journal of Diabetes Investigation*, **3**, 464-467. http://dx.doi.org/10.1111/j.2040-1124.2012.00214.x

[78] Samimi, M., Jamilian, M., Asemi, Z. and Esmaillzadeh, A. (2014) Effects of Omega-3 Fatty Acid Supplementation on Insulin Metabolism and Lipid Profiles in Gestational Diabetes: Randomized, Double-Blind, Placebo-Controlled Trial. *Clinical Nutrition*, in press.

[79] Serhiyenko, V., Serhiyenko, A. and Segin, V. (2014) The Effect of Omega-3 Polyunsaturated Fatty Acids on N-Terminal Pro-Brain Natriuretic Peptide and Lipid Concentration in Patients with Type 2 Diabetes Mellitus and Cardiovascular Autonomic Neuropathy. *Romanian Journal of Diabetes Nutrition and Metabolic Diseases*, **21**, 97-101. http://dx.doi.org/10.2478/rjdnmd-2014-0014

17

Optimization of siRNA Delivery Method into the Liver by Sequential Injection of Polyglutamic Acid and Cationic Lipoplex

Yoshiyuki Hattori*, Shohei Arai, Takuto Kikuchi, Megumi Hamada, Ryou Okamoto, Yoko Machida, Kumi Kawano

Department of Drug Delivery Research, Hoshi University, Tokyo, Japan
Email: *yhattori@hoshi.ac.jp

Abstract

Previously, we developed a novel siRNA transfer method to the liver by sequential intravenous injection of poly-L-glutamic acid (PGA) and cationic liposome/siRNA complex (cationic lipoplex). In this study, we examined the effects of the charge ratio (+/−) of cationic liposome/siRNA, molecular weight of PGA and cationic lipid of cationic liposome on the biodistribution of siRNA after sequential injection of PGA plus cationic lipoplex. When 1,2-dioleoyl-3-trimethylammonium-propane (DOTAP)/cholesterol (Chol) lipoplex was intravenously injected into mice, the accumulation of siRNA was mainly observed in the lungs. In contrast, when DOTAP/Chol lipoplex was intravenously injected at 1 min after intravenous injection of PGA, siRNA was largely accumulated in the liver. The charge ratio (+/−) of DOTAP/Chol liposome/siRNA did not affect the biodistribution of siRNA after sequential injection. As regards the molecular weight of PGA, the accumulation of siRNA was observed mainly in the liver after the sequential injection of PGA of 20.5, 38, 64 or 200 kDa plus DOTAP/Chol lipoplex. Furthermore, to examine the effect of cationic lipid of cationic liposome on the biodistribution of siRNA, we prepared other cationic liposomes composed of 1,2-di-O-octadecenyl-3-trimethylammonium propane chloride (DOTMA)/Chol, dimethyldioctadecylammonium bromide (DDAB)/Chol and O,O'-ditetradecanoyl-N-(α-trimethylammonioacetyl)di-ethanolamine chloride (DC-6-14)/Chol. For the cationic liposomes, the accumulation of siRNA was observed mainly in the liver when their cationic lipoplexes were sequentially injected after injection of PGA into mice. From these findings, sequential injection of PGA plus cationic lipoplex could deliver siRNA efficiently into the liver regardless of the charge ratio (+/−) of lipoplex, lengths of PGA and cationic lipid of liposome.

---

*Corresponding author.

Keywords

Cationic Liposome, siRNA Delivery, Polyglutamic Acid, Liver Targeting, Sequential Injection

1. Introduction

RNA interference (RNAi) is a powerful gene-silencing process that holds great promise in the field of gene therapy [1]. The liver is an important organ with a number of potential therapeutic siRNA targets, including cholesterol biosynthesis, fibrosis, hepatitis and hepatocellular carcinoma. Although none of the currently available methods of siRNA delivery is optimal for liver siRNA therapy, concerted effort from researchers has provided a wide range of choices for siRNA transfer to the liver. Generally, siRNAs fail to cross biological membranes by passive diffusion owing to their high molecular weight and anionic nature. Therefore, carriers of siRNA are required to deliver siRNA into the cytoplasm of target cells. In siRNA delivery, non-viral vectors such as cationic liposomes and cationic polymers have been more commonly used than viral vectors [2] [3]. Among all of the carriers, lipid-based formulations such as cationic liposomes are currently the most widely validated means for the systemic delivery of siRNA to the liver [4].

For efficient siRNA delivery to the liver by cationic liposomes, the cationic liposome/siRNA complex (cationic lipoplex) must be stabilized in the blood by avoiding its agglutination with blood components, and the pharmacokinetics of lipoplex after intravenous injection must be controlled because electrostatic interactions between positively charged lipoplexes and negatively charged erythrocytes cause agglutination [5], and the agglutinates contribute to high entrapment of lipoplex in the highly extended lung capillaries [6].

Poly-L-glutamic acid (PGA) is a polyamino acid having one carboxylic acid per glutamic acid unit. Previously, we developed PGA-coated lipoplex of siRNA (ternary complex of PGA, siRNA and cationic liposomes) and found that PGA coatings for cationic lipoplex prevented the accumulation of lipoplex in the lungs by inhibiting interaction with erythrocytes and could deliver siRNA to the liver [7]. Thereafter, we found that pre-treatment of erythrocytes with PGA could prevent agglutination *in vitro* after addition of cationic lipoplex [8]. Therefore, we revisited a previously reported gene transfer method [7] and developed sequential injection of PGA and cationic lipoplex for systemic gene delivery of siRNA into the liver efficiently without accumulation in the lung [8]. However, it was not clear whether siRNA delivery into the liver by sequential injection of PGA plus cationic lipoplex was affected by the molecular weight of PGA, the charge ratio (+/−) of cationic liposome/siRNA and the cationic lipid of cationic liposome. Therefore, in this study, we examined the optimal conditions of siRNA delivery into the liver by sequential injection of PGA and cationic lipoplex.

2. Materials and Methods

2.1. Materials

1,2-Dioleoyl-3-trimethylammonium-propane methyl sulfate salt (DOTAP) was obtained from Avanti Polar Lipids Inc. (Alabaster, AL, USA). 1,2-Di-*O*-octadecenyl-3-trimethylammonium propane chloride (DOTMA) was purchased from Tokyo Kasei Co., Ltd. (Tokyo, Japan). Dimethyldioctadecylammonium bromide (DDAB, product name DC-1-18) and *O,O*'-ditetradecanoyl-*N*-(*α*-trimethylammonioacetyl)diethanolamine chloride (DC-6-14) were obtained from Sogo Pharmaceutical Co., Ltd. (Tokyo, Japan). Poly-*α*-L-glutamic acid sodium salt (PGA, 20.5 kDa), poly-*α*-L-glutamic acid sodium salt (64 kDa) and poly-*α*-D-glutamic acid sodium salt (38 kDa) were purchased from Sigma-Aldrich Co. (St. Louis, MO, USA). Poly-*γ*-L-glutamic acid sodium salt (200 kDa) and cholesterol (Chol) were purchased from Wako Pure Chemical Industries, Ltd. (Osaka, Japan). All other chemicals were of the finest grade available.

2.2. siRNA

Firefly pGL3 luciferase siRNA (siRNA) and Cy5.5-labeled Luc siRNA (Cy5.5-siRNA) were synthesized by Sigma Genosys (Tokyo, Japan). The siRNA sequences of the pGL3 luciferase siRNA were as follows: sense strand: 5'-GUGGAUUUCGAGUCGUCUUAA-3', and antisense strand: 5'-AAGACGACUCGAAAUCCACAU-3'. In Cy5.5-siRNA, Cy5.5 dye was conjugated at the 5'-end of the sense strand.

2.3. Preparation of Liposome and Lipoplex

For the preparation of cationic liposomes, we used four kinds of cationic lipid, DOTAP, DOTMA, DDAB and DC-6-14 (**Figure 1**). Cationic liposomes were prepared from DOTAP/Chol, DOTMA/Chol, DDAB/Chol and DC-6-14/Chol at a molar ratio of 1/1 by a thin-film hydration method, as previously reported [7]. To prepare cationic liposome/siRNA complex (cationic lipoplex), cationic liposome suspension was mixed with siRNA by vortexing for 10 s at charge ratios (+/−) of 4/1, 6/1 and 8/1, and left for 15 min at room temperature. The theoretical charge ratio (+/−) of cationic liposome to siRNA was calculated as the molar ratio of DOTAP, DOTMA, DDAB or DC-6-14 nitrogen to siRNA phosphate.

The particle size distributions of lipoplex were measured by the cumulant method using a light-scattering photometer (ELS-Z2, Otsuka Electronics Co., Ltd., Osaka, Japan) at 25°C, after diluting the dispersion to an appropriate volume with water. The ζ-potentials were measured by electrophoresis light-scattering methods using ELS-Z2 at 25°C, after diluting the dispersion to an appropriate volume with water. When DOTAP, DOTMA, DDAB and DC-6-14 liposomes were mixed with siRNA at a charge ratio (+/−) of 4/1, their lipoplex sizes were about 340 nm, 203 nm, 418 nm and 307 nm, and their ζ-potentials were about 41 mV, 40 mV, 43 mV and 34 mV, respectively.

2.4. Biodistribution of siRNA After Intravenous Injection of Cationic Lipoplex to Mice

All animal experiments were performed with approval from the Institutional Animal Care and Use Committee of Hoshi University. At 1 min after intravenous injection of solution of 1 mg of PGA, cationic lipoplexes of 50 μg of Cy5.5-siRNA were intravenously administered *via* lateral tail veins into female BALB/c mice (8 weeks of age; Sankyo Lab. Service Corp., Tokyo, Japan). One hour after the injection of cationic lipoplex, the mice were sacrificed, and Cy5.5 fluorescent imaging of the tissues was performed using a NightOWL LB981 NC100 system (Berthold Technologies, Bad Wildbad, Germany). The excitation and emission filters were set at 630/20 and 680/30 nm, respectively. The exposure time for fluorescence was 5 seconds. A grayscale body-surface reference image was collected using a NightOWL LB981 CCD camera. The images were analyzed using the IndiGo2 software provided with the *in vivo* imaging system (Berthold Technologies). The tissues after fluorescent imaging were frozen on dry ice and sliced at 16 μm. The localization of Cy5.5-siRNA was examined using an Eclipse TS100-F microscope (Nikon, Tokyo, Japan).

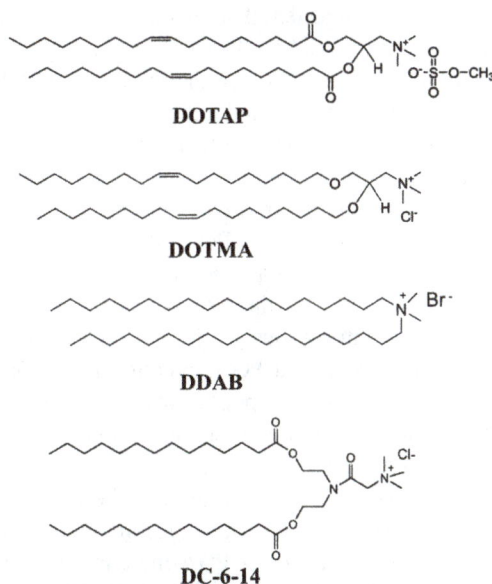

Figure 1. Chemical structure of cationic lipids for preparation of cationic liposome. 1,2-Dioleoyl-3-trimethylammonium propane methyl sulfate, DOTAP; 1,2-di-*O*-octadecenyl-3-trimethylammonium propane chloride, DOTMA; dimethyldioctadecylammonium bromide, DDAB; *O,O*'-ditetradecanoyl-*N*-(α-trimethylammonioacetyl)diethanolamine chloride, DC-6-14.

2.5. Agglutination Assay

Agglutination assay was performed according to the method described in a previous report [7]. Briefly, erythrocytes were collected from mouse blood at 4°C by centrifugation at 300 g for 3 min and resuspended in PBS as a 2% (v/v) stock suspension of erythrocytes. A total of 10 μg of PGA was added to 100 μL of erythrocyte suspension, and then the mixtures were immediately supplemented with the cationic lipoplexes of 2 μg of siRNA formed at a charge ratio (+/−) of 4/1. After incubation for 15 min at 37°C, the sample was placed on a glass plate and agglutination was observed by microscopy.

3. Results and Discussion

3.1. Effect of Order of Administration of PGA and Cationic Lipoplex on Biodistribution of siRNA

Previously, we reported that sequential injection of PGA plus cationic lipoplex of siRNA could deliver siRNA into the liver [8]. In this study, we examined the effect of charge ratio (+/−) of cationic liposome/siRNA, molecular weight of PGA and cationic lipid of cationic liposome on the biodistribution of siRNA after sequential injection of PGA plus cationic lipoplex. We decided to use DOTAP/Chol liposomes as the cationic liposomes because they had often been used for *in vivo* applications for gene delivery [9] [10], and the lipoplex of pDNA encoding tumor suppressor gene TUSC2/FUS1 had been exploited in a clinical setting for the treatment of non-small cell lung cancer (NSCLC) patients [11]. DOTAP/Chol lipoplex was formed by mixing DOTAP/Chol liposome with siRNA at a charge ratio (+/−) of 4/1. In PGA, we used poly-α-L-glutamic acid with a molecular weight of 20.5 kDa. With regard to the injected dose (mg) of PGA, 1 mg was intravenously injected because we previously found that the sequential injection of this amount plus cationic lipoplex was associated with the highest accumulation of siRNA in the liver [8], comparable to those by commercially available transfection reagent Invivofectamine2.0 and hydrodynamic injection, which can efficiently introduce siRNA into the liver by intravenous injection.

First, we evaluated the effect of the order of administration of PGA and cationic lipoplex on the biodistribution of Cy5.5-siRNA in mice. When naked siRNA was injected, strong accumulation was observed only in the kidneys (**Figure 2(a)** and **Figure 2(b)**), indicating that naked siRNA was quickly eliminated from the body by filtration in the kidneys. When DOTAP/Chol lipoplex was injected, siRNA was largely accumulated in the lungs (**Figure 2(a)** and **Figure 2(b)**). This suggested that electrostatic interactions between positively charged DOTAP/Chol lipoplexes and negatively charged erythrocytes caused agglutination, and their agglutinates were entrapped in the highly extended lung capillaries. Upon the injection of DOTAP/Chol liposomes at 1 min after the injection of naked siRNA, siRNA was accumulated mainly in the lungs, but weakly in the liver (**Figure 2(a)** and **Figure 2(b)**), indicating that most of the siRNA interacted with DOTAP/Chol liposomes in blood circulation, and their complexes were entrapped in the lungs. This result is similar to previously reported findings that sequential injection of cationic liposome plus plasmid DNA effectively transfects the lung [12]. Upon the injection of cationic lipoplex at 1 min after the injection of PGA, strong accumulation of siRNA was observed in the liver and moderately in the kidneys (**Figure 2(a)** and **Figure 2(b)**), suggesting that PGA in blood circulation might prevent the agglutination of DOTAP/Chol lipoplex with erythrocytes, and increase the accumulation in the liver. We still have no evidence that intravenously injected PGA could interact with DOTAP/Chol lipoplex in blood circulation; however, we speculated that PGA injection might prevent the agglutination of DOTAP/Chol lipoplex with erythrocytes by coating of the lipoplex with PGA in blood circulation, and increase the accumulation in the liver. However, some siRNAs might be dissociated from DOTAP/Chol lipoplexes in blood by PGA injection and be excreted by the kidneys.

In contrast, in the sequential injection of PGA at 1 min after the injection of DOTAP/Chol lipoplex, siRNA was accumulated mainly in the lungs (data not shown), suggesting that DOTAP/Chol lipoplex after intravenous injection might rapidly accumulate in the lungs before PGA injection. Moreover, upon the injection of DOTAP/Chol liposomes at 1 min after the injection of a mixture of PGA and siRNA, marked accumulation of siRNA was observed in the kidney (**Figure 2(a)** and **Figure 2(b)**), indicating that individual injection of PGA, DOTAP/Chol liposomes and siRNA could not form cationic lipoplex or ternary complex in the blood, and the most of the siRNA was rapidly eliminated from the kidneys. From these findings, the injection of PGA, followed by the injection of DOTAP/Chol lipoplex, was needed for siRNA delivery into the liver.

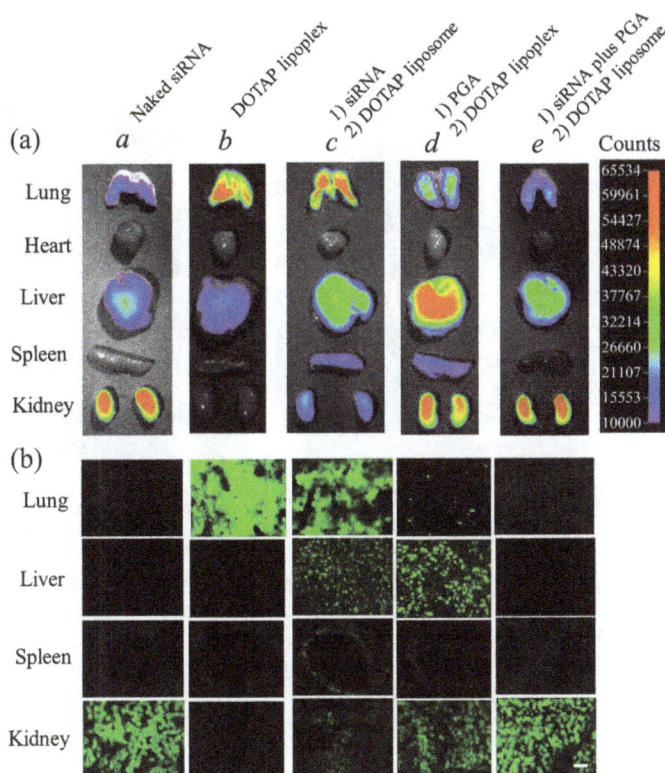

Figure 2. *Ex vivo* images of dissected tissues (a) and tissue section (b) at 1 h after the sequential injection of PGA plus DOTAP/Chol lipoplex into mice. DOTAP/Chol lipoplex was formed at a charge ratio (+/−) of 4/1. In *a* and *b*, 50 µg of naked Cy5.5-siRNA and DOTAP/Chol lipoplex of 50 µg of Cy5.5-siRNA were injected into the mice. In *c*, DOTAP/Chol liposomes were injected at 1 min after the injection of 50 µg of Cy5.5-siRNA. In *d*, DOTAP/Chol lipoplex of 50 µg of Cy5.5-siRNA was injected at 1 min after the injection of 1 mg of PGA. In *e*, DOTAP/Chol liposomes were injected at 1 min after the injection of a mixture of 50 µg of Cy5.5-siRNA and 1 mg of PGA. In (a), the exposure time for the detection of Cy5.5 fluorescence was 5 seconds. Fluorescence intensity is illustrated by a color-coded scale (red is maximum, purple is minimum). In (b), green signals indicate the localization of Cy5.5-siRNA. Scale bar = 100 µm.

3.2. Effect of Charge Ratio (+/−) of Cationic Lipoplex on the Biodistribution of siRNA

To investigate the effect of the charge ratio (+/−) of DOTAP/Chol liposomes and siRNA on the biodistribution after sequential injection of PGA plus DOTAP/Chol lipoplex, we intravenously injected DOTAP/Chol lipoplexes of Cy5.5-siRNA at charge ratios (+/−) of 6/1 and 8/1, after the injection of PGA into mice. The injection of DOTAP/Chol lipoplex at a charge ratio (+/−) of 6/1 or 8/1 after the injection of PGA exhibited high accumulation of siRNA in the liver (**Figure 3(a)** and **Figure 3(b)**), comparable to that at a charge ratio (+/−) of 4/1 (**Figure 2(a)** and **Figure 2(b)**). Although we speculated that an increased charge ratio (+/−) could reduce the exclusion of siRNA from the kidneys due to high association between cationic liposomes and siRNA *via* electrostatic interaction, siRNAs were detected in the kidneys. As a result, the charge ratio (+/−) did not largely affect the biodistribution of siRNA after the sequential injection of PGA plus DOTAP/Chol lipoplex.

3.3. Effect of Molecular Weight of PGA on Biodistribution of siRNA

Sequential injection of poly-α-L-glutamic acid of 20.5 kDa plus cationic lipoplex could deliver siRNA mainly in the liver (**Figure 2(a)** and **Figure 2(b)**). Next, we examined whether the molecular weight and isomer of PGA

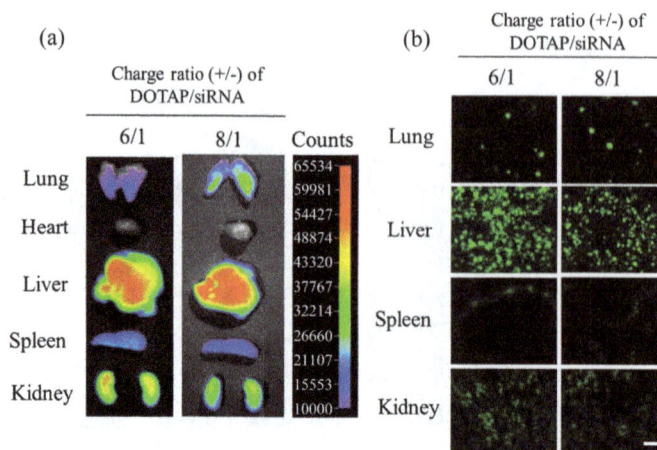

Figure 3. Effect of the charge ratio (+/−) of DOTAP/Chol lipoplex on the biodistribution of siRNA in mice after sequential injection of PGA plus DOTAP/Chol lipoplex of Cy5.5-siRNA. DOTAP/Chol lipoplexes were formed at charge ratios (+/−) of 6/1 and 8/1, and *ex vivo* images of dissected tissues (a) and tissue section (b) were obtained at 1 h after the sequential injection of 1 mg of PGA (20.5 kDa) plus DOTAP/Chol lipoplex of 50 μg of Cy5.5-siRNA into mice. In (a), the exposure time for the detection of Cy5.5 fluorescence was 5 seconds. Fluorescence intensity is illustrated by a color-coded scale (red is maximum, purple is minimum). In (b), green signals indicate the localization of Cy5.5-siRNA. Scale bar = 100 μm.

affected the biodistribution of siRNA after the sequential injection of PGA plus DOTAP/Chol lipoplex (**Figure 4(a)** and **Figure 4(b)**). In the sequential injection of poly-α-L-glutamic acid of 64 kDa, poly-α-D-glutamic acid of 38 kDa or poly-γ-L-glutamic acid of 200 kDa plus cationic lipoplex, siRNA was detected mainly in the liver (**Figure 4(b)**). However, the sequential injection of poly-γ-L-glutamic acid of 200 kDa plus DOTAP/Chol lipoplex exhibited lower accumulation of siRNA in the liver than those by other types of PGA (**Figure 4(a)**). This might indicate that large PGA (~200 kDa) could not strongly interact with DOTAP/Chol lipoplex in the blood.

3.4. Effect of Cationic Lipid of Cationic Lipoplex on Biodistribution of siRNA

Next, we examined whether cationic lipid of cationic liposome affected the biodistribution of siRNA after the sequential injection of PGA (20.5 kDa) plus cationic lipoplex. We prepared DOTMA/Chol, DDAB/Chol and DC-6-14/Chol liposomes as cationic liposomes because DOTMA, DDAB and DC-6-14 have often been used as cationic lipids in liposomal formulations for gene delivery [13]-[15]. When DOTMA lipoplex was injected into mice, siRNA was largely accumulated in the lung and liver (**Figure 5(a)**). In contrast, when DDAB/Chol and DC-6-14/Chol lipoplexes were injected, the accumulation of siRNA was observed largely in the lung. However, pre-injection of PGA could decrease the accumulation of siRNA in the lung by the injection of DOTMA/Chol, DDAB/Chol or DC-6-14/Chol lipoplex, and increased it in the liver (**Figure 5(a)**). Among the cationic liposomes, DOTAP/Chol liposomes efficiently delivered siRNA in the liver after sequential injection (**Figure 2** and **Figure 5(a)**).

Previously, we reported that the addition of PGA into erythrocyte suspension could prevent agglutination by DOTAP/Chol lipoplex [8]. Therefore, we evaluated the effect of agglutination with erythrocytes by DOTMA/Chol, DDAB/Chol and DC-6-14/Chol lipoplexes after the treatment of erythrocytes with PGA. In terms of the results, the addition of PGA into erythrocyte suspension could prevent agglutination induced by the addition of their lipoplexes (**Figure 5(b)**), indicating that PGA might interact with their lipoplexes in the blood and decrease accumulation in the lungs by preventing association with blood components.

PEGylation on the surface of cationic lipoplex (PEG-modified lipoplex) can also decrease accumulation in the lungs by preventing association with blood components; however, PEGylation abolishes the effect of gene suppression by siRNA owing to the high stability of the lipoplex. Electrostatic encapsulation of cationic lipoplex

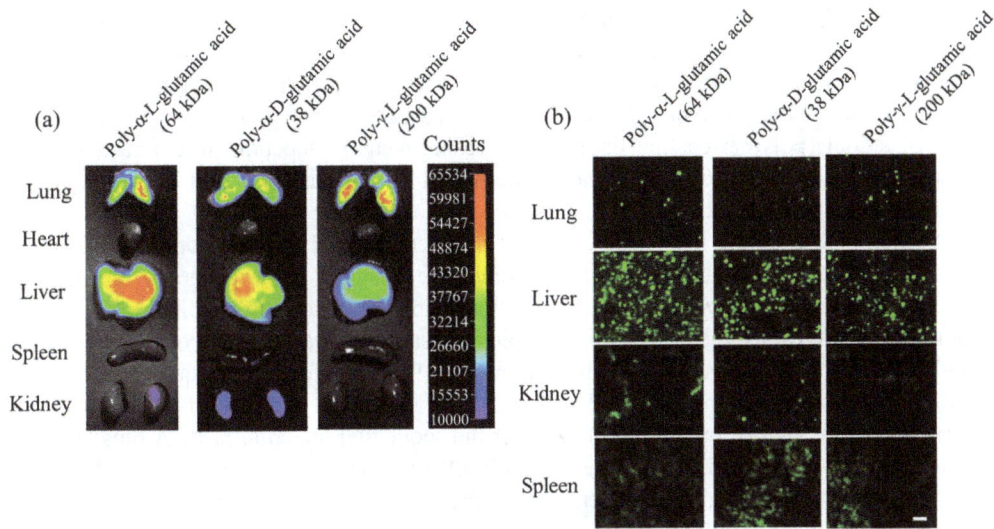

Figure 4. Effect of molecular weight of PGA on the biodistribution of siRNA in mice after the sequential injection of PGA plus DOTAP/Chol lipoplex. *Ex vivo* images of dissected tissues (a) and tissue section (b) were obtained at 1 h after sequential injection of 1 mg of PGA plus DOTAP/Chol lipoplex of 50 µg of Cy5.5-siRNA into mice. Poly-α-L-glutamic acid of 64 kDa, poly-α-D-glutamic acid of 38 kDa and poly-γ-L-glutamic acid of 200 kDa were used as a PGA. In (a), the exposure time for the detection of Cy5.5 fluorescence was 5 seconds. Fluorescence intensity is illustrated by a color-coded scale (red is maximum, purple is minimum). In (b), green signals indicate the localization of Cy5.5-siRNA. Scale bar = 100 µm.

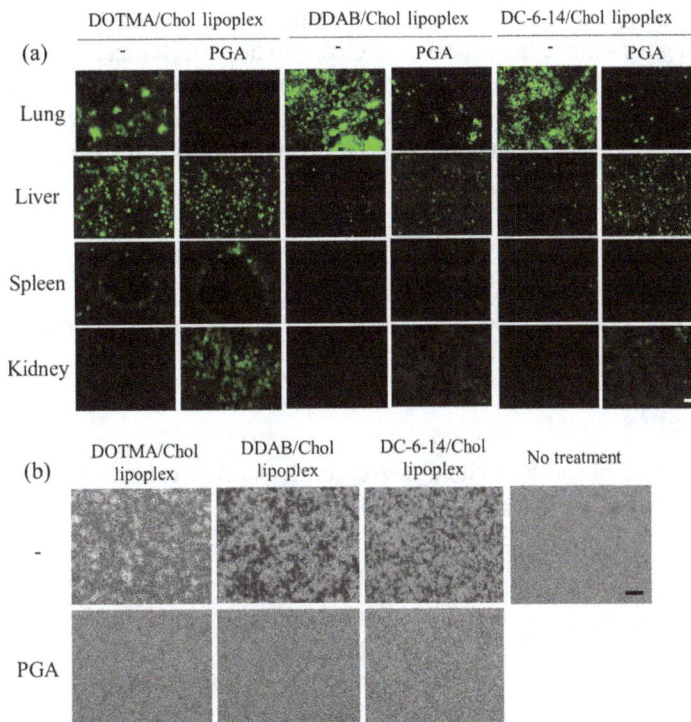

Figure 5. Effect of cationic liposomes on the biodistribution of siRNA in mice after sequential injection of PGA plus cationic lipoplex. DOTMA/Chol, DDAB/Chol and DC-6-14/Chol liposomes were used as cationic liposomes. Their cationic lipoplexes were formed by mixing with siRNA at a charge ratio (+/−) of 4/1. In (a), image of tissue section was obtained at 1 h after the sequential injection of 1 mg of PGA (20.5 kDa) plus cationic lipoplex of 50 µg of Cy5.5-siRNA into mice. Green signals indicate the localization of Cy5.5-siRNA. Scale bar = 100 µm. In (b), the agglutination of cationic lipoplexes with erythrocytes in the presence or absence of PGA (20.5 kDa) is shown. Immediately after the mixing of 10 µg of PGA with erythrocytes, cationic lipoplex of 2 µg of siRNA was added to them, and agglutination was observed by phase contrast microscopy. Scale bar = 100 µm.

with anionic biodegradable polymers such as chondroitin sulfate and PGA can also prevent the agglutination with blood components [7] [16] [17]. However, in the coating of cationic lipoplex with anionic polymer (ternary complex), the size and ζ-potential of the lipoplex were markedly affected by changing the charge ratio (+/−) of cationic lipoplex to anionic polymer [7]; therefore, this charge ratio (+/−) must be precisely controlled for the preparation of anionic polymer-coating lipoplex before intravenous injection. In contrast, sequential injection has an advantage in that cationic lipoplex can be delivered into the liver without directly coating the lipoplex with anionic polymer before injection.

Resident macrophages in the liver called Kupffer cells comprise the major population of the reticuloendothelial system (RES). Intravenously injected liposomes were shown to be generally taken up by RES [18]. Therefore, there was a possibility that most of the cationic lipoplexes accumulated in the liver might be captured by Kupffer cells. Intravenous injections of bisphosphonate such as clodronic acid or zoledronic acid (ZOL) can significantly deplete macrophages in the liver of mice [19]. Therefore, we sequentially injected PGA plus DOTAP/Chol lipoplex into the mice treated with ZOL. However, the decrease of macrophages in the liver by ZOL did not affect the biodistribution of siRNA after the sequential injection of PGA plus DOTAP/Chol lipoplex (data not shown). These findings indicated that siRNA after the sequential injection of PGA plus cationic lipoplex might not be accumulated in the liver through the uptake by Kupffer cells. However, we have no information about regions in which siRNA was localized in the liver after the sequential injection of PGA plus cationic lipoplex, but most of the siRNA in the liver was co-localized with DOTAP/Chol liposomes there (data not shown).

Previously, we reported that the sequential injection of PGA plus DOTAP/Chol lipoplex of cholesterol-conjugated ApoB siRNA could induce suppression of the ApoB mRNA level in the liver [8]. However, in unconjugated siRNA, sequential injection of PGA plus DOTAP/Chol lipoplex of ApoB siRNA did not reduce ApoB expression in the liver (unpublished data). It has also been reported that lipid conjugates of siRNAs enhance cellular uptake and gene silencing in liver cells [20]. In hepatocyte targeting by sequential injection, lipid modification of siRNA might facilitate the uptake of siRNA into hepatocytes and be able to induce a gene silencing effect. Furthermore, modification of siRNA with *N*-acetylgalactosamine ligands that target asialoglycoprotein receptors on hepatocytes is also used for targeting to hepatocytes [21]. Further study must be performed to investigate the optimal siRNA modification for the gene silencing effect in the liver after sequential injection.

4. Conclusion

In this study, we found that sequential injection of PGA plus cationic liposomes could deliver siRNA into the liver, but the charge ratio (+/−) of cationic lipoplex, molecular weight of PGA and cationic lipid of cationic liposomes did not largely affect the biodistribution of siRNA after sequential injection. Sequential injection of PGA and cationic lipoplex might produce a systemic vector of siRNA to the liver.

Acknowledgements

This project was supported in part by a Grant-in-Aid for Scientific Research (C) from the Japan Society for the Promotion of Science (KAKENHI Grant Number 26460046).

References

[1]   Kubowicz, P., Zelaszczyk, D. and Pekala, E. (2013) RNAi in Clinical Studies. *Current Medicinal Chemistry*, **20**, 1801-1816. http://dx.doi.org/10.2174/09298673113209990118

[2]   Zhang, S.B., Zhi, D.F. and Huang, L. (2012) Lipid-Based Vectors for siRNA Delivery. *Journal of Drug Targeting*, **20**, 724-735. http://dx.doi.org/10.3109/1061186X.2012.719232

[3]   Zhou, J.H., Shum, K.T., Burnett, J.C. and Rossi, J.J. (2013) Nanoparticle-Based Delivery of RNAi Therapeutics: Progress and Challenges. *Pharmaceuticals*, **6**, 85-107. http://dx.doi.org/10.3390/ph6010085

[4]   de Fougerolles, A.R. (2008) Delivery Vehicles for Small Interfering RNA *in Vivo*. *Human Gene Therapy*, **19**, 125-132. http://dx.doi.org/10.1089/hum.2008.928

[5]   Eliyahu, H., Servel, N., Domb, A.J. and Barenholz, Y. (2002) Lipoplex-Induced Hemagglutination: Potential Involvement in Intravenous Gene Delivery. *Gene Therapy*, **9**, 850-858.

[6]   Simberg, D., Weisman, S., Talmon, Y., Faerman, A., Shoshani, T. and Barenholz, Y. (2003) The Role of Organ Vas-

cularization and Lipoplex-Serum Initial Contact in Intravenous Murine Lipofection. *The Journal of Biological Chemistry*, **278**, 39858-39865. http://dx.doi.org/10.1074/jbc.M302232200

[7]   Hattori, Y., Nakamura, A., Arai, S., Nishigaki, M., Ohkura, H., Kawano, K., Maitani, Y. and Yonemochi, E. (2014) *In Vivo* siRNA Delivery System for Targeting to the Liver by Poly-L-Glutamic Acid-Coated Lipoplex. *Results in Pharma Sciences*, **4**, 1-7. http://dx.doi.org/10.1016/j.rinphs.2014.01.001

[8]   Hattori, Y., Arai, S., Okamoto, R., Hamada, M., Kawano, K. and Yonemochi, E. (2014) Sequential Intravenous Injection of Anionic Polymer and Cationic Lipoplex of siRNA Could Effectively Deliver siRNA to the Liver. *International Journal of Pharmaceutics*, **476**, 289-298. http://dx.doi.org/10.1016/j.ijpharm.2014.09.059

[9]   Song, Y.K., Liu, F., Chu, S.Y. and Liu, D.X. (1997) Characterization of Cationic Liposome-Mediated Gene Transfer *in Vivo* by Intravenous Administration. *Human Gene Therapy*, **8**, 1585-1594. http://dx.doi.org/10.1089/hum.1997.8.13-1585

[10] Templeton, N.S., Lasic, D.D., Frederik, P.M., Strey, H.H., Roberts, D.D. and Pavlakis, G.N. (1997) Improved DNA: Liposome Complexes for Increased Systemic Delivery and Gene Expression. *Nature Biotechnology*, **15**, 647-652. http://dx.doi.org/10.1038/nbt0797-647

[11] Lu, C., Stewart, D.J., Lee, J.J., Ji, L., Ramesh, R., Jayachandran, G., Nunez, M.I., Wistuba, I.I., Erasmus, J.J., Hicks, M.E., Grimm, E.A., Reuben, J.M., Baladandayuthapani, V., Templeton, N.S., McMannis, J.D. and Roth, J.A. (2012) Phase I Clinical Trial of Systemically Administered TUSC2(FUS1)-Nanoparticles Mediating Functional Gene Transfer in Humans. *PloS ONE*, **7**, e34833. http://dx.doi.org/10.1371/journal.pone.0034833

[12] Tan, Y., Liu, F., Li, Z., Li, S. and Huang, L. (2001) Sequential Injection of Cationic Liposome and Plasmid DNA Effectively Transfects the Lung with Minimal Inflammatory Toxicity. *Molecular Therapy*, **3**, 673-682. http://dx.doi.org/10.1006/mthe.2001.0311

[13] Tagami, T., Suzuki, T., Matsunaga, M., Nakamura, K., Moriyoshi, N., Ishida, T. and Kiwada, H. (2012) Anti-Angiogenic Therapy via Cationic Liposome-Mediated Systemic siRNA Delivery. *International Journal of Pharmaceutics*, **422**, 280-289. http://dx.doi.org/10.1016/j.ijpharm.2011.10.059

[14] Wollenberg, B., Kastenbauer, H.M., Schaumberg, J., Mayer, A., Andratschke, M., Lang, S., Pauli, C., Zeidler, R., Ihrler, S., Lohrs, K.N. and Rollston, R. (1999) Gene Therapy—Phase I Trial for Primary Untreated Head and Neck Squamous Cell Cancer (HNSCC) UICC Stage II-IV with a Single Intratumoral Injection of hIL-2 Plasmids Formulated in DOTMA/Chol. *Human Gene Therapy*, **10**, 141-147. http://dx.doi.org/10.1089/10430349950019273

[15] Jin, Y., Wang, S., Tong, L. and Du, L. (2015) Rational Design of Didodecyldimethylammonium Bromide-Based Nanoassemblies for Gene Delivery. *Colloids and Surfaces B: Biointerfaces*, **126**, 257-264. http://dx.doi.org/10.1016/j.colsurfb.2014.12.032

[16] Kurosaki, T., Kitahara, T., Fumoto, S., Nishida, K., Yamamoto, K., Nakagawa, H., Kodama, Y., Higuchi, N., Nakamura, T. and Sasaki, H. (2010) Chondroitin Sulfate Capsule System for Efficient and Secure Gene Delivery. *Journal of Pharmacy & Pharmaceutical Sciences*, **13**, 351-361.

[17] Kurosaki, T., Kitahara, T., Kawakami, S., Higuchi, Y., Yamaguchi, A., Nakagawa, H., Kodama, Y., Hamamoto, T., Hashida, M. and Sasaki, H. (2010) Gamma-Polyglutamic Acid-Coated Vectors for Effective and Safe Gene Therapy. *Journal of Controlled Release*, **142**, 404-410. http://dx.doi.org/10.1016/j.jconrel.2009.11.010

[18] Moghimi, S.M. and Hunter, A.C. (2001) Recognition by Macrophages and Liver Cells of Opsonized Phospholipid Vesicles and Phospholipid Headgroups. *Pharmaceutical Research*, **18**, 1-8. http://dx.doi.org/10.1023/A:1011054123304

[19] Hattori, Y., Yamashita, J., Sakaida, C., Kawano, K. and Yonemochi, E. (2015) Evaluation of Antitumor Effect of Zoledronic Acid Entrapped in Folate-Linked Liposome for Targeting to Tumor-Associated Macrophages. *Journal of Liposome Research*, in Press.

[20] Lorenz, C., Hadwiger, P., John, M., Vornlocher, H.P. and Unverzagt, C. (2004) Steroid and Lipid Conjugates of siRNAs to Enhance Cellular Uptake and Gene Silencing in Liver Cells. *Bioorganic & Medicinal Chemistry Letters*, **14**, 4975-4977. http://dx.doi.org/10.1016/j.bmcl.2004.07.018

[21] Nair, J.K., Willoughby, J.L., Chan, A., Charisse, K., Alam, M.R., Wang, Q., Hoekstra, M., Kandasamy, P., Kel'in, A.V., Milstein, S., Taneja, N., O'Shea, J., Shaikh, S., Zhang, L., van der Sluis, R.J., Jung, M.E., Akinc, A., Hutabarat, R., Kuchimanchi, S., Fitzgerald, K., Zimmermann, T., van Berkel, T.J., Maier, M.A., Rajeev, K.G. and Manoharan, M. (2014) Multivalent N-Acetylgalactosamine-Conjugated siRNA Localizes in Hepatocytes and Elicits Robust RNAi-Mediated Gene Silencing. *Journal of the American Chemical Society*, **136**, 16958-16961. http://dx.doi.org/10.1021/ja505986a

18

In Vitro Evaluation of *Sida pilosa* Retz (Malvaceae) Aqueous Extract and Derived Fractions on *Schistosoma mansoni*

Hermine Boukeng Jatsa[1,2,3*], Cintia Aparecida de Jesus Pereira[2], Ana Bárbara Dias Pereira[4], Deborah Aparecida Negrão-Corrêa[2], Fernão Castro Braga[4], Glauber Meireles Maciel[5], Rachel Oliviera Castilho[5], Pierre Kamtchouing[1], Mauro Martins Teixeira[3]

[1]Laboratory of Animal Physiology, Department of Animal Biology and Physiology, Faculty of Science, University of Yaoundé I, Yaoundé, Cameroon

[2]Laboratory of Schistosomiasis, Department of Parasitology, Institute of Biological Sciences, Federal University of Minas Gerais, Belo Horizonte, Brazil

[3]Laboratory of Immunopharmacology, Department of Biochemistry and Immunology, Institute of Biological Sciences, Federal University of Minas Gerais, Belo Horizonte, Brazil

[4]Laboratory of Phytochemistry, Department of Pharmaceutical Products, Faculty of Pharmacy, Federal University of Minas Gerais, Belo Horizonte, Brazil

[5]Laboratory of Pharmacognosy, Department of Pharmaceutical Products, Faculty of Pharmacy, Federal University of Minas Gerais, Belo Horizonte, Brazil

Email: [*]mjatsa@yahoo.fr

Abstract

Sida pilosa Retz. (Malvaceae) is a medicinal plant used in Africa for the treatment of dysmenorrhea, lower abdominal pains and intestinal helminthiasis. *S. pilosa* aqueous extract and derived fractions were investigated for their bioactivity against *Schistosoma mansoni*. The aqueous extract from *S. pilosa* aerial parts (1.25 - 40 mg/mL) and derived fractions (*n*-hexane, DCM, EtOAc and *n*-BuOH: 0.25 - 8 mg/mL) were tested on adult *S. mansoni* maintained in a GMEN culture medium. Praziquantel was used as the reference drug. After 24 h of incubation, worms were monitored for their viability and egg output. The antioxidant activity of *S. pilosa* was evaluated by the ability to scavenge the 2,2-diphenyl-1-picrylhydrazyl free radicals. The chemical composition of the *n*-BuOH fraction was investigated by HPLC-MS analysis. *S. pilosa* aqueous extract and fractions significantly increased worm mortality in a concentration-dependent manner. The *n*-BuOH fraction was the most active with a LC$_{50}$ of 1.25 mg/mL. Significant reduction of motor activity (25% to 100%) was

---

[*]Corresponding author.

recorded for surviving worms incubated in different concentrations of the extract and fractions. Incubation of *S. mansoni* in different concentrations of *S. pilosa* extract and fractions led to significant reduction of egg laying (52% to 100%). The aqueous extract and derived fractions exhibited antioxidant activity in a concentration-dependent manner. The highest antioxidant activity was found with the EtOAc fraction, followed by the DCM and *n*-BuOH fractions. HPLC-MS analysis of the *n*-butanol fraction revealed the presence of two indoloquinoline alkaloids. This study disclosed the schistosomicidal activity of the *n*-butanol fraction from *S. pilosa* aqueous extract. This activity is probably related to the indoloquinoline alkaloids identified in the fraction.

Keywords

Sida pilosa, Schistosomicidal Activity, Antioxidant Activity, Indoloquinoline Alkaloids, *Schistosoma mansoni*

1. Introduction

Schistosomiasis is a chronic and debilitating disease affecting more than 200 million people in tropical and subtropical regions. A major problem in countries where schistosomiasis is endemic is the control of the disease. While preventive chemotherapy is the most important component in schistosomiasis control, other operational components, such as health education for behavioural change, provision of safe water and sanitation, environmental management and snail control, are necessary for a comprehensive control program. Although these actions were effective to decrease mortality and morbidity, schistosomiasis remains a public health concern in most endemic countries [1]. Chemotherapy with praziquantel, a low cost anthelmintic, is still the most effective treatment. Despite its benefits, the intensive use of praziquantel has resulted in reduced cure rates, treatment failure and development of resistant schistosomes strains [2] [3]. Therefore, there is an urgent demand for new effective schistosomicidal drugs. Schistosomiasis is responsible for oxidative damages in the vertebrate host through the release of reactive oxygen species (ROS) [4]. On the other hand, different antioxidant enzymes capable of degrading ROS produced by the host innate immune response have been identified in schistosomes [5]. Therefore, plant extracts or compounds with antioxidant properties in the vertebrate host or that induce oxidative stress on parasite can have antischistosomal activity for drug development.

Considered by the World Health Organization as a neglected tropical disease, little attention has been given to the research and development of new and effective antischistosomal drugs in the last decade [6]. Plants are regarded as a rich source of bioactive molecules, which have provided a number of useful clinical agents. Recently, several *in vitro* studies have been performed to search for new active compounds from medicinal plants against *S. mansoni* and promising results have been reported [7]-[10]. Within this context, we have been evaluating the role of plants as schistosomicidal agents. *Sida pilosa* Retz. (Malvaceae) is a creeping plant founded mainly on the outskirts of dwelling areas and on wastelands. It is empirically used for the treatment of intestinal helminthiasis and lower abdominal pains. To treat intestinal helminthiasis, it is recommended to squeeze the whole plant in water and to drink the macerate as often as possible until healed [11]. Our previous studies demonstrated the schistosomicidal activity of *Sida pilosa* aqueous extract using *in vivo* models. Moreover, phytochemical screening of *S. pilosa* aqueous extract revealed the presence of terpenoids, phenols, tannins and alkaloids [12]. This study was therefore designed to investigate the *in vitro* activity of *S. pilosa* aqueous extract and derived fractions towards *Schistosoma mansoni*.

2. Materials and Methods

2.1. Plant Material

The aerial parts of *S. pilosa* Retz. (Malvaceae) (**Figure 1**) were collected in March 2009 in the locality of Leboudi 2, near Yaoundé city in Cameroon. The authenticity of the material was confirmed against the specimen n° 86/399 (Lejoly) by Prof. Louis Zapfack, botanist at the University of Yaoundé I. A voucher specimen is conserved in the National Herbarium of Yaoundé, Cameroon, under the number 53202/HNC.

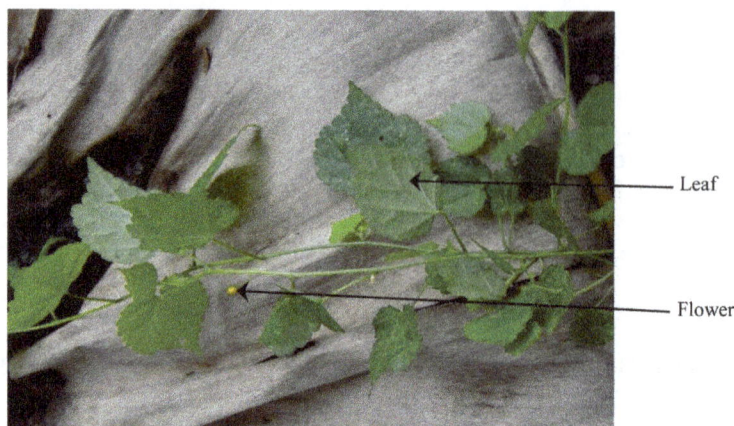

Figure 1. Aerial parts of *Sida pilosa* retz (captured by Hermine Boukeng Jatsa at Leboudi 2 in Cameroon).

2.2. Extraction and Fractionation

Air dried and powdered aerial parts of *S. pilosa* were submitted to static maceration with water (100 g/L) for 24 hours, at room temperature. The solution was filtered, frozen and then lyophilized to give aqueous extract (AE), with a recovery rate of 13.6% w/w. The aqueous extract was fractionated by partition between immiscible solvents, as follows. Portions (5 g × 13) of the *S. pilosa* lyophilized extract were suspended in MeOH/water (1:11) and sequentially partitioned with equal volumes (4 × 50 mL) of *n*-hexane, DCM, EtOAc and *n*-BuOH. Solvents were removed in a rotatory evaporator, at maximum temperature of 50˚C. The process allowed obtaining the *n*-hexane (93.30 mg), dichloromethane (345 mg), ethyl acetate (311 mg) and *n*-butanol (2760 mg) fractions.

2.3. HPLC-MS Analysis

Mass spectrometric analyses were performed at the Analytical Center from the "Universidade de São Paulo" (USP) using an Esquire 3000 plus quadrupole ion trap mass spectrometer (Bruker Daltonics, Billerica, USA). Nitrogen was used both as drying gas and as nebulizing gas (27 psi). The nebulizer temperature was set at 320˚C and a potential of 4 KV was used on the capillary. Analyses were performed at room temperature on a Gemini ODS column (250 × 4.6 mm i.d., 5 μm; Phenomenex, Torrance, CA, USA), eluted with a gradient of water and ACN (0% to 20% ACN in 30 min, 20% to 40% ACN in 5 min and return to the initial condition in 5 min), at a flow rate of 0.5 mL/min and UV detection at 210 nm. Reagents used in these analyses were of HPLC grade. A flow rate of 90 μL/min was employed for the MS analyses and positive ion mass spectra were recorded in the range *m/z* 50 - 2000. Data analysis was carried out by the interpretation of spectral data and by comparison with literature records on the chemical composition of other *Sida* species [13]-[16].

2.4. Parasite Culture and Maintenance

SWISS mice obtained from the University animal facility (CEBIO, ICB-UFMG) were subcutaneously infected with 130 cercariae of the LE strain of *S. mansoni* released from experimentally infected *Biomphalaria glabrata* at the Laboratory of Schistosomiasis (ICB/UFMG). After 7 weeks of infection, adult worms were recovered under aseptic conditions by perfusion of the mesenteric veins and liver accordingly to the method described by Pellegrino and Siqueira [17]. The experimental procedures received prior approval from the local animal ethics committee and were in accordance with the ethical principles in animal research adopted by the Brazilian National Council on Animal Experimentation (CONCEA). Adult *S. mansoni* worms (male and female) recovered from infected animals were washed three times in a Glasgow Minimum Essential Medium (GMEM-Sigma, St Louis, USA) supplemented with an antibiotic-antimycotic solution (10,000 U/mL penicillin, 10,000 μg/mL streptomycin and 25 μg/mL amphotericin B (Atlanta Biologicals, Lawrenceville, USA) and gentamicine (40 μg/mL). To test the effect of *S. pilosa* extract and derived fractions on *S. mansoni* adult worms, the bioassay followed the standard operating procedures that recommended at least 5 females and 5 males per treatment [18]. In this bioassay, 10 male and 10 female adult worms were transferred to each well of a 24-well culture plate (NUNC) containing 1800 μL of complete GMEM culture medium [GMEM medium buffered to pH 7.5 containing 20 mM of HEPES, 40 μg/mL gentamicine, 50 μg/mL penicillin, 50 μg/mL streptomycin, 100 μg/mL neomycin, 2 mM of L-glutamine and 5% heat-inactivated foetal bovine serum (GIBCO, Brazil)]. The plates were then incubated for 2 hours at 37°C in a humid atmosphere containing 5% CO_2 prior addition of products.

2.5. *In Vitro* Assays with *Schistosoma mansoni*

A wide range of concentrations (10 μg/mL to 50 mg/mL) is generally employed for *in vitro* screening of plants extracts or compounds for antischistosomal activity [7]-[10]. In this study, lyophilized crude extract of *S. pilosa* was initially dissolved in distilled water, filtered through a 0.2 μm sterile syringe filter and diluted in complete GMEM culture medium to a final concentration of 40, 20, 10, 5, 2.5 and 1.25 mg/mL. The *n*-hexane, DCM, EtOAc and *n*-BuOH fractions were dissolved in DMSO and diluted in the culture medium to final concentrations of 8, 4, 2, 1, 0.5 and 0.25 mg/mL. It is important to mention that the final volume was 2 mL/well and the maximum concentration of DMSO in each well was 0.5% v/v. Negative control for organic fractions was GMEN medium containing 0.5% of DMSO while GMEN medium was the negative control for the aqueous extract. Praziquantel was used as positive control at 100 μg/mL of final concentration. Quadruplicate measurements were carried out for each concentration and two independent experiments were performed for each sample. Culture plates were kept at 37°C for 24 h in a 5% CO_2 incubator; afterwards, worms were monitored to evaluate their viability and egg production by examination under an inverted microscope (Olympus CK × 41, Tokyo, Japan). Reduction of motor activity was defined as absence of worm motility apart from gut movements and occasional movement of head and tail of schistosome. Parasite death was defined as the absence of motor activity during 2 minutes. The median lethal concentration (LC_{50}) was calculated using the Trimmed Spearman-Karber (TSK) method [19], version 1.5 software downloaded from the US Environmental Protection Agency.

2.6. Radical Scavenging Activity—DPPH Assay

The antioxidant activity of *S. pilosa* aqueous extract and fractions was assessed using the 2, 2-diphenyl-1-picrylhydrazyl (DPPH) assay [20]. The crude extract was dissolved in distilled water and the fractions in methanol. Serial dilutions were carried out to give five concentrations in the range of 25 to 200 μg/mL for the crude extract and hexane fraction; and of 10 to 100 μg/mL for the other fractions. Each sample (2.5 mL) was mixed with 1 mL of a methanolic solution of 0.3 mMol DPPH. Rutin was employed as positive control (2.5, 10, 15, 20, and 25 μg/mL). The tests were carried out in quadruplicate. After 30 min of incubation at room temperature, in the dark, absorbance was recorded at 515 nm on a UV-VIS spectrophotometer (Hitachi U 2900, Tokyo, Japan). The antioxidant activity (AA%) was calculated according to the equation AA% = [(A_C − A_S)/A_C] × 100, where A_C is the absorbance of the control (DPPH solution) and A_S is the absorbance of the test sample. The antioxidant activity (AA%) was plotted against sample concentration, and a linear regression curve was established in order to calculate the effective concentration (EC_{50}) of the sample required to scavenge DPPH radical by 50% [20].

2.7. Statistical Analysis

Results were expressed as mean ± SEM. Data were analyzed by one-way ANOVA followed by Newman-Keuls multiple comparison test, performed using GraphPad Prism version 4.00 for Windows (GraphPad Software, San Diego, USA). The level of significance was set at $p < 0.05$.

3. Results

3.1. Mortality of Schistosomes

The mortality rate of adult *S. mansoni* worms following *in vitro* exposure to different concentrations of *S. pilosa* aqueous extract and derived fractions is shown on **Figure 2**. There was a concentration-dependent increase in mortality of adult *S. mansoni* worms after incubation with the aqueous extract and fractions. After 24 h incubation of worms with either 20 or 40 mg/mL of the extract, 100% of the worms were dead. Moreover, we recorded mortality rates of 81%, 58%, 90%, and 100% for worms incubated respectively with 8 mg/mL of the *n*-hexane, DCM, EtOAc and *n*-BuOH fractions ($p < 0.001$). Incubation of the worms with the EtOAc (0.25 mg/mL), *n*-hexane and DCM fractions (0.25 to 2 mg/mL) did not promote any worm death. No death was observed in the negative control groups (GMEN medium and 0.5% DMSO + GMEN medium). In the positive control group incubated with praziquantel (100 µg/mL), all parasites died within 24 h post-incubation. The evaluation of the median lethal concentration (LC_{50}) of *S. pilosa* aqueous extract and fractions, using the Trimmed Spearman-Karber method, disclosed the *n*-BuOH fraction as the most active one with LC_{50} of 1.25 mg/mL (0.98 - 1.62 mg/mL) (**Table 1**).

3.2. Motor Activity

Absence of worm motility apart from gut movements and minimal motor activity marked by weak movement of the suckers and occasional sway of the body were recorded in surviving worms treated with *S. pilosa* aqueous extract and various fractions. The reduction of motor activity reached 100% for all the worms exposed to GMEM medium containing 10 mg/ml of *S. pilosa* aqueous extract or 8 mg/mL of *n*-hexane and EtOAc fractions and 4 mg/mL of the *n*-BuOH fraction. The addition of 8 mg/mL of the DCM fraction also resulted in reduction of worm motility by 80%. The reduction of motor activity varied from 27% to 40% with the crude extract (1.25 to 5 mg/mL) and from 25% to 79% with the *n*-BuOH fraction (0.25 to 2 mg/mL) (**Figure 3**). Adult *S. mansoni* worms belonging to the negative control groups (GMEN medium and 0.5% DMSO + GMEN medium) showed normal motor activity marked by undulatory movements of the body and peristaltic waves along the body.

3.3. Egg Output

Oviposition was followed and the number of eggs per female evaluated after 24 h of incubation with the extract

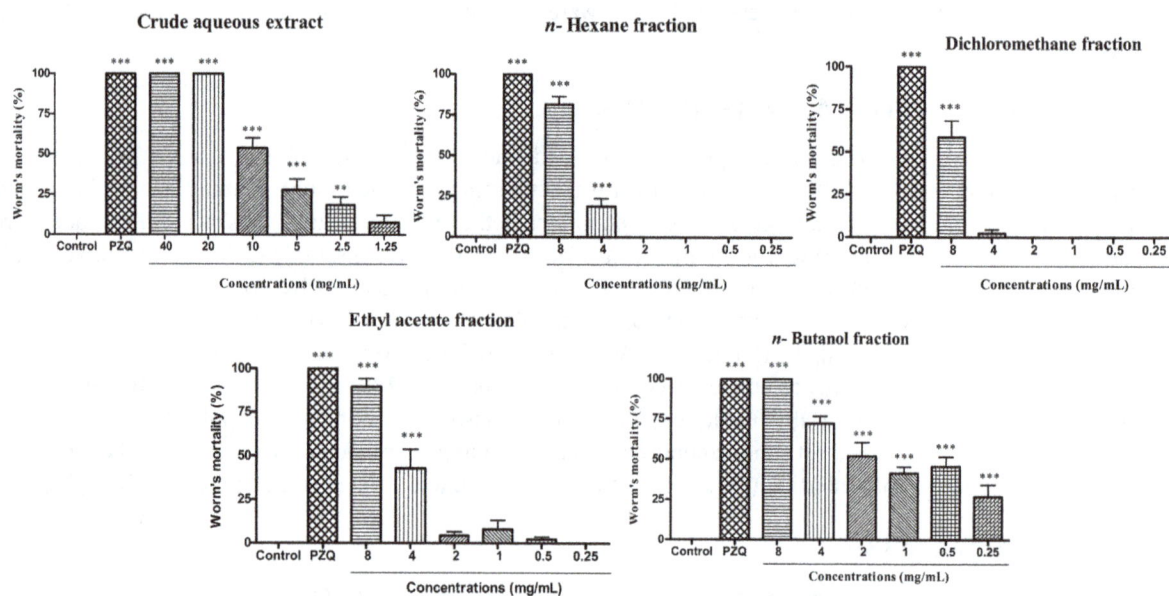

, *: values are significantly different from controls (culture medium or culture medium + 0.5% DMSO) at $p < 0.01$ and $p < 0.001$ respectively.

Figure 2. *In vitro* effect of *Sida pilosa* aqueous extract and various fractions on the mortality of *Schistosoma mansoni* after 24 h of incubation.

Table 1. Median lethal concentration (LC_{50}) values of *Sida pilosa* aqueous extract and various fractions.

Sida pilosa	LC_{50} (mg/mL)	95% low limit (mg/mL)	95% upper limit (mg/mL)
Aqueous extract	8.57	6.88	10.74
n-Hexane fraction	5.70	5.10	6.38
DCM fraction	7.03	6.27	7.88
EtOAc fraction	4.54	3.78	5.45
n-BuOH fraction	1.25	0.98	1.62

DCM fraction: dichloromethane fraction; EtOAc fraction: ethyl acetate fraction; *n*-BuOH fraction: *n*-butanol fraction.

or fractions (**Figure 4**). It generally appeared that *S. pilosa* aqueous extract and various fractions inhibited egg production. Egg laying was completely abolished by the aqueous extract at 40 mg/mL and concentrations from 20 to 2.5 mg/mL significantly reduced it by 99% to 66%. In comparison with the negative control group, treatment with the *n*-BuOH fraction from 8 to 0.25 mg/mL significantly decreased the number of eggs (97% to 85%) after 24 h of incubation ($p < 0.001$). Egg production was also reduced by the *n*-hexane, DCM and EtOAc fractions assayed at 8 mg/mL by 99%, 97% and 98% respectively. Praziquantel did not suppress the egg output, but reduced it by 98%. Reduction of oviposition was not only observed in wells containing dead worms, but also in wells where no mortality was recorded. For example, the *n*-hexane fraction (2 mg/mL) decreased egg production by 86%. The egg laying reduction also varied from 52% to 67% when worms were treated with DCM fraction (2 to 0.25 mg/mL). Significant negative correlations were established between mortality and egg output ($r = -0.60$, $r^2 = 0.36$, $p < 0.001$) and between decreased motor activity and egg output ($r = -0.42$, $r^2 = 0.18$, $p < 0.05$) for the

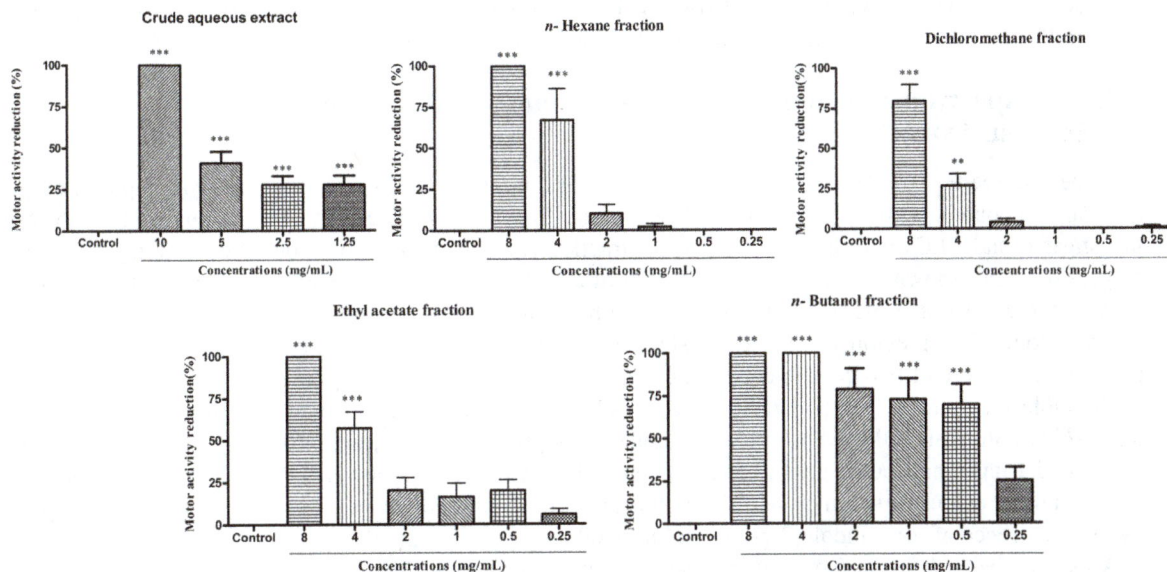

,*: values are significantly different from controls (culture medium or culture medium + 0.5% DMSO) at $p < 0.01$ and $p < 0.001$ respectively.

Figure 3. *In vitro* effect of *Sida pilosa* aqueous extract and various fractions on the motor activity of *Schistosoma mansoni* after 24 h of incubation.

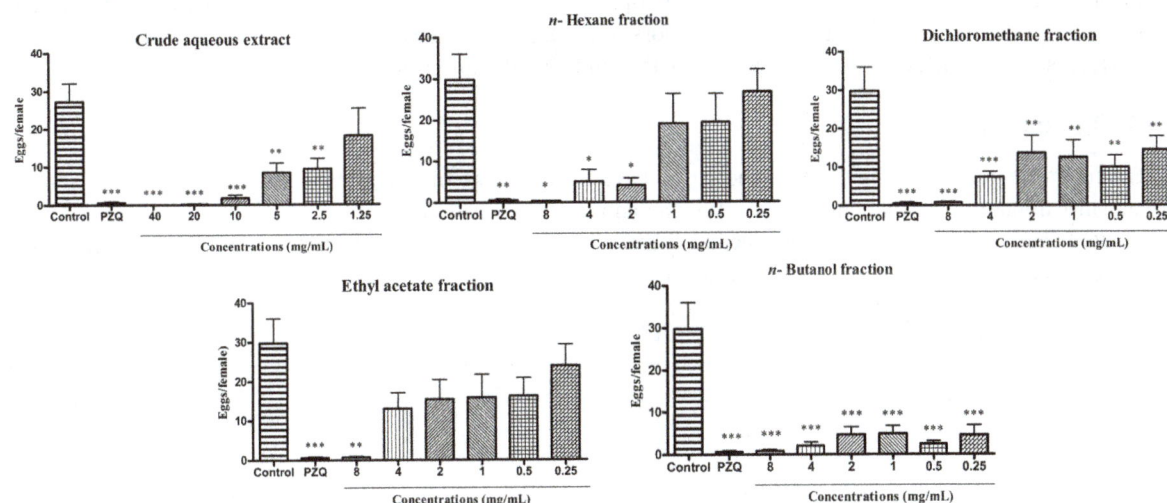

*,**,***: values are significantly different from controls (culture medium or culture medium + 0.5% DMSO) at $p < 0.05$, $p < 0.01$ and $p < 0.001$ respectively.

Figure 4. *In vitro* effect of *Sida pilosa* aqueous extract and various fractions on the egg output of *Schistosoma mansoni* after 24 h of incubation.

aqueous extract. No significant correlation between decreased motor activity and egg output was established for worms incubated with the n-BuOH fraction, but a significant negative correlation between mortality and egg output ($r = -0.45$, $r^2 = 0.20$, $p < 0.001$) was found.

3.4. DPPH Radical Scavenging Activity

The *in vitro* antioxidant activity of *S. pilosa* aqueous extract and fractions was evaluated by the capacity of samples to scavenge free radicals of DPPH. The aqueous extract and derived fractions exhibited antioxidant activity in a concentration-dependent manner. The EtOAc fraction exhibited the strongest antioxidant activity with an EC_{50} of 46.01 ± 0.63 μg/mL. The DCM and n-BuOH fractions also induced significant antioxidant response, with EC_{50} values of 60.85 ± 0.20 μg/mL and 81.14 ± 0.56 μg/mL, respectively. Although these fractions exhibited significant antioxidant activity, the EC_{50} value of the positive control rutin was 3 times lower than that of most active fraction (EtOAc fraction) (**Table 2**). The n-hexane fraction exhibited a poor radical scavenging activity (528.98 ± 3.91 μg/mL) and the aqueous extract was active at the highest concentration (150 μg/mL).

3.5. Mass Spectrometry Analysis of the *n*-Butanol Fraction from *Sida pilosa* Aqueous Extract

As expected, the HPLC-MS chromatogram recorded for the n-butanol fraction was majorly composed by peaks of polar compounds, with retention times below 20 min (**Figure 5(a)**). The chemistry of *S. pilosa* has never been investigated and TLC analyses of the n-butanol fraction revealed two major spots after spraying Dragendorff reagent (data not shown), suggesting the presence of alkaloids. Therefore, the MS data obtained for the constituents of the fraction were initially compared with literature records of alkaloids isolated from other *Sida* species. None of the previously reported alkaloids was identified in the fraction, but it was possible to conjecture the chemical nature of two constituents. Hence, the minor peak eluted at 4.6 min (compound **1**), corresponding to the molecular ion $[M + H]^+$ detected at m/z 543 (**Figure 5(b)**), was credited to a diglycoside of an indolo[3,2-*b*]quinoline alkaloid, whose putative structure is presented in **Figure 4(d)**. The proposed structure of compound **1** has a molecular mass of 542.19, compatible with the obtained HPLC-MS data. This hypothesis is based on the previous isolation of indoloquinoline alkaloids from *Sida acuta* [13] [14] [16] and is also supported by the occurrence of some indolo[3,2-*b*]quinoline alkaloid glycosides in other plant species [15].

A peak eluted at 9.3 min (compound **2**) was also present in the HPLC-MS profile of the n-butanol fraction, which produced the molecular ion $[M + H]^+$ detected at m/z 295 (**Figure 5(c)**). According to the obtained data, it was possible to infer the molecular mass of 294.14 for compound **2**. Its putative structure (**Figure 5(d)**) was proposed by comparison with the chemical structure of compound **1** and by analysis of literature data reported for indoloquinoline alkaloids from *S. acuta* [13] [14] [16]. The putative structure is supported by the fragment ion at m/z 276.9 $[M - 18]^+$ resulting from the loss of H_2O, as well as by the parent ion at m/z 248.8 $[M + H - 15 - 31]^+$, ascribed to the elimination of both a methyl and a methoxyl group (data not shown).

4. Discussion

Specie of the genus *Sida* have been reported to have a wide range of biological activities that include analgesic, anti-inflammatory, antioxidant, antibacterial and anthelmintic activities [16] [21]-[23]. Jatsa *et al.* [12] have previously shown the *in vivo* schistosomicidal activity of *S. pilosa* aqueous extract against *S. mansoni*. With the perspective of searching new active compounds against *Schistosoma* species, the activity of *S. pilosa* aqueous

Table 2. Antioxidant activity of fractions from *Sida pilosa* aqueous extract on 2, 2-diphenyl-1-picrylhydrazyl (DPPH).

Sida pilosa	EC_{50} (μg/mL)
n-Hexane fraction	528.98 ± 3.91***
Dichloromethane fraction	60.85 ± 0.20***
Ethyl acetate fraction	46.01 ± 0.63***
n-Butanol fraction	81.14 ± 0.56***
Rutin	14.81 ± 0.01

Results are mean ± SEM (n = 4). ***: values are significantly different from rutin (positive control) at $p < 0.001$.

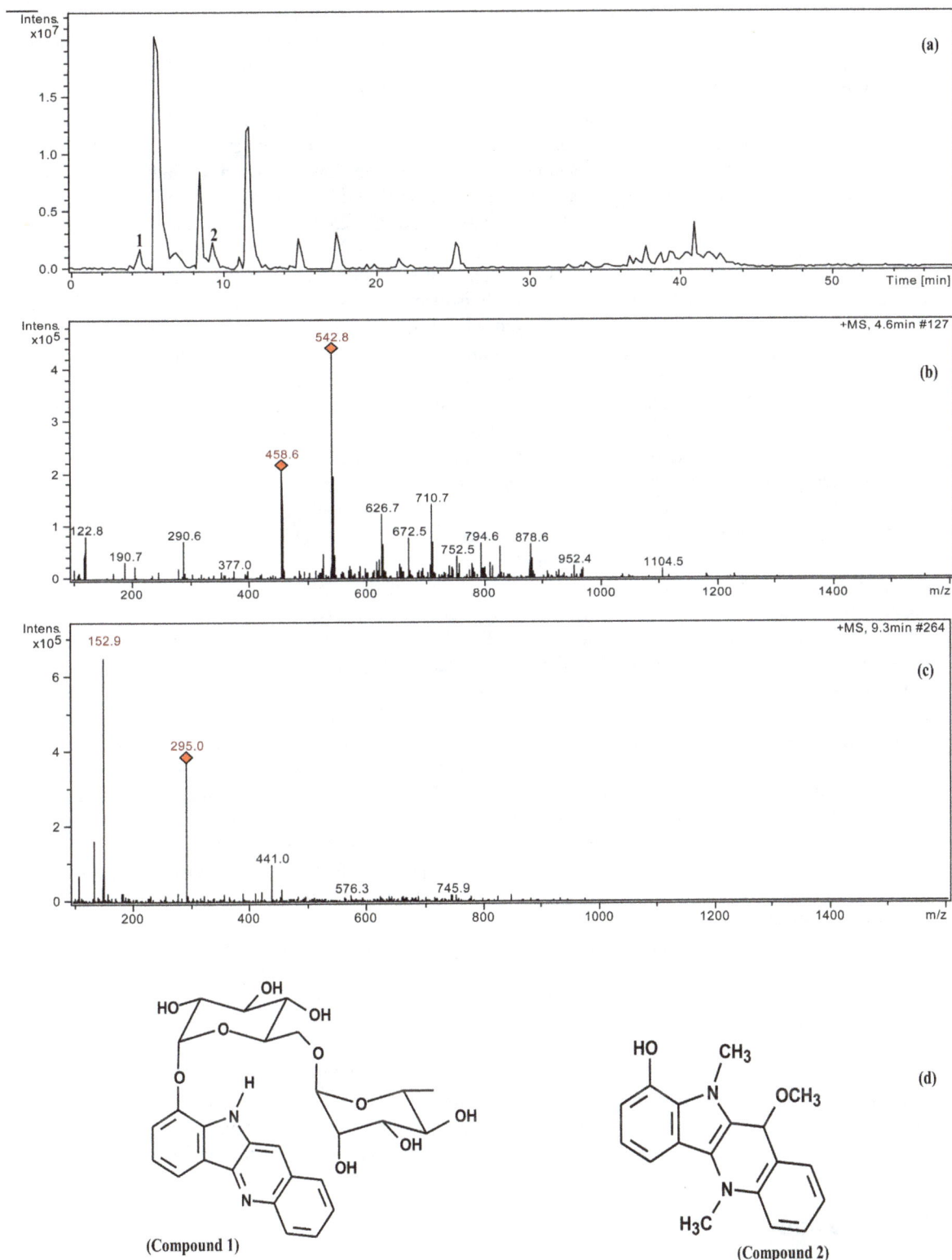

Figure 5. HPLC-MS chromatograms of the *n*-butanol fraction from *Sida pilosa* aqueous extract and the structure of indolo-quinoline alkaloids identified in the fraction. (a) HPLC chromatogram of the *n*-butanol fraction from *Sida pilosa* aqueous extract; (b) Mass spectrum of compound 1 of the *n*-butanol fraction; (c) Mass spectrum of compound 2 of the *n*-butanol fraction; (d) Structure of the two indoloquinoline alkaloids (compound **1** and compound **2**).

extract and fractions thereof were assayed *in vitro* at different concentrations.

The first parameter to consider was adult *S. mansoni* mortality. This bioassay clearly showed that the aqueous extract and various fractions were active against *S. mansoni* in a concentration-dependent manner. A similar concentration-dependent bioactivity has been reported for *Sida acuta* ethanol extract and *Sida cordifolia* aqueous and ethanol extracts against some helminths [22] [23]. Lethal concentrations of *S. pilosa* aqueous extract (20 mg/mL) and its *n*-butanol fraction (8 mg/mL) were in the range of lethal concentrations (0.6 to 25 mg/mL) of plant species popularly used against schistosomiasis in South Africa and Zimbabwe [7] [8]. In the present work, evaluation of the median lethal concentration (LC_{50}) of the aqueous extract and derived fractions disclosed the *n*-butanol fraction as the most active, with a LC_{50} of 1.25 mg/mL. Many authors have reported that biological activities displayed by some species of *Sida* are generally attributed to alkaloids present in those plants [13] [16] [24] [25]. The chemical composition of the *n*-butanol fraction was therefore characterized by HPLC-MS analyses. None of the alkaloids previously isolated from other *Sida* species was identified in the fraction by comparison with their MS data. On the other hand, it was possible to propose the putative structures of two indoloquinoline alkaloids present in the fraction. These compounds will be isolated in the future for the unambiguous elucidation of their chemical structures by spectroscopic methods. Potential biological activities of alkaloids isolated from *S. acuta* have been described by Banzouzi *et al.* [14] which identified an indoloquinoline, the cryptolepine, as an active constituent associated with the antiplasmodial activity displayed by the extract of the aerial parts of *S. acuta*. Karou *et al.* [16] [26] also associated the antimalarial and antibacterial activities of the same specie to the presence of cryptolepine and quindoline. In view of these biological activities of alkaloids, it is possible that the schistosomicidal activity displayed by the *n*-butanol fraction from *S. pilosa* aqueous extract is related to the presence of indoloquinoline alkaloids in the fraction. This fraction could be considered as a promising source for schistosomicidal compounds.

Motor activity is often evaluated as indicator of biological activity of schistosome species. A concentration-dependent reduction of worm motor activity was observed, particularly with the *n*-BuOH fraction. Absence of motility apart from guts movement, feeble motor activity and reduction of peristaltic waves along schistosomes' body after incubation in *S. pilosa* could be the consequence of the plant interference with the mechanism of contraction-relaxation of worm smooth muscles [27]. The reduction of worm motor activity was also reported after incubation of schistosomes with medicinal plants products [10] [28]-[31]. Results from this study showed that 18% of the variability of egg production was correlated to the reduction of motor activity after incubation of worms with the extract whereas worms' mortality was correlated to 36% or 20% of the variability of egg laying after incubation of worms with the extract or the fraction. The reduction of egg output could be the consequence of cytotoxic damage or specific inhibition of worm reproductive processes by one or more compounds present in medicinal plants [9]. It has been demonstrated that the inhibition of larval migration, adult worm motility and egg excretion in helminths are associated with the consumption of tannins by their hosts [32]-[34]. It then appeared that tannins present in *S. pilosa* [12] could be involved in the reduction of worm motility and reproductive processes of schistosomes.

Reactive oxygen species contribute to a large variety of diseases, including schistosomiasis [4]. Extracts or compounds that induce oxidative stress on the parasite or which have antioxidant activity on the vertebrate host might represent a potential therapeutic approach for schistosomiasis. The DPPH assay was therefore used to evaluate the scavenging capacity of *S. pilosa*. The aqueous extract and derived fractions exhibited antioxidant activity in a concentration-dependent manner. The highest antioxidant activity was found with the EtOAc fraction, followed by the DCM and *n*-BuOH fractions. When Shah *et al.* [35] studied the DPPH radical scavenging activity of the methanolic extract of *Sida cordata* (synonym of *S. pilosa*) and fractions, the ethyl acetate fraction also show the best antioxidant activity. This antioxidant potential was correlate to the phenolic and flavonoid contents of the fraction. The presence of phenols in *S. pilosa* [8] could be responsible for its antioxidant potential.

5. Conclusion

Results from this study indicate that the *n*-butanol fraction from *Sida pilosa* aqueous extract possesses *in vitro* schistosomicidal activity against *Schistosoma mansoni* adult worms and antioxidant potential. This schistosomicidal activity is probably related to indoloquinolines alkaloids present in the fraction. Further studies are needed on the isolation and bioactivity evaluation of these compounds. Moreover, *in vivo* safety and efficacy of the *n*-butanol fraction and individual compounds on schistosomiasis mansoni also need to be investigated.

In Vitro Evaluation of Sida pilosa Retz (Malvaceae) Aqueous Extract and Derived...

187

Acknowledgements

Authors are grateful to the International Foundation for Science (IFS) for financial support through grant F/3622-2F and to the CNPq-TWAS Postdoctoral Fellowship (FR 3240188106) to "Hermine Boukeng Jatsa" at the Federal University of Minas Gerais (UFMG) in Brazil.

References

[1] WHO (2013) Schistosomiasis: Progress Report 2001-2011 and Strategic Plan 2012-2020. WHO Press, Geneva, 1-74.

[2] Ismael, M., Botros, S., Metwally, A., William, S., Farchally, A., Tao, L.F., Day, T.A. and Bennett, J.L. (1999) Resistance to Praziquantel: Direct Evidence from Schistosoma mansoni Isolated from Egyptian Villagers. American Journal of Tropical Medicine and Hygiene, 60, 932-935.

[3] Cioli, D. (2000) Praziquantel: Is There Real Resistance and Are There Alternative? Current Opinion in Infectious Diseases, 13, 659-663. http://dx.doi.org/10.1097/00001432-200012000-00014

[4] Rizk, M., Fayed, T.A., Badawy, M. and El-Regal, N.S. (2006) Effect of Different Durations of Schistosoma mansoni Infection on the Levels of Some Antioxidants in Mice. Medical Journal of the Islamic World Academic of Sciences, 16, 25-34.

[5] Pal, C. and Bandyopadhyay, U. (2012) Redox-Active Antiparasitic Drugs. Antioxidants & Redox Signaling, 17, 555-582. http://dx.doi.org/10.1089/ars.2011.4436

[6] WHO (2000) General Guidelines for Methodologies on Research and Evaluation of Traditional Medicine. WHO Press, Geneva, 1-80.

[7] Sparg, S.G., van Staden, J. and Jäger, A.K. (2000) Efficiency of Traditionally Used South African Plants against Schistosomiasis. Journal of Ethnopharmacology, 73, 209-214. http://dx.doi.org/10.1016/S0378-8741(00)00310-X

[8] Molgaard, P., Nielsen, S.B., Rasmussen, D.E., Drummond, R.B., Makaza, N. and Andreassen, J. (2001) Anthelmintic Screening of Zimbabwean Plants Traditionally Used against Schistosomiasis. Journal of Ethnopharmacology, 74, 257-264. http://dx.doi.org/10.1016/S0378-8741(00)00377-9

[9] Sanderson, L., Bartlett, A. and Whitfield, P.J. (2002) In Vitro and in Vivo Studies on the Bioactivity of a Ginger (Zingiber officinale) Extract towards Adult Schistosomes and Their Egg Production. Journal of Helminthology, 76, 241-247. http://dx.doi.org/10.1079/JOH2002116

[10] de Melo, N.I., Magalhães, L.G., de Carvalho, C.E., Wakabayashi, K.A.L., Aguiar, G.P., Ramos, R.C., Mantovani, A.L.L., Turatti, I.C.C., Rodrigues, V., Groppo, M., Cunha, W.R., Veneziani, R.C.S. and Crotti, A.E.M. (2011) Schistosomicidal Activity of the Essential Oil of Ageratum conyzoides L. (Asteraceae) against Adult Schistosoma mansoni Worms. Molecules, 16, 762-773. http://dx.doi.org/10.3390/molecules16010762

[11] Adjanohoun, J.E., Aboubakar, N., Dramane, K., Ebot, M.E., Ekpere, J.A., Enow-Orock, E.G., Focho, D., Gbile, Z.O., Kamanyi, A., Kamsu Kom, J., Keita, A., Mbenkum, T., Mbi, C.N., Mbiele, A.L., Mbome, I.L., Mubiru, N.K., Naney, W.L., Nkongmeneck, B., Satabie, B., Sofowora, A., Tamze, V. and Wirmum, C.K. (1996) Traditional Medicine and Pharmacopoeia: Contribution to Ethnobotanical and Floristic Studies in Cameroon. CSTR/OUA, CNPMS, Porto-Novo.

[12] Jatsa, H.B., Endougou, A.M.E., Kemeta, D.R.A., Kenfack, C.M., Tchuem Tchuente, L.A. and Kamtchouing, P. (2009) In Vivo Antischistosomal and Toxicological Evaluation of Sida pilosa Retz on Mice BALB/c. Pharmacologyonline, 3, 531-538.

[13] Jang, D.S., Park, E.J., Kang, Y.-H., Su, B.-N., Hawthorne, M.E., Vigo, J.S., Graham, J.G., Cabieses, F., Fong, H.H.S., Mehta, R.G., Pezzuto, J.M. and Kinghorn, A.D. (2003) Compounds Obtained from Sida acuta with the Potential to Induce Quinone Reductase and to Inhibit 7,12-Dimethylbenz-[a] Anthracene-Induced Preneoplastic Lesions in a Mouse Mammary Organ Culture Model. Archives of Pharmaceutical Research, 26, 585-590. http://dx.doi.org/10.1007/BF02976704

[14] Banzouzi, J.-T., Prado, R., Menan, H., Valentin, A., Roumestan, C., Mallié, M., Banzouzi, J.-T., Prado, R., Menan, H., Valentin, A., Roumestan, C., Mallié, M., Pelissier, Y. and Blache, Y. (2004) Studies on Medicinal Plants of Ivory Coast: Investigation of Sida acuta for in Vitro Antiplasmodial Activities and Identification of an Active Constituent. Phytomedicine, 11, 338-341. http://dx.doi.org/10.1078/0944711041495245

[15] Subbaraju, G.V., Kavitha, J., Rajasekhar, D. and Jimenez, J.I. (2004) Jusbetonin, the First Indolo[3,2-b]Quinoline Alkaloid Glycoside, from Justicia betonica. Journal of Natural Products, 67, 461-462. http://dx.doi.org/10.1021/np030392y

[16] Karou, D., Savadogo, A., Canini, A., Yameogo, S., Montesano, C., Simpore, J., Colizzi, V. and Traore, A.S. (2005) Antibacterial Activity of Alkaloids from Sida acuta. African Journal of Biotechnology, 4, 1452-1457.

[17] Pellegrino, J. and Siqueira, A.F. (1968) Técnica de Perfusão Para Colheita de Schistosoma mansoni em Cobaias Experimentalmente Infestadas. Revista Brasileira de Malariologia e Doenças Tropicais, 8, 589-597.

[18] Ramirez, B., Bickle, Q., Yousif, F., Fakorede, F., Mouries, M.-A. and Nwaka, S. (2007) Schistosomes: Challenges in Compound Screening. *Expert Opinion on Drug Discovery*, **2**, S53-S61. http://dx.doi.org/10.1517/17460441.2.s1.s53

[19] Hamilton, M.A., Russo, R.C. and Thurston, R.V. (1977) Trimmed Spearman-Karber Method for Estimating Median Lethal Concentrations in Toxicity Bioassays. *Environmental Science & Technology*, **11**, 714-719. http://dx.doi.org/10.1021/es60130a004

[20] Lee, S.K., Mbwambo, Z.H., Chung, H., Luyengi, L., Gamez, E.J., Mehta, R.G., Kinghorn, A.D. and Pezzuto, J.M. (1998) Evaluation of the Antioxidant Potential of Natural Products. *Combinatorial Chemistry & High Throughput Screening*, **1**, 35-46.

[21] Franzotti, E.M., Santos, C.V.F., Rodrigues, H.M.S.L., Mourão, R.H.V., Andrade, M.R. and Antoniolli, A.R. (2000) Anti-Inflammatory, Analgesic Activity and Acute Toxicity of *Sida cordifolia* L. (Malva-Branca). *Journal of Ethnopharmacology*, **72**, 273-278. http://dx.doi.org/10.1016/S0378-8741(00)00205-1

[22] Olabiyi, T.I., Oyedunmade, E.E.A., Ibikunle, G.J., Ojo, O.A., Adesina, G.O., Adelasoye, K.A. and Ogunniran, T.A. (2008) Chemical Composition and Bio-Nematicidal Potential of Some Weed Extracts on *Meloidogyne incognita* under Laboratory Conditions. *Plant Sciences Research*, **1**, 30-35.

[23] Pawa, R.S., Jain, A., Sharma, P., Chaurasiya, P.K. and Singour, P.K. (2011) *In Vitro* Studies on *Sida cordifolia* Linn for Anthelmintic and Antioxidant Properties. *Chinese Medicine*, **2**, 47-52. http://dx.doi.org/10.4236/cm.2011.22009

[24] Gunatilaka, A.A.L., Sotheeswaran, S., Balasubramaniam, S., Chandrasekara, A.I. and Sriyani, H.T.B. (1980) Studies on Medicinal Plants of Sri Lanka. III. Pharmacologically Important Alkaloids of Some Sida Species. *Planta Medica*, **39**, 66-72. http://dx.doi.org/10.1055/s-2008-1074904

[25] Sutradhar, R.K., Rahman, A.M., Ahmad, M., Bachar, S.C., Saha, A. and Guha, S.K. (2006) Bioactive Alkaloid from *Sida cordifolia* Linn. with Analgesic and Anti-Inflammatory Activities. *Iranian Journal of Pharmacology & Therapeutics*, **5**, 175-178.

[26] Karou, D., Dicko, M.H., Sanon, S., Simpore, J. and Traore, A.S. (2003) Antimalarial Activity of *Sida acuta* Burm f. (Malvaceae) and *Pterocarpus erinaceus* Poir. (Fabaceae). *Journal of Ethnopharmacology*, **89**, 291-294. http://dx.doi.org/10.1016/j.jep.2003.09.010

[27] Doenhoff, M.J., Cioli, D. and Utzinger, J. (2008) Praziquantel: Mechanisms of Action, Resistance and New Derivatives for Schistosomiasis. *Current Opinion in Infectious Diseases*, **21**, 659-667. http://dx.doi.org/10.1097/QCO.0b013e328318978f

[28] Magalhães, L.G., Machado, C.B., Morais, E.R., de Carvalho Moreira, E.B., Soares, C.S., da Silva, S.H., da Silva Filho, A.A. and Rodrigues, V. (2009) *In Vitro* Schistosomicidal Activity of Curcumin against *Schistosoma mansoni* Adult Worms. *Parasitology Research*, **104**, 1197-1201. http://dx.doi.org/10.1007/s00436-008-1311-y

[29] Magalhães, L.G., Kapadia, G.J., da Silva Tonuci, L.R., Caixeta, S.C., Parreira, N.A., Rodrigues, V. and da Silva Filho, A.A. (2010) *In Vitro* Schistosomicidal Effects of Some Phloroglucinol Derivates from *Dryopteris* Species against *Schistosoma mansoni* Adult Worms. *Parasitology Research*, **106**, 395-401. http://dx.doi.org/10.1007/s00436-009-1674-8

[30] De Moraes, J., Nascimento, C., Lopes, P.O.M.V., Nakano, E., Yamaguchi, L.F., Kato, M.J. and Kawano, T. (2011) *Schistosoma mansoni*: *In Vitro* Schistosomicidal Activity of Piplartine. *Experimental Parasitology*, **127**, 357-364. http://dx.doi.org/10.1016/j.exppara.2010.08.021

[31] Xiao, S., Mei, J. and Jiao, P. (2009) The *in Vitro* Effect of Mefloquine and Praziquantel against Juvenile and Adult *Schistosoma japonicum*. *Parasitology Research*, **106**, 237-243. http://dx.doi.org/10.1007/s00436-009-1656-x

[32] Molan, A.L., Waghorn, G.C., Min, B.R. and Mc Nabb, W.C. (2000) The Effect of Condensed Tannins from Seven Herbages on *Trichostrongylus colubriformis* Larval Migration *in Vitro*. *Folia Parasitologica*, **47**, 39-44. http://dx.doi.org/10.14411/fp.2000.007

[33] Hoste, H., Brunet, S., Bahuaud, D., Chauveau, S., Fouraste, I. and Lefrileux, Y. (2009) Compared *in Vitro* Anthelmintic Effects of Eight Tannin-Rich Plants Browsed by Goats in the Southern Part of France. *Options Méditérranéennes*, **85**, 431-436.

[34] Paolini, V., Bergeaud, J.P., Grisez, C., Prevot, F., Dorchies, P.H. and Hoste, H. (2003) Effects of Condensed Tannins on Goats Experimentally Infected with *Haemonchus contortus*. *Veterinary Parasitology*, **113**, 253-261. http://dx.doi.org/10.1016/S0304-4017(03)00064-5

[35] Shah, N.A., Khan, M.R., Ahmad, B., Noureen, F., Rashid, U. and Khan, R.A. (2013) Investigation on Flavonoid Composition and Anti Free Radical Potential of *Sida cordata*. *BMC Complementary and Alternative Medicine*, **13**, 276-288. http://dx.doi.org/10.1186/1472-6882-13-276

19

In Vitro Anti-HIV Activity of Partially Purified Coumarin(s) Isolated from Fungal Endophyte, *Alternaria* Species of *Calophyllum inophyllum*

Melappa Govindappa[1*], Kavya C. Hemmanur[1], Shrikanta Nithin[1], Chandrappa Chinna Poojari[1], Gopalakrishna Bhat Kakunje[2], Channabasava[1]

[1]Endophytic Natural Product Laboratory, Department of Biotechnology, Shridevi Institute of Engineering & Technology, Tumkur, India
[2]Madhuca, Srinivasa Nagara, Chitpady, Udupi, India
Email: [*]dravidateja07@gmail.com, endophytessiet@gmail.com

Abstract

5 totally different endophytic fungal species were isolated from bark and leaf parts of *Calophyllum inophyllum*. Leaf part yielded *Trichoderma harzianum* and *Alternaria* species, whereas bark showed the presence of *Fusarium* species, *Aspergillus* species and unidentified fungi. Two solvents (hexane and methanol) were used for endophytic fungal extraction and the *Alternaria* species had shown the presence of coumarin whereas *Trichoderma harzianum* in methanol extract and *Fusarium* species in hexane extract had shown the coumarin(s) in all the four methods tested. The total coumarin yield was more in microwave assistance method, the methanol *Alternaria* species (3.941 ± 0.082) stood first, followed by hexane extract of *Alternaria* species (3.254 ± 0.082), *Fusarium* species (2.532 ± 0.082) and *Trichoderma harzianum* (2.294 ± 0.082), the plant extract showed 4.149 + 0.053. The methanol extract of *Alternaria* species inhibited the activity of HIV-Reverse Transcriptase (RT) (82.81 ± 1.0), integrase (98%) and protease (78) in maximum level followed by hexane extract of *Alternaria* species (71.12 ± 0.9, 89, 68), *Fusarium* species (63.92 ± 1.8, 67, 66) and *Trichoderma harzianum* (56.69 ± 0.9, 71, 63). The endophytic fungi *Alternaria* species inhibited all the three viral enzymes at maximum level and it was more than standard drug. However, in order to know possible anti-HIV, it is necessary to isolate active coumarin from the *Alternaria* species and the mechanism of action will be studied in future studies.

---

[*]Corresponding author.

Keywords

Endophytes, *Alternaria* Species, HIV-RT, Integrase, Protease, Inhibitory Activity

1. Introduction

Ayurveda is a traditional Indian medicine system being practicing by people to cure various diseases by using plant and plant based products. These practices are still continuing in Indian society. Presently various plant extracts are using in treatments of HIV [1]. Narayan *et al.* [2] have reported the importance of *C. inophyllum* in treatment of HIV by inhibiting the activity of HIV-integrase and protease. The HIV-1 encodes three multifunctional enzymes viz. protease, integrase and reverse transcriptase which are responsible for processing of viral proteins into functional enzymes and structural proteins. The RT is the functional enzyme, it transcripts viral RNA into viral DNA, where the integrase is responsible for integration of double standard DNA [3].

Development of resistant strains and side effects, the synthetic drugs are considering in failure of people interest. To find suitable remedy, the plant and plant based products are now having global importance in developing new drugs which are not having side effects. The drugs are developed for treatments of HIV and are able to inhibit the replication of virus and its replicating enzymes activities.

Calophyllum inophyllum is ornamental plant wood which is hard and strong and has been used in construction or boat building. Among the medicinal uses the oil is used to treat diabetic sores, psoriasis, sun burn and heal blisters. In southern Africa, it is useful for rheumatism, arthritis and lesions due to herpes. It is also used for problems of scalp and hair. The leaves are used for skin care and eye inflammations. The plant has important biological compounds, viz. coumarins, xanthones, truterpenes and it shows antitumor, cytotoxic, antibacterial, analgesic activities. The *C. inophyllum* also shows antiviral activity, especially the anti-HIV activity by inhibiting antiviral replicating and functional enzymes [4]. For continuous use of plant and plant based drugs, in the future the plants may be vanished. To safeguard the plants and continue to derive medicinal important drugs, endophyte is one of the important organisms to exploit the above same things and we can produce the compounds at higher concentration within short duration. The present work is aimed to isolate different endophytes of *Calophyllum inophyllum* and evaluated their extracts for anti-HIV activities (by inhibiting three enzymes viz., RT, intrgrase and protease).

2. Materials and Methods

2.1. Reagents/Chemicals

All the chemicals and media were purchased from Sigma-Aldrich, Merck and all the reagents were of AR grade.

2.2. Collection of Plant Material

Plant *Calophyllum inophyllum* was collected from Western Ghat region of Udupi, Karnataka during February 2015. Plant was identified with the help of taxonomist, Dr Gopal Krishna Bhat, Udupi.

2.3. Isolation, Identification and Mass Multiplication of Fungal Endophytes

2.3.1. Mass Culture of Fungal Endophytes

Mass cultured the each fungal endophytes using potato dextrose broth for 8 days at room temperature ($26°C \pm 2°C$) in separately. After incubation, the fungal mycelium mat was taken for extraction using hexane and methanol. Based on the earlier report of Umashankar *et al.* [5], Microwave Assisted Extraction (MAE) method was used, the endophytic fungal mat mixed with methanol was kept for extraction in microwave method at 2 cycles of 5 minutes each at $100°C$ and analyzed the percentage of coumarin.

2.3.2. Identification of Coumarin in Isolated Endophytic Fungal Species

Test 1. 3 ml of ethanol extract was evaporated to dryness in a vessel and the residue was dissolved in hot distilled water. It was then cooled and divided into two test portions, one was the reference, the other was the test. To the second test tube, 0.5 ml of 10 NH_4OH was added. The occurrence of intense/fluorescence under UV light was a positive test for the presence of coumarins and derivatives. The experiment was carried out for all the experiments in three replicates [6].

Test 2. 5 ml of the extract was evaporated to dryness and the residue was dissolved in 2 ml of distilled water. The aqueous solution was divided into two equal parts in test tubes. One part was the reference. To the other test tube, 0.5 ml of 10% ammonia solution was added and the test tubes were observed under UV light indicated. The occurrence of a bluish green fluorescence under UV light indicated the presence of coumarin derivatives [6].

Test 3. To the concentrated alcoholic extract of drug few drops of alcohol $FeCl_3$ solution was added. Development of deep green colour, which turned yellow on addition of conc. HNO_3, indicated presence of coumarins.

Test 4. The alcoholic extract was mixed with 1N NaOH solution (one ml each). Development of blue-green fluorescence formation indicated presence of coumarins.

Test 5, detection of phenols. In beakers, 5 ml of each previous filtered extract were taken and 1ml of $FeCl_3$ (1%) and 1 ml $K_3(Fe(CN)_6)$ (1%) were added. The appearance of fresh radish blue color indicated the presence of polyphenols.

2.4. Anti-HIV Activities

2.4.1. HIV-1 Reverse Transcriptase Inhibition Assay

The HIV reverse transcriptase enzyme inhibition was done with endophytic fungal extracts of *C. inophyllum* using HIV-RT inhibition method with slight modification of Rege *et al.* [7]. 25 µl of each endophytic fungal extract (final concentration 5 mg/ml) was added to the reaction mixture. The final mixture was 100 µl (50 mM Tris, pH 7.8), 150 mM KCl, 5 mM $MgCl_2$, 0.05% NP-40, 0.5 mM EGTA, 5 mM DTT, 20 µM dTTP, 0.3 M Glutathione, 2.5 µg/ml BSA, 0.5 µCi (microcurrie) of [³H]TTP, 2.5 µg/ml poly (rA).p(dT). The reaction was started by adding of 0.5 units of recombinant reverse transcriptase enzyme, the mixture was incubated for 3 h at 37°C and terminated the reaction by adding of 25 µl of 0.1 EGTA by chilling the mixture on ice. 100 µl of each reaction mixture was spotted uniformly onto circular 2.5 cm DE-81 Whatmann filters and kept at ambient temperature for 15 min. The dried filters were washed four times with 5% aqueous $Na_2HPO_4 \cdot 7H_2O$ followed by two or three washed with double distilled water. Finally, the filters were thoroughly dried and subjected to scintillation counting. Negative control was set up in parallel and AZT (Azidothymidine/Zidovudine) was used as positive control. Inhibition was calculated as follow,

$$\text{Inhibition percentage} = \left[(\text{CPM of negative control} - \text{CPM of test}) / \text{CPM of negative control} \right] \times 100,$$

where CPM is count per minute.

2.4.2. Assay of HIV-1 Protease Inhibitory Activity

This assay was modified from the previously reported method [8]. In brief, the recombinant HIV-1 PR solution was diluted with a buffer composed of a solution containing 50 mM of sodium acetate (pH 5.0), 1 mM ethylenediamine disodium (EDTA.2Na) and 2 mM 2-mercaptoethanol (2-ME) and mixed with glycerol in the ratio 3:1. The substrate peptides Arg-Val-Nle-NH2 was diluted with a buffer solution of 50 mM sodium acetate (pH 5.0). Two microliters of plant extract and four microliters of HIV-1 PR solution (0.025 mg/ml) were added to a solution containing 2 µl of substrate solution (2 mg/ml) and the reaction mixture of 10 µl was incubated at 37°C for 1 h. A control reaction was performed under the same condition, but without the plant extract. The reaction was stopped by heating the reaction mixture at 90°C for 1 min. Subsequently, 20 µl of sterile water was added and an aliquot of 10 µl was analyzed by HPLC using RP-18 column (4.6 mm × 150 mm i.d., Supelco 516 C-18-DB 5 µm, USA). Ten microliters of the reaction mixture was injected to the column and gradiently eluted with acetonitrile (15% - 40%) and 0.2% trifluoroacetic acid (TFA) in water, at a flow rate of 1.0 ml/min. The elution profile was monitored at 280 nm. The retention times of the substrate and p-NO_2-Phe-bearing hydrolysate were 4.709 and 2.733 min, respectively. The inhibitory activity of HIV-1 PR was calculated as follows,

$$\% \text{ inhibition} = \left(A_{\text{control}} - A_{\text{sample}} \right) \times 100 / A_{\text{control}}$$

whereas A is the relative peak of the product hydrolysate. Acetyl pepstatin was used as a positive control.

2.4.3. Assay of HIV-IN Inhibitory Activity

Oligonucleotide substrates. Oligonucleotides of long terminal repeat donor DNA (LTR-D) and target substrate

(TS) DNA were purchased from QIAGEN Operon, USA and stored at −25°C before use. The sequence of bio-tinylated LTR donor DNA and its unlabelled complement were 5'-biotin-ACCCTTTTAGTCAGTGTGGA AAATCTCTAGCAGT-3'(LTR-D1) and 3'-GAAAATCAGTCACACCTTTTAGAGATCGTCA-5' (LTR-D2), respectively. Those of the target substrate DNA (digoxigenin-labelled target DNA, TS-1) and its 3'-labelled complement were 5'-TGACCAAGGGCTAATTCACT-digoxigenin and digoxigenin-ACTGGTTCCCGATTAA GTGA-5' (TS-2), respectively.

2.4.4. Multiplate Integration Assay (MIA)

The integration reaction was evaluated according to the method previously described [9]. Briefly, a mixture (45 μl) composed of 12 μl of IN buffer [containing 150 mM 3-(N-morpholino) propane sulfonic acid, pH 7.2 (MOPS), 75 mM MnCl$_2$, 5 mM dithiothritol (DTT), 25% glycerol and 500 μg/ml bovine serum albumin], 1 μl of 5 pmol/ml digoxigenin-labelled target DNA and 32 μl of sterilized water were added into each well of a 96 well plate. Subsequently, 6 μl of sample solution and 9 μl of 1/5 dilution of integrase enzyme was added to the plate and incubated at 37°C for 80 min. Wells were washed with PBS four times, 100 μl of 500 mU/ml alkaline phosphatase (AP) labelled anti-digoxigenin antibody were added and incubated at 37°C for 1 h. The plate was washed again with washing buffer containing 0.05% Tween 20 in PBS four times and with PBS four times. Then, AP buffer (150 μl) containing 100 mM Tris-HCl (pH 9.5), 100 mM NaCl, 5 mM MgCl$_2$ and 10 mM p-nitrophenyl phosphate was added to each well and incubated at 37°C for 1 h. Finally, the plate was measured with a microplate reader at a wavelength of 405 nm. A control composed of a reaction mixture, 50% DMSO and an integrase enzyme, while a blank is buffer-E containing 20 mM MOPS (pH 7.2), 400 mM potassium gluta-mate, 1 mM ethylenediamine tetra acetate disodium salt (EDTA.2Na), 0.1% Nonidet-P40 (NP-40), 20% glyce-rol, 1 mM DTT and 4 M urea without the integrase enzyme. Suramin, a polyanionic HIV-1 IN inhibitor was used as a positive control.

$$\text{Percent inhibition of integrase} = \% \text{ inhibition} = \left(A_{control} - A_{sample}\right) \times 100 \big/ A_{control}$$

where A is the optical density detected from each well.

2.4.5. Assay of Gp120 Binding Inhibition

Binding of Gp120 to CD4 was analysed using a commercially available Gp120 capture ELISA kit using stan-dard procedure of Rege et al. [7]. To check, our fungal endophytic extracts could interfere with the binding of CD4 to Gp120 by interaction with soluble Gp120, each fungal extract (5 mg/ml) was mixed with 25 ng of puri-fied Gp120 in a total volume of 100 μl and incubated at room temperature (26°C ± 2°C) for 1h. Each mixture was added to microtiter plate wells separately coated with CD4 ligand and incubated at room temperature for 1 h. The solutions were aspirated and the wells were washed 3 times with buffer. The Gp120 binding to CD4 was assessed by using detector reagent provided in the kit. Negative and positive control (heparin) was set up in pa-rallel.

The percent inhibition was calculated by,

$$\text{Percent inhibition} = \left[\left(A_{control} - A_{sample}\right)\big/A_{control}\right] \times 100 \,,$$

A is the optical density.

3. Results and Discussion

Table 1 predicts that two parts (leaf and bark) of *Calophyllum inophyllum* yielded five different endophytic fungal species. The leaf part exhibited only two fungi (*Trichoderma harzianum* and *Alternaria* species) and *Al-ternaria* species, *Fusarium* species and unidentified fungi were noticed from the bark part. The *Alternaria* spe-cies was identified in two parts.

The coumarin(s) identification tests were conducted to all endophytic fungi using separate two different sol-vent. The coumarin presence was observed in methanol extracts of *T. harzianum* and in hexane extract of *Fusa-rium* species. Both hexane and methanol extract of *Alternaria* species had shown the presence of coumarin (**Table 2**). The methanol extract of *Alternaria* species had shown highe activity of integrase followed by hexane extract of *Alternaria* species. The total coumarin yield was more in microwave assistance method, the methanol

Table 1. Presence of fungal endophytes in different parts of *Calophyllum inophyllum*.

Fungal endophytes	Parts used	
	Leaf	Bark
Trichoderma harzianum	+	−
Fusarium species	−	+
Aspergillus flavus	−	+
Alternaria species	+	−
Unidentified fungi	−	+

+: presence, −: not presence, data based on three replicates of each.

Table 2. Identification of coumarin(s) in two solvent extracts of endophytic fungal species of *C. inophyllum*.

Fungal endophytes	Solvents used	
	Hexane	Methanol
Trichoderma harzianum	−	+
Fusarium species	+	−
Aspergillus flavus	−	−
Alternaria species	+	+
Unidentified fungi	−	−

+: presence, −: not presence, data based on three replicates of each.

Alternaria species (3.941 ± 0.082) stood first, followed by hexane extract of *Alternaria* species (3.254 ± 0.082), *Fusarium* species (2.532 ± 0.082) and *Trichoderma harzianum* (2.294 ± 0.082), the plant extract showed 4.149 ± 0.053 (**Table 3**). The highest amount of coumarins was obtained from microwave assistance method, 2 cycles of 5 min at 100°C. Similar results were noticed by Umashankar *et al*. (2012) by using same method.

Evaluated all the two solvent endophytic fungal extracts against HIV-RT, the highest activity was observed with methanol extract of *Alternaria* species (82.81 ± 1.0) followed by hexane extract of *Alternaria* species (71.12 ± 0.9), *Fusarium* species (54.32 ± 1.4) and *Trichoderma harzianum* extracts (48.81 ± 1.3) were compared with standard heparin (74.54 ± 0.8) (**Table 4**). The methanol and hexane extract of *Alternaria* species inhibited the RT at maximum level, it was more than standard (heparin). The more inhibition of integrase was observed in methanol extract of *Alternaria* species (98), it was greater than the standard drug followed by same endophytic hexane extract (89) (**Figure 1**). Pepsin or Gp 120 binding assay was also greatly inhibited by methanol extract of *Alternaria* species (86.38 ± 1.9), the activity was more than to standard drug (72.51 ± 1.4) (**Table 5**). The protease activity was strongly inhibited by methanol extract of *Alternaria* species (78) followed by hexane extract of *Alternaria* species (68) followed by *Fusarium* species (66) and *Trichoderma harzianum* (63) and these data was compared with standard drug acetylpepstain (81). The plant extract had shown 73% of inhibition of the enzyme protease (**Figure 2**). Similar results are reported by Narayan *et al*. [2] by using plant *C. inophyllum* different solvent extract. Our results were also confirmatory with the findings of Rege *et al*. [7], Govindappa *et al*. [10], Estari *et al*. [11] and Rege and Chowdhury [12]. Some of endophytic crude extracts or isolated compounds possessed the anti-HIV activity by inhibiting these enzymes [13]-[15]. This is the first report of endophytic fungal species of *C. inophyllum*, presence coumarin(s) and their *in vitro* anti-HIV activity and further research has to be carried out to find out exact anti-HIV coumarin molecule.

Table 3. Yield of total coumarin(s) from different endophytic fungal species in microwave assistance method.

Endophytic fungal species extracts	Inhibition percentage of RT
Trichoderma harzianum	2.294 ± 0.082
Fusarium species	2.532 ± 0.082
Alternaria species (HE)	3.254 ± 0.082
Alternaria species (ME)	3.941 ± 0.052
Plant extract	4.149 ± 0.053

Table 4. Effect of endophytic fungal coumarin(s) on HIV-RT inhibition.

Endophytic fungal species extracts	Inhibition percentage of RT
Trichoderma harzianum	48.81 ± 1.3
Fusarium species	54.32 ± 1.4
Alternaria species (HE)	71.12 ± 0.9
Alternaria species (ME)	82.81 ± 1.0
Heparin (control) (12.5 units)	74.54 ± 0.8

HE: Hexane extract, ME: Methanol extract, data based on three replicates of each. Note: inhibition > 50% is considered as significant.

Table 5. Effect of endophytic fungal coumarin(s) extracts on Gp120 binding inhibition.

Endophytic fungal species extracts	Inhibition of Gp120 binding
Trichoderma harzianum	56.69 ± 0.9
Fusarium species	63.92 ± 1.8
Alternaria species (HE)	78.41 ± 1.2
Alternaria species (ME)	86.38 ± 1.9
AZT (control) (0.0016 mg/ml)	72.51 ± 1.4

HE: Hexane extract, ME: Methanol extract, data based on three replicates of each. Note: inhibition > 50% is considered as significant.

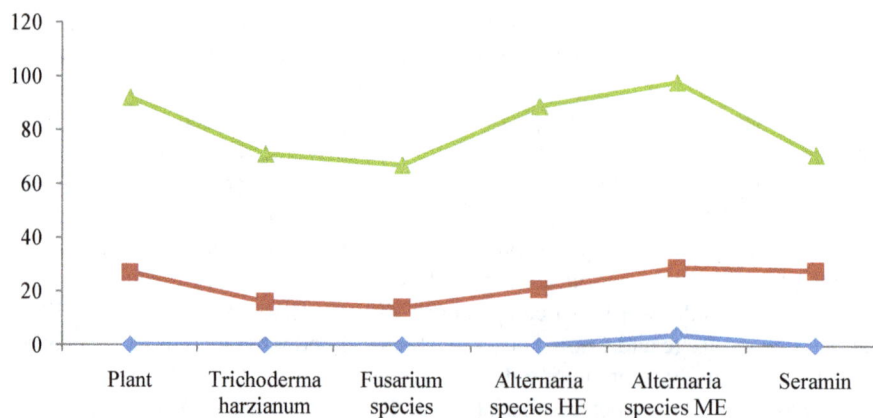

Figure 1. Effect of endophytic extracts in inhibition of integrase enzyme.

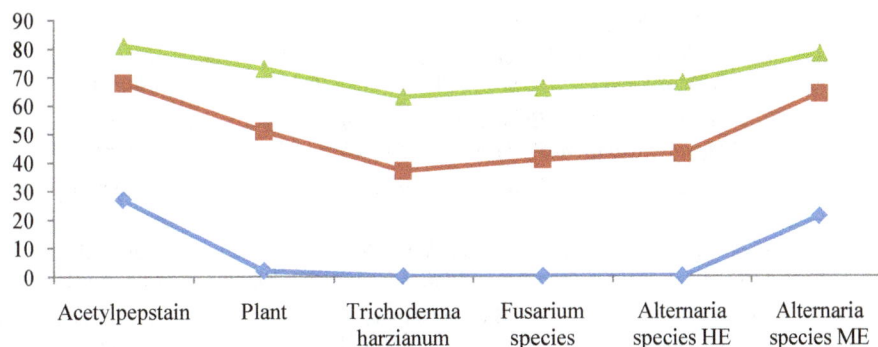

Figure 2. Inhibition of protease activity by different endophytic fungal extracts.

4. Conclusion

Five different endophytic fungal species were identified from bark and leaf part of *Calophyllum inophyllum* and the methanol extract of *Alternaria* species yielded more coumarin compared to other endophytic fungal species and solvent extract. The methanol extract of *Alternaria* species inhibited the activity of HIV-RT, integrase and protease in maximum level by inhibiting their activity. The coumarin(s) present in the endophytic fungi, *Alternaria* species can be identified in further research and the exact coumarin their role role in inhibiting the HIV replicating enzymes can also be identified.

Acknowledgements

The authors wish to thank, SERB-DST, New Delhi and Dr. Amitava Roy, Scientist "F", SERB, for supporting the financial assistance for the project (SB/MEO-355/2013 dated 29-10-2013).

Conflict of Interest

The authors confirm that this article content has no conflict of interest.

References

[1]   Jassim, S.A.A. and Naji, M.A. (2003) Novel Antiviral Agents: A Medicinal Plant Perspective. *Journal of Applied Microbiology*, **95**, 412-427. http://dx.doi.org/10.1046/j.1365-2672.2003.02026.x

[2]   Narayan, C.L. and Rai, R.V. (2011) A Screening Strategy for Selection of Anti-HIV Integrase and anti-HIV Protease Inhibiotors from Plant Extracts of Indian Medicinal Plants. *International Journal of Phytomedicine*, **3**, 312-318.

[3]   Tewtrakul, S., Nakamura, N., Hattori, M., Fujiwara, T. and Supavita, T. (2002) Flavanone and Flavonol Glycosides from the Leaves of *Thevetia peruviana* and Their HIV-1 Reverse Transcriptase and HIV-1 Integrase Inhibitory Activities. *Chemical and Pharmaceutical Bulletin*, **50**, 630-635.

[4]   Sundur, S., Shrivastava, B., Sharma, P., Raj, S.S. and Jayasekhar, V.L. (2014) A Review Article of Pharmacological Activities and Biological Importance of *Calophyllum inophyllum*. *International Journal of Advanced Research*, **2**, 599-603.

[5]   Umashankar, T., Govindappa, M. and Ramachandra, Y.L. (2014) *In Vitro* Antioxidant and Antimicrobial Activity of Partially Purified Coumarins from Fungal Endophytes of *Crotalaria pallid*. *International Journal of Current Microbiology and Applied Sciences*, **3**, 58-72.

[6]   Jagessar, R.C. and Cox, M. (2010) Phytochemical Screening of the CHCl$_3$ and CH$_3$CH$_2$OH Extract of Stems, Twigs, Roots and Barks of *Conocarpus erectus* L. *International Journal of Academic Research*, **2**, 36-45.

[7]   Rege, A.A., Ambaye, R.Y. and Deshmukh, R.A. (2010) *In Vitro* Testing of Anti-HIV Activity of Some Medicinal Plants. *Indian Journal of Natural Products and Resources*, **1**, 193-199.

[8]   Tewtrakul, S., Subhadhirasakul, S. and Kummee, S. (2003) HIV-1 Protease Inhibitory Effects of Medicinal Plants Used as Self Medication by AIDS Patients. *Songklanakarin Journal of Science and Technology*, **25**, 239-243.

[9]   Tewtrakul, S., Miyashiro, H., Hattori, M., Yoshinaga, T., Fujiwara, T., Tomimori, T., *et al.* (2001) Inhibitory Effects of Flavonoids on Human Immunodeficiency Virus Type-1 Integrase. *Journal of Traditional Medicines*, **18**, 229-238.

[10]   Govindappa, M., Kumar, N.V.A. and Santoyo, G. (2011) *Crotalaria pallida* Extracts as a Putative HIV-Protease Inhi-

bitors. *Journal of Research in Biology*, **4**, 285-291.

[11] Estari, M., Venkanna, L., Sripriya, D. and Lalitha, R. (2012) Human Immunodeficiency Virus (HIV-1) Reverse Transcriptase Inhibitory Activity of *Phyllanthus emblica* Plant Extract. *Biology and Medicine*, **4**, 178-182.

[12] Rege, A.A. and Chowdhury, A.S. (2014) Evaluation of *Ocimum sanctum* and *Tinospora cordifolia* as Probable HIV Protease Inhibitors. *International Journal of Pharmaceutical Sciences Review and Research*, **25**, 315-318.

[13] Xiang, Z.C., Jiang, Y. and Guo, S.X. (2006) *In Vitro* Anti-HIV Activity of a Chinese Fungus Extract. *Biomedical and Environmental Sciences*, **19**, 169-172.

[14] Umashankar, T., Govindappa, M. and Ramachandra, Y.L. (2012) *In Vitro* Antioxidant and Anti-HIV Activity of Endophytic Coumarin from *Crotalaria pallida* Aiton. *Planta Medica*, **78**, 102. http://dx.doi.org/10.1055/s-0032-1307610

[15] Wellensiek, B.P., Ramakrishnan, R., Bashyal, B.P., Eason, Y., Gunatilaka, A.A.L. and Ahmad, N. (2013) Inhibition of HIV-1 Replication by Secondary Metabolites from Endophytic Fungi of Desert Plants. *The Open Virology Journal*, **7**, 72-80. http://dx.doi.org/10.2174/1874357920130624002

20

Epidermal Growth Factor Enhances Orthovanadate-Induced Contraction via Src and Myosin Phosphatase Target Subunit 1 in Rat Vascular Smooth Muscle

Tomoya Sasahara, Natsumi Ohkura, Mariko Shin, Akira Onodera, Katsutoshi Yayama[*]

Laboratory of Cardiovascular Pharmacology, Department of Biopharmaceutical Sciences, Kobe Gakuin University, Kobe, Japan
Email: [*]yayama@pharm.kobegakuin.ac.jp

Abstract

Inhibition of protein tyrosine phosphatase by orthovanadate induces vasoconstriction, which is mediated by the Rho kinase-dependent inactivation of myosin light chain phosphatase (MLCP) via signaling downstream of Src-induced activation of the epidermal growth factor (EGF) receptor. The present study investigated the potential role of EGF in orthovanadate (OVA)-dependent vasoconstriction. OVA-induced aortic contraction significantly increased in the presence of EGF, and was abolished by inhibitors of Rho kinase (Y27632), extracellular signal-regulated kinase 1 and 2 (Erk1/2) (FR180204), Erk1/2 kinase (PD98059), EGF receptor (AG1478), and Src (PP2). Treatment of the rat endothelium-denuded thoracic aorta with either EGF or OVA augmented the phosphorylation of myosin phosphatase target subunit 1 (MYPT1) at Thr-853 and of the EGF receptor at Tyr-1173. The phosphorylation of MYPT1 was further increased by co-stimulation with EGF and OVA. EGF receptor phosphorylation at Tyr-845 was also increased by EGF or OVA; this effect was augmented by co-stimulation with EGF and OVA, and was abolished by Src inhibition. In addition, Erk1/2 was phosphorylated by EGF or by co-treatment with EGF and OVA; this was abolished by an EGF receptor inhibitor, but not by Src inhibition. These results suggested that OVA-induced EGF-related contraction was mediated by the Rho kinase-dependent inactivation of MLCP via two different signaling cascades: Src-dependent phosphorylation of the EGF receptor at Tyr-845 and EGF-dependent phosphorylation of Erk1/2.

Keywords

Epidermal Growth Factor, Myosin Light Chain Phosphatase, Mitogen-Activated Kinase,

---

[*]Corresponding author.

Orthovanadate

1. Introduction

Smooth muscle contraction is regulated by Ca^{2+}-dependent and Ca^{2+}-independent pathways. The increase in cytosolic Ca^{2+} in smooth muscle cells activates myosin light chain kinase (MLCK), which phosphorylates myosin light chain (MLC), leading to smooth muscle contraction [1]. Phosphorylated MLC is dephosphorylated by MLC phosphatase (MLCP), allowing the contracted smooth muscle to return to the relaxed state [2]. MLCP consists of three subunits: a 37-kDa catalytic subunit, a 20-kDa variable subunit, and a 110 - 130-kDa myosin phosphatase target subunit 1 (MYPT1) [3]. Phosphorylation of MYPT1 by activated Rho kinase reduces MLCP activity, leading to prolonged smooth muscle contraction [4] [5].

The function of vascular smooth muscle is also regulated by the balance of protein tyrosine kinases and protein tyrosine phosphatases. Disruption of the cellular tyrosine phosphorylation equilibrium causes several diseases, and the activities of both protein tyrosine kinases and phosphatases are therefore tightly controlled [6]. Vanadium compounds such as sodium orthovanadate (OVA) are well-characterized inhibitors of protein tyrosine phosphatase [7]. In addition, vanadates have several other biochemical and pharmacological properties, such as the inhibition of ATPases [8], epidermal growth factor (EGF)-like mitogenic activity [9], insulin-mimetic properties [10], anti-apoptotic activities [11], and antitumor or carcinogenic properties [12] [13]. Vanadium compounds can affect signaling pathways in cells, including phospholipase D, focal adhesion kinase, phospholipase C-γ, Src, phosphatidyl inositol 3-kinase, and extracellular signal-regulated kinase 1 and 2 (Erk1/2) [14]-[19]. In the vasculature, vanadium compounds also enhance the production of vasoactive metabolites such as prostaglandin I, nitric oxide (NO), and endothelium-derived hyperpolarizing factor, leading to relaxation of vascular smooth muscle [20]-[23]. In contrast, several studies reported that vanadates induced vascular and non-vascular smooth muscle contraction; this was observed in the guinea pig taenia coli, trachea, and gallbladder smooth muscle [24]-[26] and in the rat gastric longitudinal muscle and myometrium [27] [28]. Vanadate-induced contraction of guinea pig ileal longitudinal smooth muscle was regulated by the activation of a Rho kinase-dependent pathway, resulting in an increase in MLC phosphorylation [29]. Recently, we reported that OVA caused Rho kinase-dependent contraction of the rat thoracic aorta and phosphorylation of MYPT1 in vascular smooth muscle cells [30]. These reports showed that inhibition of protein tyrosine phosphatases by vanadates induced smooth muscle contraction through Rho kinase-dependent inactivation of MLCP. We have shown that OVA-induced vasoconstriction was mediated by the Rho kinase-dependent inactivation of MLCP via signaling downstream of Src-induced transactivation of the EGF receptor (EGFR) [30]. We also showed that EGF caused Ca^{2+} sensitization in the rat thoracic aorta by Rho kinase-dependent inactivation of MLCP through the Erk1/2 kinase (MEK) pathway [31]. However, EGF did not induce contraction of the normotensive rat thoracic aorta. In addition, the relationships amomg Src, EGF, and tyrosine phosphatase involved in smooth muscle contraction were unclear. The present study therefore assessed whether activation of Src by OVA-mediated inhibition of tyrosine phosphatase was involved in EGF-related contraction of rat vascular smooth muscle.

2. Materials and Methods

2.1. Inhibitors

The inhibitors used in this study are described in **Table 1** and were purchased from Merck-Millipore (Tokyo, Japan). OVA was purchased from Nacalai Tesque (Kyoto, Japan). The concentration of inhibitors were selected based our previous studies [30] [31].

2.2. Organ Chamber Experiments

All animal experiments were performed in accordance with the Guidelines of the Kobe Gakuin University Experimental Animal Care. Male Wistar rats, 7 - 8 weeks old and weighing 170 - 200 g, were anesthetized with diethyl ether. The thoracic aorta was excised, placed in Krebs-Henseleit solution (118.4 mM NaCl, 4.7 mM KCl, 2.5 mM $CaCl_2$, 1.2 mM KH_2PO_4, 1.2 mM $MgSO_4$, 25.0 mM $NaHCO_3$, and 11.1 mM glucose; pH 7.4), and then

Table 1. Inhibitors used in this study.

Product Name	Target	Chemical Name	Used Concentration (μM)
AG1478	EGFR	(4-[3-chloroanilino]-6,7-dimethoxyquinazoline)	10
AS601245	JNK	([Z]-2-[benzo{d}thiazol-2{3H}-ylidene]-2-[2-{(2-[pyridin-3-yl]ethyl)amino}pyrimidin-4-yl]acetonitrile)	10
FR180204	Erk1/2	(5-[2-phenyl-pyrazolo{1,5-a}pyridin-3-yl]-1H-pyrazolo[3,4-c]pyridazin-3-ylamine)	10
ML-7	MLCK	(1-[5-iodonaphthalene-1-sulfonyl]homopiperazine)	10
PD98059	MEK	(2'-amino-3'-methoxyflavone)	10
PP2	Src	(4-amino-3-[4-chlorophenyl]-1-[t-butyl]-1H-pyrazolo[3,4-d]pyrimidine)	3
SB203580	MAPK p38	(4-[4-fluorophenyl]-2-[4-methylsulfinylphenyl]-5-[4-pyridyl]1H-imidazole)	10
Y27632	Rho kinase	(R-[+]-trans-N-[4-pyridyl]-4-[1-aminoethyl]-cyclohexanecarboxamide)	10

cleaned of adherent tissue. The aorta was cut into 5-mm rings, and the endothelium was removed by carefully rotating a manipulator inside the lumen of the rings. Six rings, obtained from one animal, were fixed vertically under a resting tension of 1.0 g in 5-ml organ chambers (UC-5A; Medical Kishimoto, Kyoto, Japan) filled with Krebs-Henseleit solution (37°C, pH 7.4) and aerated continuously with a gaseous mixture of 95% O_2 and 5% CO_2 for 60 min. Isometric tension changes were measured by a force displacement transducer (AP-5; Medical Kishimoto) coupled to a dual-channel chart recorder (SS-250F; SEKONIC, Tokyo, Japan). All tissue rings were exposed to 60 mM KCl for 30 min for measurement of the maximal contractile force.

Prior to isotonic measurements of vascular contractility, arteries were allowed to equilibrate for another 60 min. After equilibration, OVA was added to the bath solution to achieve a final concentration of 0.01 - 1 mM. EGF (1 or 10 nM) was dissolved in Krebs-Henseleit solution supplemented with 5% trehalose; this was then added to the organ bath 5 min prior to the addition of OVA.

The inhibitors used in the present study were dissolved in dimethyl sulfoxide and added to the organ chambers in 10-μL volumes 20 min before the addition of OVA. The contractile effect of OVA was expressed as a percentage of the maximal force evoked by 60 mM KCl.

2.3. Western Blotting

Aortic rings were equilibrated as described above and then treated with EGF (10 nM) and/or OVA (0.5 mM) for 5 min. In some experiments, inhibitors were added to the organ bath 20 min before EGF and/or OVA treatment. The rings were homogenized in 50 μL lysis buffer, comprised of 50 mM Tris-HCl (pH7.4), 25 mM CHAPS, protease inhibitor cocktail (Nacalai Tesque), and phosphatase inhibitor cocktail (Nacalai Tesque). Samples were centrifuged at 15,000 × g for 10 min at 4°C, and the concentration of soluble protein in the supernatant was determined using a BCA Protein Assay Kit (Thermo Scientific, Waltham, MA, USA). Equal amounts of protein (1.5 μg/lane) were separated by sodium dodecyl sulfate-polyacrylamide gel electrophoresis and transferred to polyvinyldifluoride (PVDF) membranes (Immobilon-P; Millipore, Billerica, MA, USA). The blots were then blocked in 5% skimmed milk in Tris-buffered saline (0.1% Tween 20 in 10 mM Tris-HCl, pH 7.5, containing 100 mM NaCl) and incubated overnight at 4°C in Tris-buffered saline with rabbit antibodies against MYPT1 (1:200; Santa Cruz Biotechnology, Santa Cruz, CA, USA), Thr-853-phosphorylated MYPT1 (1:200; Santa Cruz Biotechnology), Erk1/2 (1:1000; Cell Signaling, Danvers, MA, USA), Thr-202/Tyr-204-phosphorylated Erk1/2 (1:1000; Cell Signaling), EGFR (1:1000; Cell Signaling), and EGFR that was phosphorylated at Tyr-1173 (1:1000; Cell Signaling) and at Tyr-845 (1:1000; Cell Signaling). The PVDF membranes were then washed with Tris-buffered saline, and incubated with horseradish peroxidase-conjugated goat anti-rabbit antibodies (1:2000; Bio-Rad, Hercules, CA, USA) in Tris-buffered saline for 1 h at room temperature. After washing twice in Tris-buffered saline, the blots were visualized using an enhanced chemiluminescence detection system (GE Healthcare Japan, Tokyo, Japan). Immunoblots were quantified using densitometry with Versa Doc 5000 MP (Bio-Rad) and Quantity One software (Bio-Rad).

2.4. Statistical Analysis

All data are expressed as the mean ± the standard error of the mean (SEM). Statistical comparisons were performed using one-way analysis of variance with pair-wise comparisons made using the Bonferroni-Dunn method. Comparisons of concentration-response curves were made using repeated-measures analysis of variance followed by the Bonferroni-Dunn test using the Graph Pad Prism 6 software. Differences were considered statistically significant at P < 0.05.

3. Results

3.1. EGF Enhanced OVA-Induced Contraction of Rat Endothelium-Denuded Thoracic Aorta

OVA activates endothelial NO synthase [23] and it is likely that endothelium-derived NO attenuates the contractile effects of OVA in aortic rings. Since the aim of this study was to evaluate the roles of OVA and EGF in rat aortic smooth muscle contraction, we measured the contractile force in endothelium-denuded aortic rings in order to remove any NO-induced effects. The concentration-response curves for OVA significantly increased in endothelium-denuded rings exposed to stepwise increases in the concentration of OVA (**Figure 1**). Pretreatment of endothelium-denuded aortic rings with EGF (1 or 10 nM) further increased vasoconstriction, as compared with OVA alone. However, EGF alone (1 or 10 nM) did not induce contraction of endothelium-denuded rat thoracic aorta (data not shown).

3.2. Effects of Src, EGFR, and Rho Kinase Inhibitors on OVA- and EGF-Induced Aortic Contraction

To explore the signaling pathways involved in vasoconstriction induced by co-stimulation with EGF and OVA, the effects of various inhibitors on the contractile force generated in the presence of EGF (10 nM) and OVA (0.5 mM) were investigated in endothelium-denuded aortic rings. OVA was previously shown to activate Src, EGFR, and Rho kinase in rat thoracic smooth muscle, resulting in increased contraction [30]. Therefore, we studied the effects of Rho kinase inhibitors on aortic contraction induced by EGF and OVA. As shown in **Figure 2**, the contractile effects of EGF and OVA were abolished by the Rho kinase inhibitor, Y27632. The specific Src inhibitor, PP2, or the EGFR inhibitor, AG1478, also significantly attenuated the contractile effects of EGF and OVA (**Figure 2**). However, the MLCK inhibitor, ML-7, did not affect the contraction of endothelium-denuded thoracic aortic rings induced by EGF and OVA.

3.3. Effects of MEK, Erk1/2, p38 Mitogen Activated Protein Kinase (MAPK p38), and c-Jun N-Terminal Kinase (JNK) Inhibitors on OVA- and EGF-Induced Aortic Contraction

EGF was previously reported to induce MLCP inactivation through Erk1/2 dependent Rho kinase activation [31].

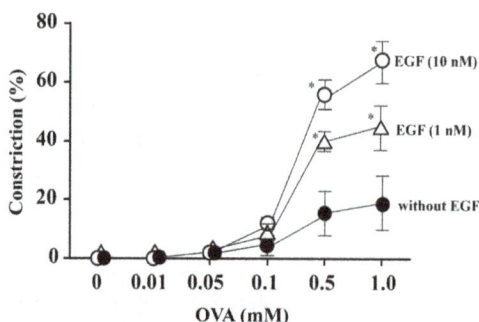

Figure 1. Effect of epidermal growth factor (EGF) on sodium orthovanadate (OVA)-induced contraction of endothelium-denuded rat thoracic aortic ring preparations. OVA concentration-response curves were constructed by measuring the force after each stepwise increase in the OVA concentration and are shown in the absence or presence of EGF (as indicated), added to the organ bath 5 min before OVA. Contractile force was expressed as a percentage of the maximal force evoked by 60 mM KCl. Data are presented as mean ± SEM for aortic rings from 5 rats; *P < 0.05 vs. control (without EGF).

Therefore, we assessed whether the enhancement of the vasoconstrictive effects of OVA (0.5 mM) by EGF (10 nM) was affected by MEK or Erk1/2 inhibitors. We observed that treatment of these aortic rings with a MEK inhibitor (PD98059) or an Erk1/2 inhibitor (FR180204) significantly reduced the effects of EGF on OVA-induced contraction (**Figure 3**). However, inhibitors of JNK (AS601245) and MAPK p38 (SB203580) did not significantly affect the vasoconstriction observed in the presence of EGF (10 nM) and OVA (0.5 mM) (**Figure 3**).

3.4. Effects of Various Inhibitors on EGF- and/or OVA-Induced MYPT1 Phosphorylation

To determine whether Rho kinase is a downstream effector of Src and/or EGFR during EGF (10 nM)-mediated enhancement of OVA (0.5 mM)-induced vasoconstriction, we measured the levels of phosphorylated MYPT1

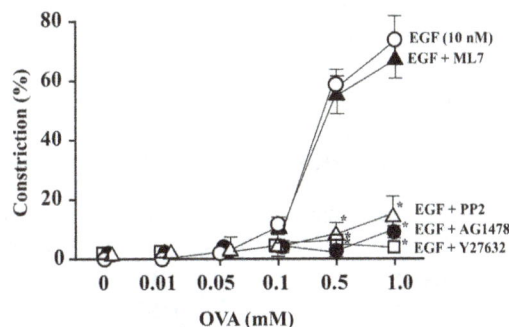

Figure 2. Effect of inhibitors of myosin light chain kinase (ML-7), Src (PP2), epidermal growth factor (EGF) receptor (AG1478), or Rho kinase (Y27632) on sodium orthovanadate (OVA)-induced contraction of EGF-treated rat endothelium-denuded thoracic aortic ring preparations. EGF (10 nM) was added 5 min before the addition of OVA, and ML-7 (10 μM), PP2 (3 μM), AG1478 (10 μM) or Y27632 (10 μM) was added to the organ bath 20 min before the addition of OVA. The concentration-response curves for OVA were constructed by measuring the force after each stepwise increase in the OVA concentration. Contractile force was expressed as a percentage of the maximal force evoked by 60 mM KCl. Data are expressed as mean ± SEM for aortic rings taken from 5 animals; $^*P < 0.05$ vs. EGF only.

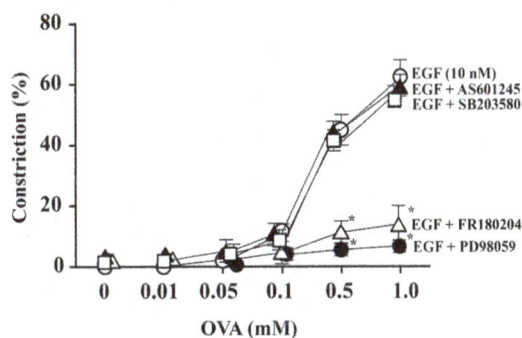

Figure 3. Effects of inhibitors of mitogen-activated protein kinase (MAPK p38), extracellular signal-regulated kinases 1 and 2 (Erk1/2), Erk1/2 kinase (MEK), or c-jun N-terminal kinase (JNK) on sodium orthovanadate (OVA)-induced contraction of epidermal growth factor (EGF)-treated rat endothelium-denuded thoracic aortic ring preparations. EGF (10 nM) was added 5 min before the addition of OVA, and inhibitors of MEK (PD98059; 10 μM), Erk1/2 (FR180204; 10 μM), MAPK p38 (SB203580; 10 μM), or JNK (AS601245; 10 μM) were added to the organ bath 20 min before the addition of OVA. The concentration-response curves for OVA were constructed by measuring the force after each stepwise increase in the OVA concentration. Contractile force was expressed as a percentage of the maximal force evoked by 60 mM KCl. Data are expressed as mean ± SEM for aortic rings taken from 5 animals; $^*P < 0.05$ vs. EGF only.

(Thr-853) in rat endothelium-denuded thoracic aorta after stimulation in the presence or absence of various inhibitors. Since co-stimulation with EGF and OVA produced rapid contraction of endothelium-denuded aortic rings, presenting as a hyperbolic rise in tension development for 5 min followed by linear rise (data not shown) and treating aortic rings with OVA or EGF increased the ratio of phosphorylated to total EGFR, Erk1/2, and MYPT1 rapidly within 2 min, and the increased levels were maintained for 10 min [30] [31], we measured the levels of phosphorylated MYPT1 5 min after exposure to OVA. When rings were treated with only EGF, we measured phosphorylation levels of proteins 5 min after stimulation of EGF. As shown in **Figure 4**, the ratio of phosphorylated to total MYPT1 was increased after treatment with 10 nM EGF or 0.5 mM OVA ($P < 0.05$ for both treatments, as compared with control), and further increased by co-treatment with 10 nM EGF and 0.5 mM OVA ($P < 0.05$ versus EGF only and versus OVA only). The increased phosphorylation of MYPT1 induced by co-stimulation with EGF and OVA was significantly reduced by inhibitors specific for Src (PP2), EGFR (AG1478), Rho kinase (Y27632), MEK (PD98059), and Erk1/2 (FR180204). However, inhibitors of JNK (AS601245) and MAPK p38 (SB203580) did not affect the phosphorylation of MYPT1 induced by EGF and OVA. These results suggested that this EGF- and OVA-induced phosphorylation of MYPT1 in rat endothelium-denuded thoracic aorta was mediated by Src-, EGFR-, MEK-, and Erk1/2-dependent activation of Rho kinase.

3.5. Effects of Various Inhibitors on EGF- and/or OVA-Induced Erk1/2 Phosphorylation

To determine whether Erk1/2 is the downstream effector of EGFR during EGF-mediated enhancement of OVA-induced Rho kinase activation, we measured the level of Erk1/2 that was phosphorylated at Thr-202/Tyr-204 in rat endothelium-denuded thoracic aortic rings in the presence or absence of various inhibitors. As shown in Figure 5, the ratio of phosphorylated to total Erk1/2 was increased following exposure to 10 nM EGF or 0.5 mM OVA ($P < 0.05$ for both treatments, as compared with control). Erk1/2 phosphorylation was further increased by co-stimulation with EGF and OVA, as compared with OVA only ($P < 0.05$). The increase in Erk1/2 phosphorylation induced by co-stimulation with EGF and OVA was significantly reduced in the presence of inhibitors of EGFR (AG1478), MEK (PD98059), and Erk1/2 (FR180204), but not by inhibition of Src, JNK, MAPK p38, and Rho kinase (**Figure 5**).

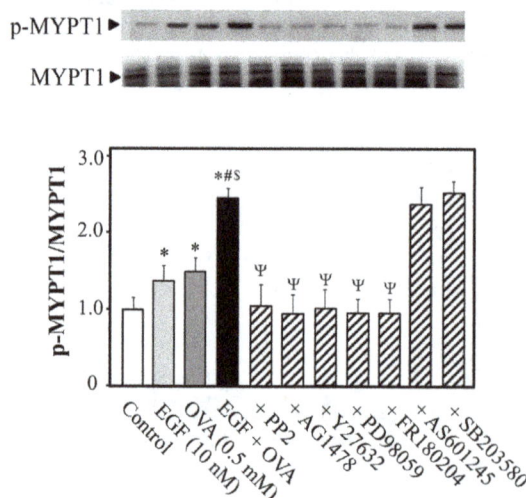

Figure 4. Inhibitor effects on sodium orthovanadate (OVA)- and/or epidermal growth factor (EGF)-induced phosphorylation of myosin phosphatase target subunit 1 (MYPT1) in rat endothelium-denuded thoracic aortic rings. Phosphorylated (Thr-853) and total MYPT1 were measured by western blotting 5 min after treatment with EGF (10 nM) and/or OVA (0.5 mM). The aortic rings were exposed to PP2 (3 µM), AG1478 (10 µM), Y27632 (10 µM), PD98059 (10 µM), FR180204 (10 µM), AS601245 (10 µM), SB203580 (10 µM), or control (10 µL dimethyl sulfoxide) for 15 min prior to EGF and/or OVA treatment. The bar graphs show the densitometric data as the ratio of Thr-853-phosphorylated MYPT1 to total MYPT1. Data are presented as mean ± SEM from 4 independent experiments; $^*P < 0.05$ vs. control; $^#P < 0.05$ vs. EGF, $^\$P < 0.05$ vs. OVA; $^\Psi P < 0.05$ vs. EGF plus OVA.

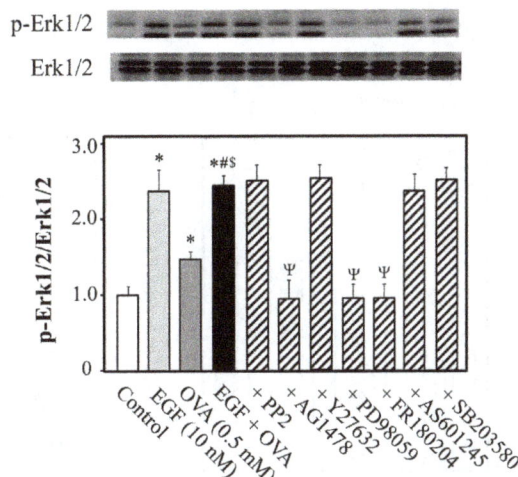

Figure 5. Inhibitory effects on sodium orthovanadate (OVA)- and/or epidermal growth factor (EGF)-induced phosphorylation of extracellular signal-regulated kinases 1 and 2 (Erk1/2) in rat endothelium-denuded thoracic aortic rings. Phosphorylated (p-Erk1/2; Thr-202/Tyr-204) and total Erk1/2 were measured by western blotting 5 min after treatment with EGF (10 nM) and/or OVA (5 mM). The aortic rings were exposed to Y27632 (10 μM), AG1478 (10 μM), PP2 (3 μM), PD98059 (10 μM), FR180204 (10 μM), or control (10 μL dimethyl sulfoxide) for 15 min prior to EGF and/or OVA treatment. The bar graphs show the densitometric data as the ratio of p-Erk1/2 to total Erk1/2. Data are presented as the mean ± SEM of 4 independent experiments; $^*P < 0.05$ vs. control; $^\#P < 0.05$ vs. EGF, $^\$P < 0.05$ vs. OVA; $^\Psi P < 0.05$ vs. EGF plus OVA.

3.6. EGF and OVA Induced EGFR Phosphorylation

We investigated whether the combination of EGF (10 nM) and OVA (0.5 mM) induced phosphorylation of the EGFR at Tyr-845 and Tyr-1173. Western blotting using a phospho-specific antibody for EGFR Tyr-1173 revealed a significantly increased signal in endothelium-denuded rat thoracic aortic rings treated with EGF or OVA, and in tissue co-treated with EGF and OVA (**Figure 6(a)**). The phosphorylation of EGFR at Tyr-845 was also significantly increased following exposure of the thoracic aortic rings to EGF or OVA ($P < 0.05$ for both treatments, as compared with control). This Tyr-845 phosphorylation was further increased by co-treatment with EGF and OVA ($P < 0.05$ versus EGF only and versus OVA only; **Figure 6(b)**). The increase in EGFR Tyr-845 phosphorylation induced by co-stimulation with EGF and OVA was significantly reduced in the presence of the Src inhibitor, PP2 (**Figure 6(b)**).

4. Discussion

In the present study, we demonstrated that EGF enhanced OVA-induced contraction of the rat endothelium-denuded thoracic aorta and that this effect was mediated by Src, EGFR, MEK, Erk1/2, and Rho kinase. Treatment of the rat endothelium-denuded thoracic aorta with EGF or OVA augmented the phosphorylation of MYPT1. This was further increased by co-stimulation with EGF and OVA, and was blocked by pretreatment with inhibitors of Src, EGFR, MEK, and Erk1/2. The phosphorylation of EGFR at Tyr-1173 in rat endothelium-denuded thoracic aorta was increased by treatment with EGF or OVA, and by co-treatment with EGF and OVA. Phosphorylation of EGFR at Tyr-845 was also augmented by exposure to EGF or OVA. This was further increased by co-stimulation with EGF and OVA, and was reduced by inhibition of Src.

Vanadium compounds such as OVA are tyrosine phosphatase inhibitors, which induce contraction of several tissues including guinea pig ileal longitudinal smooth muscle [29] and rat thoracic arteries [30]. The present study indicated that OVA-induced aortic smooth muscle contraction was mediated by the EGFR, because an EGFR inhibitor (AG1478) abolished this effect. Previous research has demonstrated that vanadium compound-induced smooth muscle contraction was mediated by Rho kinase activation [24]-[27] [32]-[36]. Mori and Tsushima identified a role for Rho kinase in OVA-induced smooth muscle contraction in guinea pig ileal longitudinal smooth muscle, where a Rho kinase inhibitor (Y27632) blocked OVA-induced contraction and MLC

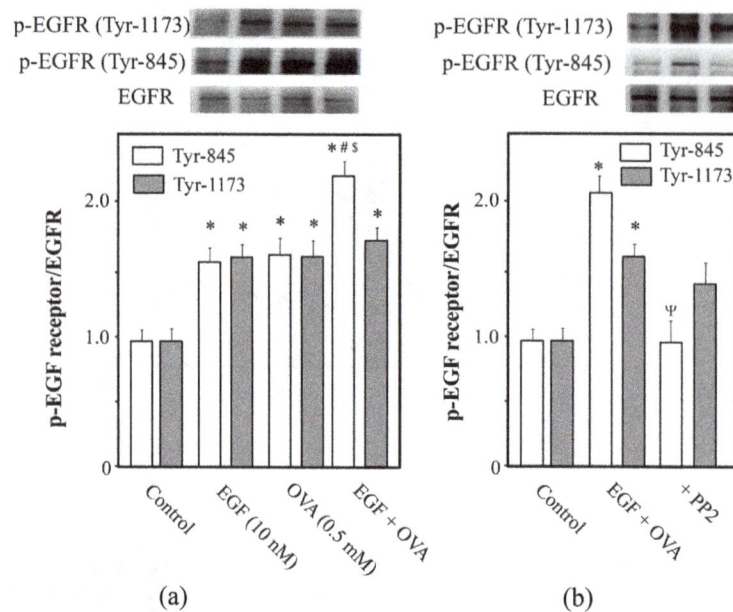

Figure 6. Effect of sodium orthovanadate (OVA)- and/or epidermal growth factor (EGF)-induced phosphorylation of EGF receptor (EGFR) at Tyr-845 and at Tyr-1173 in the rat endothelium-denuded thoracic aorta. (a) Rat endothelium-denuded thoracic aortic rings were treated with EGF (10 nM) and/or OVA (0.5 mM) for 5 min prior to analysis of phosphorylated EGFR (p-EGFR) at Tyr-845 and at Tyr-1173 by western blotting. (b) PP2 (3 μM) was added 15 min before treatment with EGF (10 nM) and/or OVA (0.5 mM) for 5 min and subsequent analysis of p-EGFR by western blotting. The bar graphs show the densitometric quantification of the ratio of p-EGFR to total EGFR. Data are presented as the mean ± SEM of four independent experiments; $^*P < 0.05$ vs. control; $^\#P < 0.05$ vs. EGF, $^\$P < 0.05$ vs. OVA; $^\Psi P < 0.05$ vs. EGF plus OVA.

phosphorylation [29]. This was consistent with our earlier study, where we showed that OVA-induced smooth muscle contraction was Rho kinase-dependent, since Rho kinase inhibition abolished OVA-induced aortic contraction, whereas MLCK inhibition by ML-7 did not affect this process [30]. In addition, several studies have reported that OVA- or pervanadate-induced contraction of smooth muscle cells was not accompanied by a rise in cytosolic Ca^{2+}, but instead occurred as a result of an increased Ca^{2+} sensitivity of the contractile apparatus [36]-[38]. Activation of Rho kinase inhibits MLCP by phosphorylating MYPT1; this causes Ca^{2+} sensitization and thereby enhances contraction in the absence of a change in the cytosolic Ca^{2+} levels [29].

OVA-induced contraction of the rat thoracic aorta is mediated by Rho kinase-dependent inactivation of MLCP via signaling downstream of Src-induced transactivation of EGFR [30]. The binding of EGF to the EGFR induces receptor dimerization, which triggers autophosphorylation of five specific tyrosine residues (Tyr-1173, -1148, -1086, -1068, and -992) in the intracellular carboxy-terminal region of the EGFR. EGFR at Tyr-1173 represents the major autophosphorylation site [39]. Src functions as a co-transducer of transmembrane signals emanating from a variety of polypeptide growth factor receptors, including the EGFR [40]. Src can activate the EGFR either directly, by phosphorylation of EGFR at Tyr-845 in the cytoplasm [40] [41], or indirectly via the metalloproteinase-catalyzed release of heparin-binding (HB)-EGF from pro-HB-EGF [42]. In our previous study, OVA increased the phosphorylation of Src at Tyr-416 in rat vascular smooth muscle cells and this effect was blocked in the presence of a Src inhibitor. Furthermore, two inhibitors of pro-EGF shedding (TAPI-0 and CRM 197) blocked not only OVA-induced contraction of the rat endothelium-denuded thoracic aorta, but also OVA-induced phosphorylation of MYPT1 and of EGFR at Tyr-1173 and at Tyr-845 in rat vascular smooth muscle cells [30]. The observation that OVA-induced EGF phosphorylation at Tyr-1173 and Tyr-845 was blocked by Src inhibition suggests that the transactivation of EGF via pro-HB-EGF processing depends on Src kinase activity in vascular smooth muscle cells [30]. In the present study, we showed that EGF and/or OVA induced EGFR phosphorylation at Tyr-845 and Tyr-1173 in rat endothelium-denuded thoracic aorta. The contraction and the phosphorylation of EGFR at Tyr-845 were further increased by co-treatment with EGF and OVA, and were abolished by treatment with a Src inhibitor. The aortic contraction and the phosphorylation of MYPT1 induced by OVA or EGF were further augmented by co-stimulation with EGF and OVA, and inhibited by Src inhibition. The phosphorylation of EGFR at Tyr-845 is a major Src-dependent phosphorylation site that is associated with increased receptor function. Src-catalyzed phosphorylation of EGFR at this residue is thought to be essential for mitogenic signaling via the EGFR, since cells expressing Y845F mutant EGFR showed markedly decreased DNA synthesis in response to EGF [40] [43] [44]. Therefore, it is likely that the activation of Src by inhibitors of protein tyrosine phosphatase (such as OVA) induces phosphorylation of EGFR at Tyr-845, which in turn results in increased signaling via the EGFR and activation of Rho kinase dependent MYPT1 phosphorylation in rat endothelium-denuded thoracic aorta.

The MAPK family members, such as Erk1/2, MAPK p38, and JNK, are the major transducers of signals generated by EGF [45]. We used inhibitors to explore the role of MAPKs in EGF- and OVA-induced aortic contraction and Rho kinase-dependent MYPT1 phosphorylation. The increase in MYPT1 phosphorylation was abolished by inhibitors of Src, EGFR, MEK, Erk1/2, and Rho kinase, but not of JNK or MAPK p38. Subsequently, we showed that OVA and/or EGF induced Erk1/2 phosphorylation in endothelium-denuded rat thoracic aorta, an effect that was abolished by inhibitors targeting the EGFR, MEK, and Erk1/2, but not by Src and Rho kinase inhibition. Binding of EGF to EGFR leads to the phosphorylation of Erk1/2 [46]. Src can phosphorylate the EGFR either directly or indirectly [40]-[42], resulting in vascular smooth muscle contraction [30]. The vasoconstrictive effects of co-stimulation of rat endothelium-denuded thoracic aorta with EGF and OVA were blocked by Src and Erk1/2 inhibitors. Src inhibition also blocked the EGF and OVA-induced EGFR phosphorylation at Tyr-845 in this preparation, but failed to inhibit Erk1/2 phosphorylation. Taken together, OVA-induced Src activated the phosphorylation of MYPT1 by phosphorylating the EGFR at Tyr-845, leading to smooth muscle contraction, whereas EGF activated MYPT1 phosphorylation through Erk1/2 phosphorylation. Thus, it seems that two different pathways regulate MYPT1 phosphorylation in smooth muscle exposed to EGF and OVA.

Vascular smooth muscle contraction in response to EGF was observed in thoracic aorta preparations from deoxycorticosterone acetate (DOCA)-salt hypertensive rats [47] and from a one kidney, one-clip hypertensive rat model [48]. Kim *et al.* reported that EGF-induced aortic contraction in DOCA-salt hypertensive rats was regulated by Erk1/2 and Rho kinase. However, EGF did not induce contraction of vascular smooth muscle from normotensive rats [49]. These reports suggested that EGF-induced vascular smooth muscle contraction was regulated by MEK, Erk1/2, and Rho kinase in hypertensive rats, but not in normotensive rats [49]. The phosphorylation of Src, EGFR, and Erk1/2 was significantly higher in vascular smooth muscle cells from spontaneously hypertensive rats, as compared to those in Wistar-Kyoto rats [50] [51]. Touyz *et al.* reported that angiotensin II increased the synthesis of DNA in vascular smooth muscle cells derived from small peripheral resistance arteries from hypertensive patients, but not in those from normotensive patients. Inhibition of Src reduced Erk1/2 activity and normalized Erk1/2 responses in normotensive patients [52]. These studies and our recent findings suggest that Src plays an important role in the regulation of vascular smooth muscle functions.

In summary, the present study provides the novel finding that Src phosphorylates the EGFR at Thr-845, which in turn activates MYPT1 phosphorylation via an unknown signaling cascade, leading to smooth muscle contraction and vessel constriction. On the other hand, EGF activates Erk1/2 phosphorylation, which phosphorylates MYPT1, resulting in smooth muscle contraction. Although EGF alone does not induce vascular smooth muscle contraction, it enhances OVA-induced contraction. Interestingly, both the activation of Src by OVA and of Erk1/2 by EGF result in MLCP inactivation via MYPT1 phosphorylation, leading to smooth muscle contraction via different signaling pathways. However, the OVA target molecule involved in Src-dependent vessel contraction is unclear, as it is the signaling cascade involved in Rho kinase dependent MYPT1 phosphorylation. Further studies are required to comprehensively elucidate the role of protein tyrosine phosphatase regulation in the mechanisms underlying vasoconstriction.

Acknowledgments

This study was partially supported by a Grant-in-Aid for Scientific Research (C) (No. 15K07984) from the Ministry of Education, Culture, Sports, Science and Technology of Japan.

Conflict of Interest

There are no conflicts of interest to declare.

References

[1]   Kamm, K.E. and Stull, J.T. (1985) The Function of Myosin and Myosin Light Chain Kinase Phosphorylation in Smooth Muscle. *Annual Review of Pharmacology and Toxicology*, **25**, 593-620. http://dx.doi.org/10.1146/annurev.pa.25.040185.003113

[2]   Lin, G., Fandel, T.M., Shindel, A.W., Wang, G., Banie, L., Ning, H., Lue, T.F. and Lin, C.S. (2011) Modulation of Smooth Muscle Tonus in the Lower Urinary Tract: Interplay of Myosin Light-Chain Kinase (MLCK) and MLC Phosphatase (MLCP). *BJU International*, **108**, E66-E70. http://dx.doi.org/10.1111/j.1464-410x.2010.09819.x

[3]   Arimura, T., Suematsu, N., Zhou, Y.B., Nishimura, J., Satoh, S., Takeshita, A., Kanaide, H. and Kimura, A. (2001) Identification, Characterization, and Functional Analysis of Heart-Specific Myosin Light Chain Phosphatase Small Subunit. *The Journal of Biological Chemistry*, **276**, 6073-6082. http://dx.doi.org/10.1074/jbc.M008566200

[4]   Somlyo, A.P. and Somlyo, A.V. (2003) Ca^{2+} Sensitivity of Smooth Muscle and Nonmuscle Myosin II: Modulated by G Proteins, Kinases, and Myosin Phosphatase. *Physiological Reviews*, **83**, 1325-1358. http://dx.doi.org/10.1152/physrev.00023.2003

[5]   Sward, K., Mita, M., Wilson, D.P., Deng, J.T., Susnjar, M. and Walsh, M.P. (2003) The Role of RhoA and Rho-Associated Kinase in Vascular Smooth Muscle Contraction. *Current Hypertension Reports*, **5**, 66-72. http://dx.doi.org/10.1007/s11906-003-0013-1

[6]   Tiganis, T. and Bennett, A.M. (2007) Protein Tyrosine Phosphatase Function: The Substrate Perspective. *Biochemical Journal*, **402**, 1-15. http://dx.doi.org/10.1042/BJ20061548

[7]   Swarup, G., Cohen, S. and Garbers, D.L. (1982) Inhibition of Membrane Phosphotyrosyl-Protein Phosphatase Activity by Vanadate. *Biochemical and Biophysical Research Communications*, **107**, 1104-1109. http://dx.doi.org/10.1016/0006-291X(82)90635-0

[8]   Cantley Jr., L.C. Josephson, L., Warner, R., Yanagisawa, M., Lechene, C. and Guidotti, G. (1977) Vanadate Is a Potent (Na,K)-ATPase Inhibitor Found in ATP Derived from Muscle. *The Journal of Biological Chemistry*, **252**, 7421-7423.

[9]   Chen, Y. and Chan, T.M. (1993) Orthovanadate and 2,3-Dimethoxy-1,4-naphthoquinone Augment Growth Factor-Induced Cell Proliferation and c-fos Gene Expression in 3T3-L1 Cells. *Archives of Biochemistry and Biophysics*, **305**, 9-16. http://dx.doi.org/10.1006/abbi.1993.1387

[10] Mehdi, M.Z., Pandey, S.K., Theberge, J.F. and Srivastava, A.K. (2006) Insulin Signal Mimicry as a Mechanism for the Insulin-Like Effects of Vanadium. *Cell Biochemistry and Biophysics*, **44**, 73-81. http://dx.doi.org/10.1385/CBB:44:1:073

[11] Morita, A., Yamamoto, S., Wang, B., Tanaka, K., Suzuki, N., Aoki, S., Ito, A., Nanao, T., Ohya, S., Yoshino, M., Zhu, J., Enomoto, A., Matsumoto, Y., Funatsu, O., Hosoi, Y. and Ikekita, M. (2010) Sodium Orthovanadate Inhibits p53-Mediated Apoptosis. *Cancer Research*, **70**, 257-265. http://dx.doi.org/10.1158/0008-5472.CAN-08-3771

[12] Wozniak, K. and Blasiak, J. (2004) Vanadyl Sulfate Can Differentially Damage DNA in Human Lymphocytes and HeLa Cells. *Archives of Toxicology*, **78**, 7-15. http://dx.doi.org/10.1007/s00204-003-0506-3

[13] Sabbioni, E., Pozzi, G., Pintar, A., Casella, L. and Garattini, S. (1991) Cellular Retention, Cytotoxicity and Morphological Transformation by Vanadium(IV) and Vanadium(V) in BALB/3T3 Cell Lines. *Carcinogenesis*, **12**, 47-52. Http://Dx.Doi.Org/10.1093/Carcin/12.1.47

[14] Soeda, S., Shimada, T., Koyanagi, S., Yokomatsu, T., Murano, T., Shibuya, S. and Shimeno, H. (2002) An Attempt to Promote Neo-Vascularization by Employing a Newly Synthesized Inhibitor of Protein Tyrosine Phosphatase. *FEBS Letters*, **524**, 54-58. http://dx.doi.org/10.1016/S0014-5793(02)03002-8

[15] Carr, A.N., Davis, M.G., Eby-Wilkens, E., Howard, B.W., Towne, B.A., Dufresne, T.E. and Peters, K.G. (2004) Tyrosine Phosphatase Inhibition Augments Collateral Blood Flow in a Rat Model of Peripheral Vascular Disease. *AJP: Heart and Circulatory Physiology*, **287**, H268-H276. http://dx.doi.org/10.1152/ajpheart.00007.2004

[16] Natarajan, V., Scribner, W.M. and Vepa, S. (1997) Phosphatase Inhibitors Potentiate 4-Hydroxynonenal-Induced Phospholipase D Activation in Vascular Endothelial Cells. *American Journal of Respiratory Cell and Molecular Biology*, **17**, 251-259. http://dx.doi.org/10.1165/ajrcmb.17.2.2623

[17] Yuan, Y., Meng, F.Y., Huang, Q., Hawker, J. and Wu, H.M. (1998) Tyrosine Phosphorylation of Paxillin/pp125FAK and Microvascular Endothelial Barrier Function. *American Journal of Physiology*, **275**, H84-H93.

[18] Garcia, J.G., Schaphorst, K.L., Verin, A.D., Vepa, S., Patterson, C.E. and Natarajan, V. (1985) Diperoxovanadate Alters Endothelial Cell Focal Contacts and Barrier Function: Role of Tyrosine Phosphorylation. *Journal of Applied Physiology*, **89**, 2333-2343.

[19] Suzuki, E., Nagata, D., Yoshizumi, M., Kakoki, M., Goto, A., Omata, M. and Hirata, Y. (2000) Reentry into the Cell Cycle of Contact-Inhibited Vascular Endothelial Cells by a Phosphatase Inhibitor. Possible Involvement of Extracellular Signal-Regulated Kinase and Phosphatidylinositol 3-Kinase. *The Journal of Biological Chemistry*, **275**, 3637-3644. http://dx.doi.org/10.1074/jbc.275.5.3637

[20] Shimizu, H., Takayama, H., Lee, J.D., Satake, K., Taniguchi, T., Yamamura, H. and Nakamura, T. (1994) Effects of Vanadate on Prostacyclin and Endothelin-1 Production and Protein-Tyrosine Phosphorylation in Human Endothelial Cells. *Thrombosis and Haemostasis*, **72**, 973-978.

[21] Helgadottir, A., Halldorsson, H., Magnusdottir, K., Kjeld, M. and Thorgeirsson, G. (1997) A Role for Tyrosine Phosphorylation in Generation of Inositol Phosphates and Prostacyclin Production in Endothelial Cells. *Arteriosclerosis, Thrombosis, and Vascular Biology*, **17**, 287-294. http://dx.doi.org/10.1161/01.ATV.17.2.287

[22] Hellermann, G.R., Flam, B.R., Eichler, D.C. and Solomonson, L.P. (2000) Stimulation of Receptor-Mediated Nitric Oxide Production by Vanadate. *Arteriosclerosis, Thrombosis, and Vascular Biology*, **20**, 2045-2050. http://dx.doi.org/10.1161/01.ATV.20.9.2045

[23] Nakaike, R., Shimokawa, H., Owada, M.K., Tokunaga, O., Yasutake, H., Kishimoto, T., Imada, C., Shiraishi, T., Egashira, K. and Takeshita, A. (1996) Vanadate Causes Synthesis of Endothelium-Derived NO via Pertussis Toxin-Sensitive G Protein in Pigs. *American Journal of Physiology*, **271**, H296-H302.

[24] Di Salvo, J., Semenchuk, L.A. and Lauer, J. (1993) Vanadate-Induced Contraction of Smooth Muscle and Enhanced Protein Tyrosine Phosphorylation. *Archives of Biochemistry and Biophysics*, **304**, 386-391. http://dx.doi.org/10.1006/abbi.1993.1366

[25] Nayler, R.A. and Sparrow, M.P. (1983) Mechanism of Vanadate-Induced Contraction of Airways Smooth Muscle of the Guinea-Pig. *British Journal of Pharmacology*, **80**, 163-172. http://dx.doi.org/10.1111/j.1476-5381.1983.tb11062.x

[26] Alcon, S., Camello, P.J., Garcia, L.J. and Pozo, M.J. (2000) Activation of Tyrosine Kinase Pathway by Vanadate in Gallbladder Smooth Muscle. *Biochemical Pharmacology*, **59**, 1077-1089. http://dx.doi.org/10.1016/S0006-2952(00)00237-9

[27] Laniyonu, A., Saifeddine, M., Ahmad, S. and Hollenberg, M.D. (1994) Regulation of Vascular and Gastric Smooth Muscle Contractility by Pervanadate. *British Journal of Pharmacology*, **113**, 403-410. http://dx.doi.org/10.1111/j.1476-5381.1994.tb17003.x

[28] Boulven, I., Robin, P., Desmyter, C., Harbon, S. and Leiber, D. (2002) Differential Involvement of Src Family Kinases in Pervanadate-Mediated Responses in Rat Myometrial Cells. *Cellular Signalling*, **14**, 341-349. http://dx.doi.org/10.1016/S0898-6568(01)00269-8

[29] Mori, M. and Tsushima, H. (2004) Vanadate Activates Rho A Translocation in Association with Contracting Effects in Ileal Longitudinal Smooth Muscle of Guinea Pig. *Journal of Pharmacological Sciences*, **95**, 443-451. http://dx.doi.org/10.1254/jphs.FP0030576

[30] Yayama, K., Sasahara, T., Ohba, H., Funasaka, A. and Okamoto, H. (2014) Orthovanadate-Induced Vasocontraction Is Mediated by the Activation of Rho-Kinase through Src-Dependent Transactivation of Epidermal Growth Factor Receptor. *Pharmacology Research & Perspectives*, **2**, Article ID: e00039. http://dx.doi.org/10.1002/prp2.39

[31] Sasahara, T., Ohkura, N., Kobe, A. and Yayama, K. (2015) Epidermal Growth Factor Induces Ca^{2+} Sensitization through Rho-Kinase-Dependent Phosphorylation of Myosin Phosphatase Target Subunit 1 in Vascular Smooth Muscle. *European Journal of Pharmacology*, **762**, 89-95. http://dx.doi.org/10.1016/j.ejphar.2015.05.042

[32] Rapp, J.P. (1981) Aortic Responses to Vanadate: Independence from (Na,K)-ATPase and Comparison of Dahl Salt-Sensitive and Salt-Resistant Rats. *Hypertension*, **3**, 1168-1172. http://dx.doi.org/10.1161/01.HYP.3.3_Pt_2.I168

[33] Sanchez-Ferrer, C.F., Marin, J., Lluch, M., Valverde, A. and Salaices, M. (1988) Actions of Vanadate on Vascular Tension and Sodium Pump Activity in Cat Isolated Cerebral and Femoral Arteries. *British Journal of Pharmacology*, **93**, 53-60. http://dx.doi.org/10.1111/j.1476-5381.1988.tb11404.x

[34] Fox, A.A., Borchard, U. and Neumann, M. (1983) Effects of Vanadate on Isolated Vascular Tissue: Biochemical and Functional Investigations. *Journal of Cardiovascular Pharmacology*, **5**, 309-316. http://dx.doi.org/10.1097/00005344-198303000-00024

[35] Shimada, T., Shimamura, K. and Sunano, S. (1986) Effects of Sodium Vanadate on Various Types of Vascular Smooth Muscles. *Journal of Vascular Research*, **23**, 113-124. http://dx.doi.org/10.1159/000158628

[36] Spurrell, B.E., Murphy, T.V. and Hill, M.A. (2000) Tyrosine Phosphorylation Modulates Arteriolar Tone but Is Not Fundamental to Myogenic Response. *The American Journal of Physiology—Heart and Circulatory Physiology*, **278**, H373-H382.

[37] Masui, H. and Wakabayashi, I. (2000) Tyrosine Phosphorylation Increases Ca^{2+} Sensitivity of Vascular Smooth Muscle Contraction. *Life Sciences*, **68**, 363-372. http://dx.doi.org/10.1016/S0024-3205(00)00942-5

[38] Murphy, T.V., Spurrell, B.E. and Hill, M.A. (2002) Mechanisms Underlying Pervanadate-Induced Contraction of Rat Cremaster Muscle Arterioles. *European Journal of Pharmacology*, **442**, 107-114. http://dx.doi.org/10.1016/S0014-2999(02)01498-X

[39] Voldborg, B.R., Damstrup, L., Spang-Thomsen, M. and Poulsen, H.S. (1997) Epidermal Growth Factor Receptor (EGFR) and EGFR Mutations, Function and Possible Role in Clinical Trials. *Annals of Oncology*, **8**, 1197-1206. http://dx.doi.org/10.1023/A:1008209720526

[40] Biscardi, J.S., Maa, M.C., Tice, D.A., Cox, M.E., Leu, T.H. and Parsons, S.J. (1999) C-Src-Mediated Phosphorylation of the Epidermal Growth Factor Receptor on Tyr[845] and Tyr[1101] Is Associated with Modulation of Receptor Function. *The Journal of Biological Chemistry*, **274**, 8335-8343. http://dx.doi.org/10.1074/jbc.274.12.8335

[41] Sato, K., Sato, A., Aoto, M. and Fukami, Y. (1995) C-Src Phosphorylates Epidermal Growth Factor Receptor on Tyrosine 845. *Biochemical and Biophysical Research Communications*, **215**, 1078-1087. http://dx.doi.org/10.1006/bbrc.1995.2574

[42] Pai, R., Soreghan, B., Szabo, I.L., Pavelka, M., Baatar, D. and Tarnawski, A.S. (2002) Prostaglandin E2 Transactivates EGF Receptor: A Novel Mechanism for Promoting Colon Cancer Growth and Gastrointestinal Hypertrophy. *Nature Medicine*, **8**, 289-293. http://dx.doi.org/10.1038/nm0302-289

[43] Tice, D.A., Biscardi, J.S., Nickles, A.L. and Parsons, S.J. (1999) Mechanism of Biological Synergy between Cellular Src and Epidermal Growth Factor Receptor. *Proceedings of the National Academy of Sciences of the United States of America*, **96**, 1415-1420. http://dx.doi.org/10.1073/pnas.96.4.1415

[44] Haskell, M.D., Slack, J.K., Parsons, J.T. and Parsons, S.J. (2001) C-Src Tyrosine Phosphorylation of Epidermal Growth Factor Receptor, P190 RhoGAP, and Focal Adhesion Kinase Regulates Diverse Cellular Processes. *Chemical Reviews*, **101**, 2425-2440. http://dx.doi.org/10.1021/cr0002341

[45] Cowan, K.J. and Storey, K.B. (2003) Mitogen-Activated Protein Kinases: New Signaling Pathways Functioning in Cellular Responses to Environmental Stress. *Journal of Experimental Biology*, **206**, 1107-1115. http://dx.doi.org/10.1242/jeb.00220

[46] Zhang, Y., Wang, L.Y., Zhang, M.M., Jin, M.L., Bai, C.X. and Wang, X.D. (2012) Potential Mechanism of Interleukin-8 Production from Lung Cancer Cells: An Involvement of EGF-EGFR-PI3K-Akt-Erk Pathway. *Journal of Cellular Physiology*, **227**, 35-43. http://dx.doi.org/10.1002/jcp.22722

[47] Florian, J.A. and Watts, S.W. (1999) Epidermal Growth Factor: A Potent Vasoconstrictor in Experimental Hypertension. *American Journal of Physiology*, **276**, H976-H983.

[48] Northcott, C., Florian, J.A., Dorrance, A. and Watts, S.W. (2001) Arterial Epidermal Growth Factor Receptor Expression in Deoxycorticosterone Acetate-Salt Hypertension. *Hypertension*, **38**, 1337-1341. http://dx.doi.org/10.1161/hy1201.096815

[49] Kim, J., Lee, C.K., Park, H.J., Kim, H.J., So, H.H., Lee, K.S., Lee, H.M., Roh, H.Y., Choi, W.S., Park, T.K. and Kim, B. (2006) Epidermal Growth Factor Induces Vasoconstriction through the Phosphatidylinositol 3-Kinase-Mediated Mitogen-Activated Protein Kinase Pathway in Hypertensive Rats. *Journal of Pharmacological Sciences*, **101**, 135-143. http://dx.doi.org/10.1254/jphs.FP0060021

[50] Li, Y., Levesque, L.O. and Anand-Srivastava, M.B. (2010) Epidermal Growth Factor Receptor Transactivation by Endogenous Vasoactive Peptides Contributes to Hyperproliferation of Vascular Smooth Muscle Cells of SHR. *AJP: Heart and Circulatory Physiology*, **299**, H1959-H1967. http://dx.doi.org/10.1152/ajpheart.00526.2010

[51] Sandoval, Y.H., Li, Y. and Anand-Srivastava, M.B. (2011) Transactivation of Epidermal Growth Factor Receptor by Enhanced Levels of Endogenous Angiotensin II Contributes to the Overexpression of Gialpha Proteins in Vascular Smooth Muscle Cells from SHR. *Cellular Signalling*, **23**, 1716-1726. http://dx.doi.org/10.1016/j.cellsig.2011.06.006

[52] Touyz, R.M., Wu, X.H., He, G., Salomon, S. and Schiffrin, E.L. (2002) Increased Angiotensin II-Mediated Src Signaling via Epidermal Growth Factor Receptor Transactivation Is Associated with Decreased C-Terminal Src Kinase Activity in Vascular Smooth Muscle Cells from Spontaneously Hypertensive Rats. *Hypertension*, **39**, 479-485. http://dx.doi.org/10.1161/hy02t2.102909

21

Investigation of *in Vitro* and *in Vivo* Metabolism of Schisandrin B from Schisandrae Fructus by Liquid Chromatography Coupled Electrospray Ionization Tandem Mass Spectrometry

Tianxiu Qian[1,2], Pou Kuan Leong[3], Kam Ming Ko[3], Wan Chan[1*]

[1]Department of Chemistry, The Hong Kong University of Science and Technology, Hong Kong SAR, China
[2]Institute of Medicinal Plant Development, Chinese Academy of Medical Sciences & Peking Union Medical College, Beijing, China
[3]Division of Life Science, The Hong Kong University of Science and Technology, Hong Kong SAR, China
Email: *chanwan@ust.hk

Abstract

Schisandrin B (Sch B) is one of the active dibenzocyclooctadiene lignans found in the Schisandrae Fructus. Experimental studies have shown that Sch B possesses various pharmacological properties, including anti-cancer, neuroprotective and nephroprotective activities. However, no detailed information on its biotransformation was reported in the literature. Here, we investigated the *in vitro* and *in vivo* metabolism of Sch B by using ultra-performance liquid chromatography coupled with tandem mass spectrometry. *In vitro* study detected and identified one oxygenated metabolite. Four metabolites were detected and identified from the *in vivo* study. The results indicated that the metabolism of Sch B mainly involved the demethylation of methoxy groups, the opening of five-member ring and the glucuronidation of metabolites in rats. The metabolites were identified for the first time by MS/MS analyses.

Keywords

Schisandrin B, Metabolism, Disposition, UPLC-MS/MS

---

*Corresponding author.

1. Introduction

Schisandrin B (Sch B, **Figure 1**) is the most abundant active dibenzocyclooctadiene lignan isolated from Schisandrae Fructus, the fruit of *Schisandra chinensis* (Turcz) Baillon (Wu-Wei-Zi in Chinese), which grows wild in Russia, Northeast China, Korea and Japan. The herb is commonly used in Chinese medicine for therapeutic (clinically prescribed for the treatment of viral and chemical hepatitis [1]) and health-promoting purposes. Given the broad range of therapeutic application of Schisandrae Fructus, scientists have attempted to isolate the active ingredient in Schisandrae Fructus. In 1950s, an active principle, schisandrin (a dibenzocyclooctadiene lignan) was first successfully isolated in form of crystal [2]. Then more than 30 lignans have been subsequently isolated, including Sch B. A growing body of experimental evidence has shown that Sch B possesses a wide spectrum of biological activities. It has been demonstrated that Sch B produces anti-cancer action *in vitro* and *in vivo* by inhibiting cancer invasion and metastasis or enhancing doxorubicin-induced apoptosis of cancer cells [3]-[6]. Sch B was also found to protect against carbon tetrachloride-induced hepatotoxicity [7]-[11] and enhance the hepatoprotection against various toxicants in rodents [12]-[16]. In addition, a number of studies showed that Sch B protected against nephrotoxicity induced by cisplatin [17] [18], cyclosporine A [19], gentamicin [20] and mercury in rodents [21] [22]. Other biological activities of Sch B included antioxidation [23]-[27], anti-inflammation [28] [29] and cytoprotection *in vitro* [30].

Lee *et al.* demonstrated that Sch B produced neuroprotective effect on rats subjected to transient focal cerebral ischemia, presumably by inhibiting inflammation and preventing metalloproteinase degradation [31]. Recently, it has been reported that Sch B produced anti-neuroinflammatory action in lipopolysaccharide-induced microglia [32]. Sch B also produced protection against $A\beta_{1-42}$-induced neurotoxicity *in vitro* [33]. Furthermore, it has recently been reported that Sch B is able to prevent age-related neurodegeneration [34], cerebral ischemia/reperfusion injury *in vivo* [35] and cerebral toxicity induced by hydroperoxide *in vivo* [36].

The tissue non-specific protective action of Sch B has made it a promising lead compound for new drug development. In this regard, *in vivo* pharmacokinetics and tissue distribution study of Sch B has been reported [37]. Sun *et al.* determined the metabolites of Sch B *in vivo* by measuring the accurate mass of the predicted metabolite using Q-TOF [38]. However, there was no precise identification of Sch B metabolites. For a better understanding of the biochemical mechanism underlying the tissue protection afforded by Sch B, we endeavored to investigate the metabolism of Sch B *in vitro* and *in vivo* by MS/MS analyses which enabled the identification of key metabolites.

Mass spectrometry analysis can provide information such as molecular weight, fragment ions and other chemical structural parameters on the analyte. Liquid chromatography coupled with tandem mass spectrometry (LC-MS^n) is a powerful technique for determining and identifying the compound of interest. The high sensitivity of MS used as a LC detector facilitates the detection of new minor constituents, which is otherwise not detectable by classical means. HPLC-MS [39]-[41] and UPLC-MS [42] methods have been used to determine the level of Sch B in biological samples. The results indicated that mass spectrometry was highly specific and sensitive for identifying Sch B from biological matrix. In these studies, LC-MS was proved to be a rapid, specific and sensitive method to detect the presence of Sch B. In the present study, a rapid, sensitive and specific UPLC-MS/MS method was developed to study the *in vitro* and *in vivo* metabolism of Sch B.

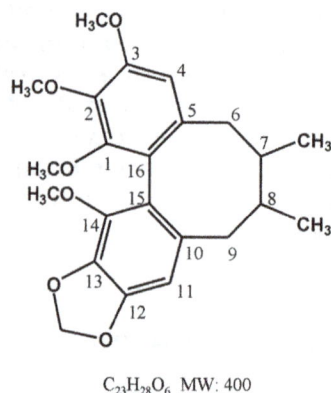

$C_{23}H_{28}O_6$ MW: 400

Figure 1. Chemical structure of schisandrin B.

2. Materials and Methods

2.1. Reagents

Sch B (purity > 99%) was isolated from the fruit of *Schisandra chinensis* (Turcz) Baillon. Rat S9 fraction, NADPH and glucose-6-phosphate (G-6-P) were purchased from Sigma Company (St. Louis, MO, USA). Acetonitrile of HPLC grade was purchased from Duksan Pure Chemicals (Kyunkido, Korea). Methanol was purchased from Tedia (Fairfield, OH, USA). All other reagents were of highest purity available. Potassium phosphate solution is prepared in-house using the aforementioned reagents. Deionized water used in the experiments was produced from a Milli-Q system (Millipore, Milford, MA, USA).

2.2. *In Vitro* Study of Sch B in Rat S9 Fraction

Five microliters of 10 mM Sch B solution was incubated with a 1 mL potassium phosphate solution (100 mM, pH 7.4) containing rat liver S9 fraction (1 mg/mL), cofactors NADPH (1 mM), G-6-P (10 mM) and activator $MgCl_2$ (3 mM). The incubation was carried out for 2 h at 37°C. The incubation mixture was then collected and 4 mL cold methanol was used to quench the metabolic reaction by precipitating all proteins as well as to extract Sch B and its metabolites. The methanol extract was then centrifuged at $8000 \times g$ for 10 min. The supernatant was dried under nitrogen stream and the residue was dissolved in 3 mL 20% methanol in H_2O (w/w). The reconstituted solution was pretreated by solid phase extraction before the UPLC-MS analysis. Negative control incubations containing no Sch B were conducted under the same experimental conditions, and the samples were also pretreated by solid phase extraction prior to UPLC-MS analysis.

2.3. *In Vivo* Study of the Metabolism of Sch B in Rats

Male Sprague-Dawley rats were obtained from the Animal and Plant Care Facilities in the Hong Kong University of Science & Technology. The experimental protocol was approved by the Research Practice Committee in HKUST. Sch B was orally administered (50 mg/kg) to male Sprague Dawley rats (body weight 200 - 220 g, prior fasting but with water for 12 h). Rats were housed in metabolic cages that allowed the separated collection of urine and feces samples. Urine and feces samples were collected from 0 to 48 hours post-dosing with Sch B.

2.4. Solid Phase Extraction Procedure

All samples from rat liver S9 fraction incubation as well as urine and feces samples were pretreated by solid phase extraction (SPE) prior to UPLC-MS analysis. Waters Sep-Pak C_{18} SPE column (1 mL, 50 mg) was first preconditioned with 2 mL methanol and then equilibrated with 2 mL pure water. Samples were loaded onto the preconditioned SPE columns directly. After being washed with 2 mL pure water, the SPE column was eluted using 2 mL methanol solution. The eluted methanol solution was dried with nitrogen stream, and the residue was reconstituted in 1 mL methanol and centrifuged at $8000 \times g$ for 10 min. The supernatant was injected into the UPLC-MS system for analysis.

2.5. Sample Preparation

Urine samples were filtered and then pretreated by solid phase extraction, as described above. Ten microliter of the supernatant was analyzed by using UPLC-MS and UPLC-MS/MS for Sch B and its metabolites.

　　Feces samples were suspended in pure water and then the mixture was sonicated for 30 min. The feces suspension was filtered and then pretreated by solid phase extraction. Ten microliter of the supernatant was analyzed by using UPLC-MS and UPLC-MS/MS for Sch B and its metabolites.

2.6. UPLC-ESI-MS Analysis

The UPLC-ESI-MS system consisted of a Waters Acquity ultra performance LC and a Waters Xevo G2 Q-Tof mass spectrometer (Waters, Singapore). Positive ESI ion mode was used to analyze Sch B and its metabolites in biological samples. The following parameters of the mass tune for positive ion mode were used: capillary voltage 3.0 KV, sampling cone 20, extraction cone 4.0, the source temperature at 150°C and desolvation temperature at 400°C, the desolvation gas flow at 800 L/h. Full-scan mass spectra at a mass range of *m/z* 50 - 1000 were acquired. Mass chromatogram for protonated molecular $[M + H]^+$ ions of Sch B and its metabolites were used for the determination. Molecular ion masses of potential metabolites were examined and the corresponding extracted mass chromatograms were recorded. Chromatographic separation was achieved on a Waters Acquity UPLC BEH C_{18} column (2.1 mm × 50 mm, 1.7 μm, Ireland). The mobile phase consisted of 0.1% formic acid in water (A) and acetonitrile (B). The gradient program was from 30% B, changed to 100% B within 2 min and held at 100% B for 4 min, then back to 30% B within 1 min and held 30% B till 10 min at a flow rate of 0.35 mL/min. B. The acquired UPLC-MS data were processed using Marker Lynx (Waters, Singapore).

3. Results

3.1. UPLC-MS and UPLC-MS/MS Analyses of Sch B

Conditions for UPLC and MS analysis were optimized with standard Sch B and the MS chromatogram and MS/MS spectrum of Sch B were shown in **Figure 2**. Sch B was eluted at about 5.27 min under the present

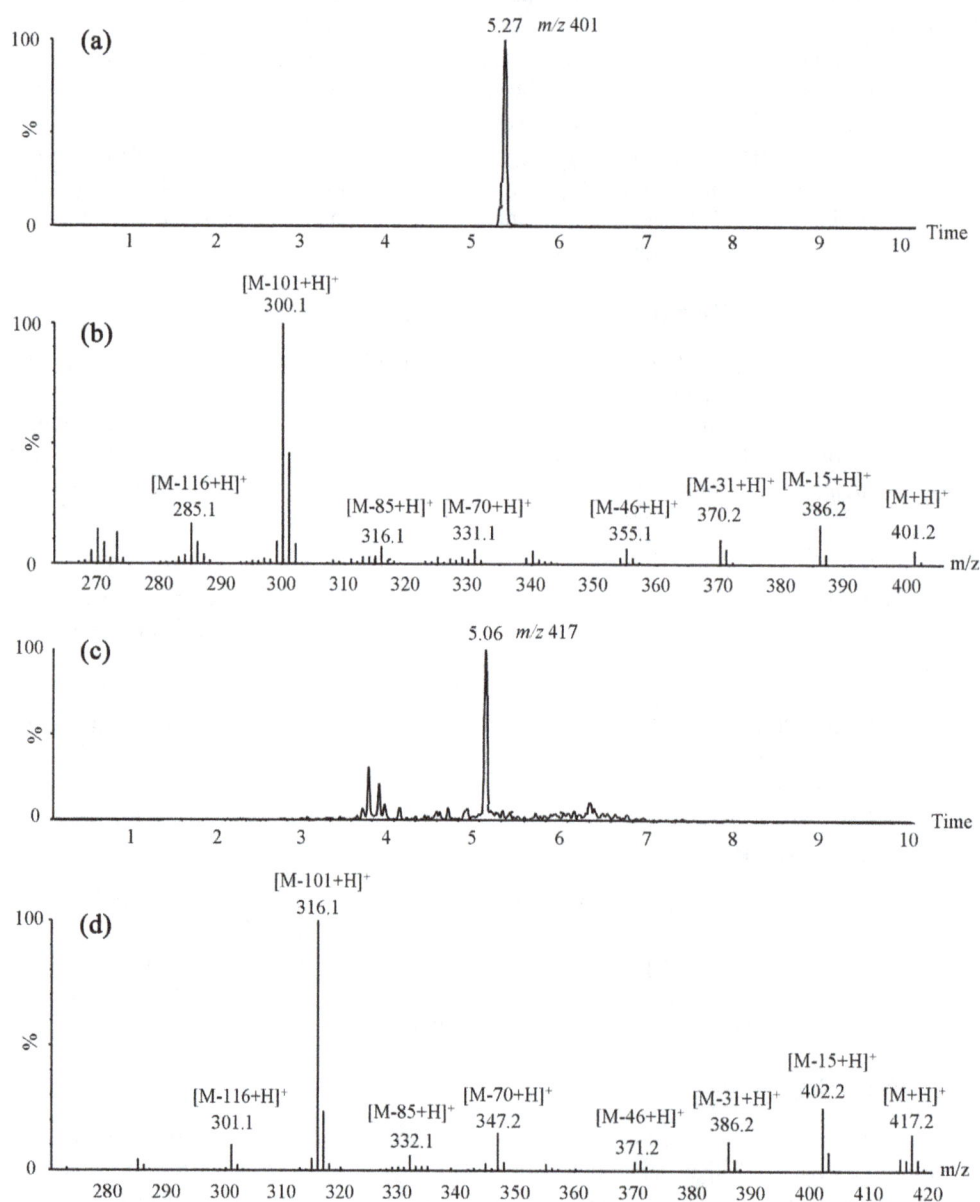

Figure 2. Full scan UPLC-MS chromatogram and MS/MS spectrum of standard Sch B ((a) Raw chromatogram data; (b) MS/MS spectrum) and metabolite M1 ((c) Raw chromatogram data; (d) MS/MS spectrum) detected from the *in vitro* incubation sample with rat S9.

experimental conditions with the protonated molecular ion at m/z 401 (**Figure 2(a)**). **Figure 2(b)** shows the MS/MS spectrum of standard Sch B, with the fragment ions at m/z 386 (M + H − 15), 370 (M + H − 31), 355 (M + H − 46), 331 (M + H − 70), 316 (M + H − 85), 300 (M + H − 101, base peak) and 285 (M + H − 116).

3.2. Determination of Sch B Metabolites from Rat S9 Fraction Incubation

By comparing with the negative control of *in vitro* incubation, the metabolite detection was achieved by UPLC-MS analysis and confirmed with UPLC-MS/MS experiments in positive ESI mode. One metabolite was detected from the incubation sample, namely, M1. **Figure 2(c)** and **Figure 2(d)** show the UPLC-MS chromatogram and the MS/MS spectrum of the metabolite M1, respectively. The extract ion of M1 was detected at m/z 417 (**Figure 2(c)**). **Figure 2(d)** shows the UPLC-MS/MS spectrum of metabolite M1. MS/MS analysis of M1 revealed the same fragment pattern as the parent Sch B (**Figure 2(b)**).

3.3. UPLC-MS/MS Analyses of Metabolites in Feces Collected Sch B-Treated Rats

Similar to the *in vitro* study, the metabolite detections were achieved by UPLC-MS analyses and confirmed with MS/MS experiments in positive ESI mode. After comparing with blank feces sample, four metabolites, namely, M1, M2, M3 and M4 (m/z 471, 387, 389 and 565, respectively), were detected in rat feces samples collected during the period of 0 - 48 h following the oral administration of Sch B (**Figure 3**). As shown in **Figure 3(a)**, both UPLC-MS data and MS/MS spectra of the peak at 5.06 (min) were identical to those of M1, whereas the other two peaks at 4.81 and 3.63 were also detected in the blank feces sample. Thus, the peak at 5.06 was identified as M1. Four demethylated metabolites at m/z value of 387 were identified at retention times of 4.82, 4.74, 4.68, 3.66 min from the UPLC-MS analysis of the feces sample (**Figure 3(b)**, M2). The peaks at 5.52 and 3.99 also existed in blank feces sample. Three peaks for the extracted ion at m/z 389 (M3, **Figure 3(c)**, peak at 3.38 also existed in blank sample) revealed the existence of isomer status for M3. However, the metabolite M4 at m/z 565 (M4, **Figure 3(d)**) showed the peak at 3.47.

Figure 4 shows the MS/MS spectrum of M2, M3 and M4. The MS/MS spectra of M2 at 4.82, 4.74, 4.68 and 3.66 in the chromatogram were shown in **Figure 3(b)**. Based on the protonated molecular ion at m/z 387 (**Figure 4(a)**), the fragment ions at m/z 372, 355 and 340, as well as fragment ions at m/z 317, 302, 286 (base peak) and 271 produced a similar fragmentation pattern to that of the parent Sch B (**Figure 2(b)**). While **Figure 4(b)** shows the MS/MS spectrum of M3 at 4.04 and 3.47 in the chromatogram shown in **Figure 3(c)**, **Figure 4(c)** shows the MS/MS spectrum of M4 at 3.47 in the chromatogram shown in **Figure 3(d)**.

3.4. UPLC-MS/MS Analyses of Metabolites in Rat Urine Collected from Sch B-Dosed Rats

Similar to the feces sample, the metabolite detection in urine sample was achieved by UPLC-MS analyses and confirmed with MS/MS experiments in positive ESI mode. When comparing with blank urine sample, three metabolites were detected in rat urine sample collected during the period of 0 - 48 h following the oral administration of Sch B. MS/MS analyses showed that the data were consistent with those of M2-M4, which were identified metabolites in rat feces. UPLC-MS chromatogram and MS/MS spectrum were not described here. The high resolution MS data and accurate MS error of Sch B and the metabolites were shown in **Table 1**. The high accuracy of MS data confirmed the identification of metabolites.

4. Discussion

In the MS/MS spectrum of standard Sch B (**Figure 2(b)**), based on the protonated molecular ion at m/z 401, the fragment ions at m/z 386 (M + H − 15), 370 (M + H − 31) and 355 (M + H − 46) indicated the loss of CH_3, OCH_3 and OCH_3 + CH_3 moieties, respectively, while the fragment ions at m/z 331 (M + H − 70), 316 (M + H − 85), 300 (M + H − 101, base peak) and 285 (M + H − 116) evidenced the loss of C_5H_{10}, C_5H_{10} + CH_3, C_5H_{10} + OCH_3 and C_5H_{10} + OCH_3 + CH_3 moieties, respectively. The results suggested that fragment pathways of Sch B under ESI-MS involved the loss of CH_3 and OCH_3 from the methoxy groups of the structure, as well as opening of the octa-member ring and the loss of C_5H_{10}. The fragment pattern of Sch B, as observed in the present study, was consistent with that reported by He *et al.* [43].

The UPLC-MS chromatogram of metabolite M1 (**Figure 2(c)**) demonstrated that the extract ion of M1 was detected at m/z 417 (**Figure 2(c)**), which was 16 Da larger than the parent Sch B (at m/z 401) (**Figure 2(a)**), suggesting that M1 was a mono-oxygenated Sch B. In the UPLC-MS/MS spectrum of metabolite M1 (**Figure 2(d)**), MS/MS analysis of M1 revealed the same fragment pattern as the parent Sch B (**Figure 2(b)**), suggesting that M1 was an oxygenated metabolite of Sch B. The fragment ion at m/z 347 $[M - 70 + H]^+$ indicated that the oxygenation site was at C_4 or C_{11}. The identification was further confirmed by high-accuracy MS analysis, with the mass error between the theoretical (417.1913) and measured (417.1923) m/z values of the $[M + H]^+$ ion being less than 2.5 ppm (**Table 1**).

Table 1. Molecular formula, accurate mass, measured mass and mass error of Sch B and its metabolites in rat.

Name	Molecular formula	Accurate $[M + H]^+$	Measured $[M + H]^+$	Mass error (ppm)
Sch B	$C_{23}H_{28}O_6$	401.1964	401.1989	6.23
M1	$C_{23}H_{28}O_7$	417.1913	417.1923	2.39
M2	$C_{22}H_{26}O_6$	387.1808	387.1809	0.26
M3	$C_{22}H_{28}O_6$	389.1964	389.1983	4.88
M4	$C_{28}H_{36}O_{12}$	565.2285	565.2281	−0.71

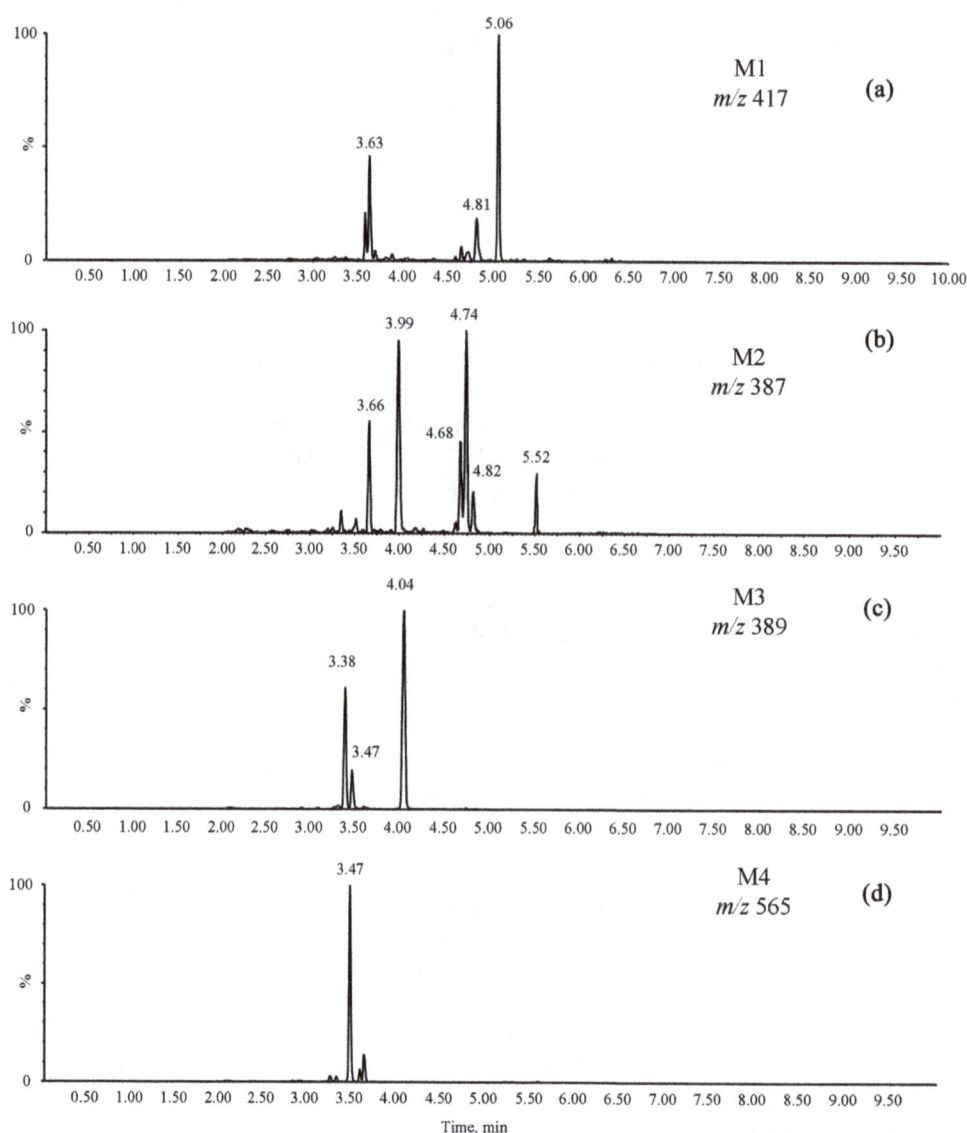

Figure 3. Extracted UPLC-MS chromatogram of M1-M4 m/z 417 (a), 387 (b), 389 (c), 565 (d) detected from rat feces sample after oral administration of Sch B.

When we examined the metabolites in feces collected Sch B-treated rats using UPLC-MS/MS four metabolites, namely, M1, M2, M3 and M4, were detected (**Figure 3**). These four isomeric demethylated metabolites (M2, **Figure 3(b)**) may have resulted from the enzymatic hydrolysis of the methoxy groups in Sch B. Three peaks for the extracted ion at m/z 389 (M3, **Figure 3(c)**) revealed the existence of isomer status for M3. However, the metabolite M4 at m/z 565 (M4, **Figure 3(d)**) showed the peak at 3.47, which was 176 Da larger than the metabolite M3 at m/z 389 (**Figure 3(c)**), suggestive of a product derived from the glucuronidation of M3.

The UPLC-MS/MS spectrum of metabolite M2, M3 and M4 were also analyzed in the present study. The MS/MS spectra of M2 (**Figure 4(a)**) at 4.82, 4.74, 4.68 and 3.66 in the chromatogram were shown in **Figure 3(b)**. MS/MS spectra at the four retention times were identical, indicating that four isomeric metabolites existed and their structures were similar, *i.e.* demethylated site was on methoxy groups. Based on the protonated molecular ion at m/z 387 (**Figure 4(a)**), the fragment ions at m/z 372, 355 and 340, as well as fragment ions at m/z 317, 302, 286 (base peak) and 271 produced a similar fragmentation pattern to that of the parent Sch B (**Figure 2(b)**). Thus, M2 was identified as the demethylated Sch B. **Figure 4(b)** shows the MS/MS spectrum of M3 at 4.04

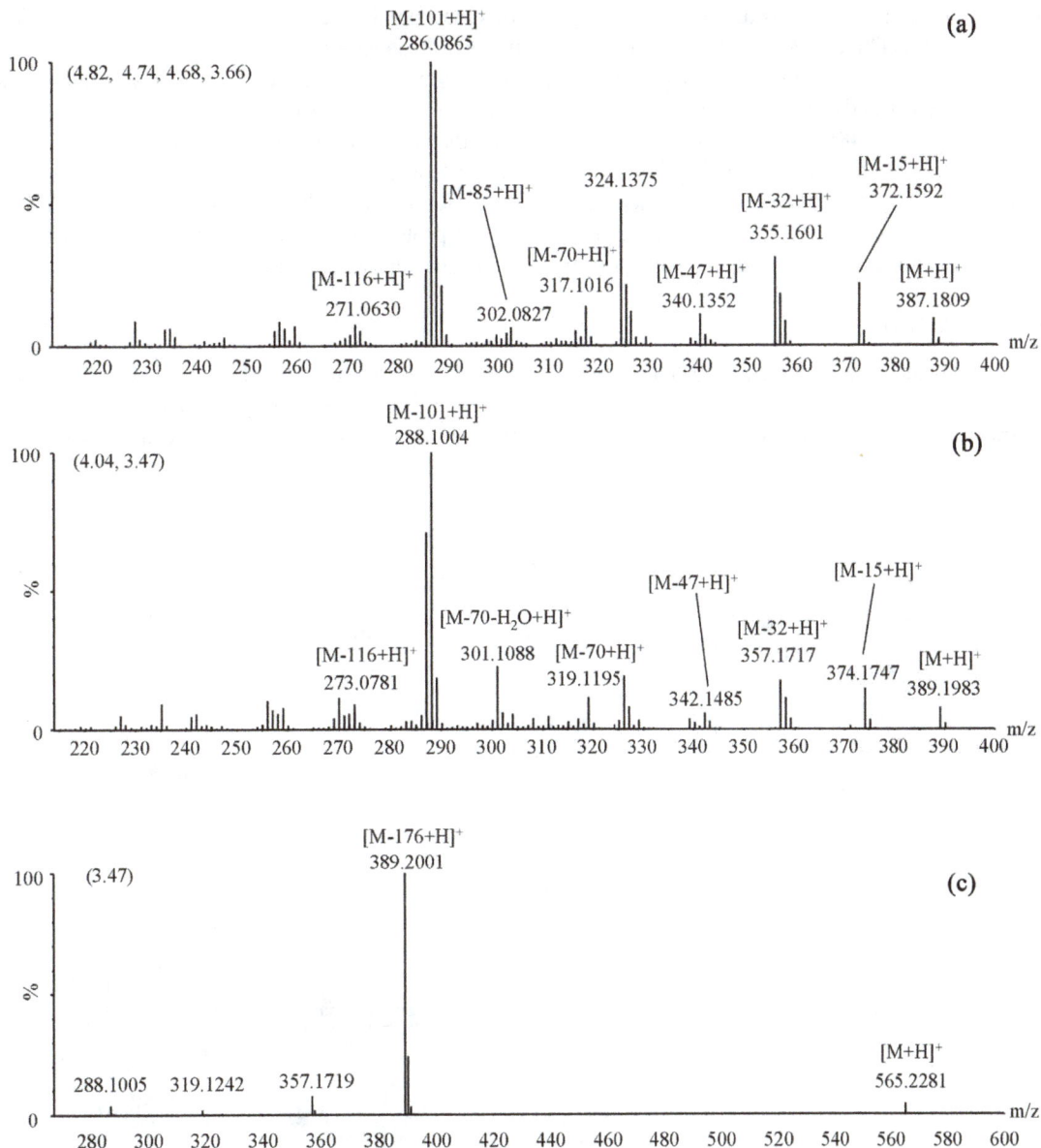

Figure 4. UPLC-MS/MS spectrum of metabolite M2 ((a) Peak at 4.82, 4.74, 4.68 and 3.66 min), M3 ((b) Peak at 4.04 and 3.47 min) and M4 ((c) Peak at 3.47 min).

and 3.47 in the chromatogram shown in **Figure 3(c)**. Similarly, based on the protonated molecular ion at m/z 389, the fragment ions at m/z 374, 357 and 342, as well as the fragment ions at m/z 319, 301, 288 (base peak) and 273 produced a similar fragmentation pattern as the parent Sch B (**Figure 2(b)**), which was identified as the opened five-member ring metabolite of Sch B. **Figure 4(c)** shows the MS/MS spectrum of M4 at 3.47 in the chromatogram shown in **Figure 3(d)**. The fragment ion at m/z 389 (base peak) evidenced the loss of 176 Da from the protonated molecular ion at m/z 565, other fragment ions were fragmented from the ion at m/z 389 and the fragmentation pattern was as same as the metabolite M3. Thus M4 was the glucuronidated form of M3. Conceivably, the peak at 3.47 in **Figure 3(c)** should be M4, which dissociated at ESI source before entered the MS detector. The peak at 4.04 in **Figure 3(c)** should represent M3, which was identified as the opened five-member ring metabolite. Taken together, the metabolic pathway of Sch B in rats was summarized in **Figure 5**.

Results from some recent studies have shed light on the underlying mechanism of how Sch B induces a tissue non-specific antioxidant response [8] [34]. They revealed that the cocomitant production of reactive oxygen species (ROS) during the cytochrome P450 (CYP)-catatlzyed metabolism of Sch B can activate the antioxidant signal transduction pathway with a resultant induction of antioxidant response [8]. However, the metabolite(s) of Sch B which can cause the production ROS is yet to be determined. In the present study, among the four metabolites of Sch B (**Figure 5**), Sch B-M1 was found to possess a catechol moiety. In this connection, some studies also demonstrated that demethylenation of methylendioxy group resulted in the formation of catechol [44]-[46], which is a redox active moiety. Catechol can be oxidized into quinone which undergoes redox cycling and generates ROS [47] [48]. A recent study has also proposed that ROS from quinone redox cycling can elicit antioxidant response via redox signaling [49]. These findings lend a strong support to the involvement of CYP-catalyzed metabolism of the methylenedioxy group in the Sch B molecule in eliciting the antioxidant response and hence tissue protection. An increased understanding the protective mechanism of Sch B has offered a promising prospect of using Sch B as an agent for mitigating the age-related diseases in humans.

5. Conclusion

The method of UPLC coupled to QTOF mass spectrometry was developed and applied to study the metabolic fate of Sch B *in vitro* and *in vivo*. One mono-oxygenated metabolite was found after incubating Sch B with rat S9 fraction *in vitro*. Four metabolites of Sch B were identified from rat feces and urine following the oral

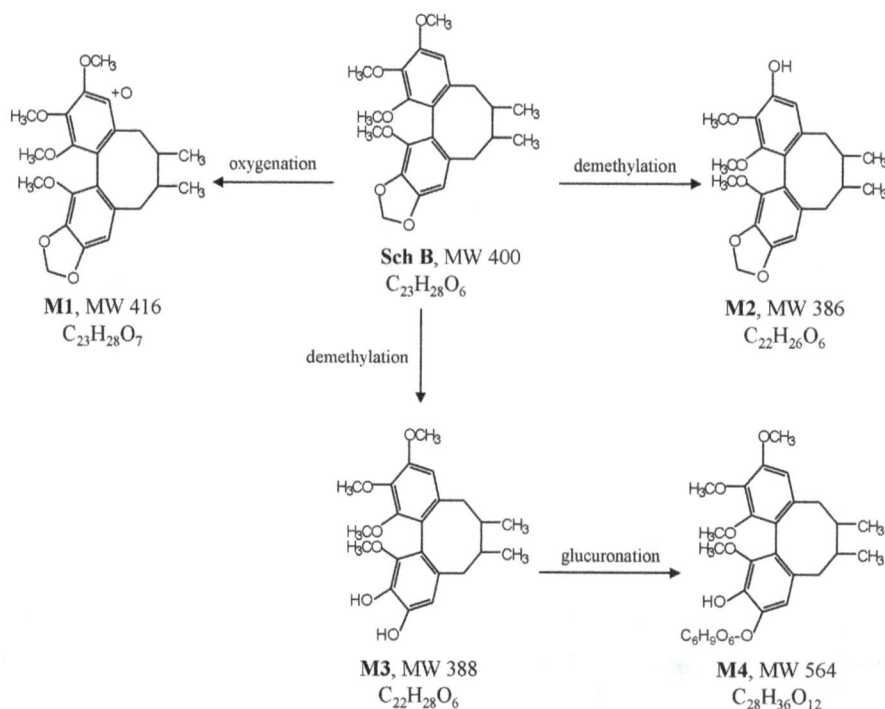

Figure 5. Proposed metabolic pathways of Sch B in rats.

administration of Sch B. The structures of metabolites were elucidated by high-accuracy MS and MS/MS analyses. The metabolic reactions of Sch B were found to mainly involve the mono-oxygenation of C_4 or C_{11}, the demethylation of methoxy groups, the opening of five-member ring and the glucuronidation of metabolites in rats.

Acknowledgements

Dr Wan Chan expresses his sincere thanks the Hong Kong University of Science and Technology for supporting this research (grant R9310). TX Qian was partially supported by a Postdoctoral Fellowship from the Provost office, HKUST.

References

[1]   Hancke, J.L., Burgos, R.A. and Ahumada, F. (1999) *Schisandra chinensis*. (Turcz.) Baill. *Fitoterapia*, **70**, 451-471. http://dx.doi.org/10.1016/S0367-326X(99)00102-1

[2]   Balandin, D.A. (1951) Schizandrin—A New Stimulant from Schizandra Fruits. In: Lazarev, N.V., Ed., *Materials for the Study of Stimulants and Tonics from Ginseng and Schizandra Roots*, Far East Branch of USSR Academy of Science, Vladivotok, 45-50.

[3]   Liu, X., Zhang, C., Jin, X., Li, Y., Zheng, X. and Li, L. (2007) Inhibitory Effect of Schisandrin B on Gastric Cancer Cells *in Vitro*. *World Journal of Gastroenterology*, **13**, 6506-6511. http://dx.doi.org/10.3748/wjg.13.6506

[4]   Li, L., Lu, Q., Shen, Y. and Hu, X. (2006) Schisandrin B Enhances Doxorubicin-Induced Apoptosis of Cancer Cells but Not Normal Cells. *Biochemical Pharmacology*, **71**, 584-595. http://dx.doi.org/10.1016/j.bcp.2005.11.026

[5]   Li, L., Wang, T., Xu, Z., Yu, Y., Chen, W. and Chen, F. (2005) Effects of Schisandrin B on Reversing Multidrug Resistance in Human Breast Cancer Cells Transfected with mdr1 Gene. *Chinese Medical Journal*, **85**, 1633-1637.

[6]   Xu, Y., Liu, Z., Sun, J., Pan, Q., Sun, F., Yan, Z. and Hu, X. (2011) Schisandrin B Prevents Doxorubicin-Induced Chronic Cardiotoxicity and Enhances Its Anticancer Activity *in Vivo*. *PLoS ONE*, **6**, e28335. http://dx.doi.org/10.1371/journal.pone.0028335

[7]   Chen, Y., Ip, S.P., Ko, K.M., Poon, T.C., Ng, E.W., Lai, P,B., Mao, Q.Q., Xian, Y.F. and Che, C.T. (2011) A Proteomic Approach in Investigating the Hepatoprotective Mechanism of Schisandrin B: Role of Raf Kinase Inhibitor Protein. *Journal of Proteome Research*, **10**, 299-304. http://dx.doi.org/10.1021/pr100871h

[8]   Leong, P.K., Chiu, P.Y., Leung, H.Y. and Ko, K.M. (2012) Cytochrome P450-Catalysed Reactive Oxygen Species Production Mediates the (−)Schisandrin B-Induced Glutathione and Heat Shock Responses in AML12 Hepatocytes. *Cell Biology International*, **36**, 321-326. http://dx.doi.org/10.1042/CBI20090451

[9]   Pu, H.J., Cao, Y.F., He, R.R., Zhao, Z.L., Song, J.H., Jiang, B., Huang, T., Tang, S.H., Lu, J.M. and Kurihara, H. (2012) Correlation between Antistress and Hepatoprotective Effects of Schisandra Lignans Was Related with Its Antioxidative Actions in Liver Cells. *Evidence-Based Complementary and Alternative Medicine*, **2012**, Article ID: 161062. http://dx.doi.org/10.1155/2012/161062

[10] Chiu, P.Y., Leung, H.Y., Siu, A.H., Poon, M.K. and Ko, K.M. (2007) Schisandrin B Decreases the Sensitivity of Mitochondria to Calcium Ion-Induced Permeability Transition and Protects against Carbon Tetrachloride Toxicity in Mouse Livers. *Biological and Pharmaceutical Bulletin*, **30**, 1108-1112. http://dx.doi.org/10.1248/bpb.30.1108

[11] Pan, S.Y., Han, Y.F., Carlier, P.R., Pang, Y.P., Mak, D.H., Lam, B.Y. and Ko, K.M. (2002) Schisandrin B Protects against Tacrine- and Bis(7)-Tacrine-Induced Hepatotoxicity and Enhances Cognitive Function in Mice. *Planta Medica*, **68**, 217-220. http://dx.doi.org/10.1055/s-2002-23145

[12] Chiu, P.Y., Tang, M.H. and Ko, K.M. (2003) Hepatoprotective Mechanism of Schisandrin B: Role of Mitochondrial Glutathione Antioxidant Status and Heat Shock Proteins. *Free Radical Biology and Medicine*, **35**, 368-380. http://dx.doi.org/10.1016/S0891-5849(03)00274-0

[13] Stacchiotti, A., Volti, G.L. and Rodella, L.F. (2009) Schisandrin B Stimulates a Cytoprotective Response in Rat Liver Exposed to Mercuric Chloride. *Food and Chemical Toxicology*, **47**, 2834-2840. http://dx.doi.org/10.1016/j.fct.2009.09.003

[14] Li, L., Zhang, T., Zhou, L., Xing, G., Chen, Y. and Xin, Y. (2013) Schisandrin B Attenuates Acetaminophen-Induced Hepatic Injury through Overexpression of Heat Shock Protein 27 and 70 in Mice. *Journal of Gastroenterology and Hepatology*, **23**, 640-647.

[15] Pan, S.Y., Jia, Z.H., Zhang, Y., Yu, Q., Wang, X.Y., Sun, N., Zhu, P.L., Yu, Z.L. and Ko, K.M. (2013) A Novel Mouse Model of Combined Hyperlipidemia Associated with Steatosis and Liver Injury by a Single-Dose Intragastric Administration of Schisandrin B/Cholesterol/Bile Salts Mixture. *Journal of Pharmacological Sciences*, **123**, 110-119. http://dx.doi.org/10.1254/jphs.13087FP

[16] Pao, T.T., Hsu, K.F., Liu, K.T., Chang, L.G., Chuang, C.H. and Sung, C.Y. (1977) Protective Action of Schizandrin B on Hepatic Injury in Mice. *Chinese Medical Journal (English Edition)*, **3**, 173-179.

[17] Bunel, V., Antoine, M.H., Nortier, J., Duez, P. and Stévigny, C. (2013) Protective Effects of Schizandrin and Schizandrin B towards Cisplatin Nephrotoxicity *in Vitro*. *Journal of Applied Toxicology*, **34**, 1311-1319. http://dx.doi.org/10.1002/jat.2951

[18] Li, M., Jin, J., Li, J., Guan, C.W., Wang, W.W., Qiu, Y.W. and Huang, Z.Y. (2012) Schisandrin B Protects against Nephrotoxicity Induced by Cisplatin in HK-2 Cells via Nrf2-ARE Activation. *Acta Pharmaceutica Sinica*, **47**, 1434-1439.

[19] Zhu, S., Wang, Y., Chen, M., Jin, J., Qiu, Y., Huang, M. and Huang, Z. (2012) Protective Effect of Schisandrin B against Cyclosporine A-Induced Nephrotoxicity *in Vitro* and *in Vivo*. *The American Journal of Chinese Medicine*, **40**, 551-566. http://dx.doi.org/10.1142/S0192415X12500425

[20] Chiu, P.Y., Leung, H.Y. and Ko, K.M. (2008) Schisandrin B Enhances Renal Mitochondrial Antioxidant Status, Functional and Structural Integrity, and Protects against Gentamicin-Induced Nephrotoxicity in Rats. *Biological and Pharmaceutical Bulletin*, **31**, 602-605. http://dx.doi.org/10.1248/bpb.31.602

[21] Stacchiotti, A., Volti, G., Lavazza, A., Schena, I., Aleo, M.F., Rodella, L.F. and Rezzani, R. (2011) Different Role of Schisandrin B on Mercury-Induced Renal Damage *in Vivo* and *in Vitro*. *Toxicology*, **286**, 48-57. http://dx.doi.org/10.1016/j.tox.2011.05.005

[22] Liu, W., Xu, Z., Yang, H., Deng, Y., Xu, B. and Wei, U. (2011) The Protective Effects of Tea Polyphenols and Schisandrin B on Nephrotoxicity of Mercury. *Biological Trace Element Research*, **143**, 1651-1665. http://dx.doi.org/10.1007/s12011-011-8996-y

[23] Chiu, P.Y., Lam, P.Y., Yan, C.W. and Ko, K.M. (2011) Schisandrin B Protects against Solar Irradiation-Induced Oxidative Injury in BJ Human Fibroblasts. *Fitoterapia*, **82**, 682-691. http://dx.doi.org/10.1016/j.fitote.2011.02.010

[24] Ip, S.P. and Ko, K.M. (1996) The Crucial Antioxidant Action of Schisandrin B in Protecting against Carbon Tetrachloride Hepatotoxicity in Mice: A Comparative Study with Butylated Hydroxytoluene. *Biochemical Pharmacology*, **52**, 1687-1693. http://dx.doi.org/10.1016/S0006-2952(96)00517-5

[25] Xue, J., Liu, G., Wei, H. and Pan, Y. (1992) Antioxidant Activity of Two Dibenzocyclooctene Lignans on the Aged and Ischemic Brain in Rats. *Free Radical Biology and Medicine*, **12**, 127-135. http://dx.doi.org/10.1016/0891-5849(92)90006-3

[26] Zhang, T.M., Wang, B.E. and Liu, G.T. (1989) Action of Schizandrin B, an Antioxidant, on Lipid Peroxidation in Primary Cultured Hepatocytes. *Acta Pharmacologica Sinica*, **10**, 353-356. (Article in Chinese)

[27] Giridharan, V.V., Thandavarayan, R.A., Sato, S., Ko, K.M. and Konishi, T. (2011) Prevention of Scopolamine-Induced Memory Deficits by Schisandrin B, an Antioxidant Lignan from *Schisandra chinensis* in Mice. *Free Radical Research*, **45**, 950-958. http://dx.doi.org/10.3109/10715762.2011.571682

[28] Lam, P.Y., Yan, C.W. and Ko, K.M. (2011) Schisandrin B Protects against Solar Irradiation-Induced Oxidative Stress in Rat Skin Tissue. *Fitoterapia*, **82**, 393-400. http://dx.doi.org/10.1016/j.fitote.2010.11.018

[29] Checker, R., Patwardhan, R.S. and Sandur, S.K. (2012) Schisandrin B Exhibits Anti-Inflammatory Activity through Modulation of the Redox-Sensitive Transcription Factors Nrf2 and NF-kB. *Free Radical Biology and Medicine*, **53**, 1421-1430. http://dx.doi.org/10.1016/j.freeradbiomed.2012.08.006

[30] Lam, P.Y. and Ko, K.M. (2012) Beneficial Effect of (-)Schisandrin B against 3-Nitropropionic Acid-Induced Cell Death in PC12 Cells. *Biofactors*, **38**, 219-225. http://dx.doi.org/10.1002/biof.1009

[31] Lee, T.H., Jung, C.H. and Lee, D.H. (2012) Neuroprotective Effects of Schisandrin B against Transient Focal Cerebral Ischemia in Sprague-Dawley Rats. *Food and Chemical Toxicology*, **50**, 4239-4245. http://dx.doi.org/10.1016/j.fct.2012.08.047

[32] Zeng, K., Zhang, T., Fu, H., Liu, G. and Wang, X. (2012) Schisandrin B Exerts Anti-Neuroinflammatory Activity by Inhibiting the Toll-Like Receptor 4-Dependent MyD88/IKK/NF-κB Signaling Pathway in Lipopolysaccharide-Induced Microglia. *European Journal of Pharmacology*, **692**, 29-37. http://dx.doi.org/10.1016/j.ejphar.2012.05.030

[33] Wang, B. and Wang, X. (2009) Schisandrin B Protects Rat Cortical Neurons against Abeta1-42-Induced Neurotoxicity. *Pharmazie*, **64**, 450-454.

[34] Lam, P.Y. and Ko, K.M. (2012) Schisandrin B as a Hormetic Agent for Preventing Age-Related Neurodegenerative Diseases. *Oxidative Medicine and Cellular Longevity*, **2012**, Article ID: 250825. http://dx.doi.org/10.1155/2012/250825

[35] Chen, N., Chiu, P.Y. and Ko, K.M. (2008) Schisandrin B Enhances Cerebral Mitochondrial Antioxidant Status and Structural Integrity, and Protects against Cerebral Ischemia/Reperfusion Injury in Rats. *Biological and Pharmaceutical Bulletin*, **31**, 1387-1391. http://dx.doi.org/10.1248/bpb.31.1387

[36] Ko, K.M. and Lam, B.Y. (2002) Schisandrin B Protects against Tert-Butylhydroperoxide Induced Cerebral Toxicity by Enhancing Glutathione Antioxidant Status in Mouse Brain. *Molecular and Cellular Biochemistry*, **238**, 181-186. http://dx.doi.org/10.1023/A:1019907316129

[37] Zhu, H., Zhang, X., Guan, J., Cui, B., Zhao, L. and Zhao, X. (2013) Pharmacokinetics and Tissue Distribution Study of Schisandrin B in Rats by Ultra-Fast Liquid Chromatography with Tandem Mass Spectrometry. *Journal of Pharmaceutical and Biomedical Analysis*, **78-79**, 136-140. http://dx.doi.org/10.1016/j.jpba.2013.01.041

[38] Sun, H., Wu, F., Zhang, A., Wei, W., Han, Y. and Wang, X. (2013) Profiling and Identification of the Absorbed Constituents and Metabolites of *Schisandra* Lignans by Ultra-Performance Liquid Chromatography Coupled to Mass Spectrometry. *Biomedical Chromatography*, **27**, 1511-1519. http://dx.doi.org/10.1002/bmc.2951

[39] Wang, B.L., Hu, J.P. and Li, Y. (2008) Simultaneous Quantification of Four Active *Schisandra* Lignans from a Traditional Chinese Medicine *Schisandra chinensis* (Wuweizi) in Rat Plasma Using Liquid Chromatography/Mass Spectrometry. *Journal of Chromatography B*, **865**, 114-120. http://dx.doi.org/10.1016/j.jchromb.2008.02.016

[40] Huang, X., Song, F., Liu, Z. and Liu, S. (2007) Studies on Lignan Constituents from *Schisandra chinensis* (Turcz.) Baill. Fruits Using High-Performance Liquid Chromatography/Electrospray Ionization Multiple-Stage Tandem Mass Spectrometry. *Journal of Mass Spectrometry*, **42**, 1148-1161. http://dx.doi.org/10.1002/jms.1246

[41] Tang, J., Shao, B., Liu, Y., Liu, H., Ji, H., Zhu, D. and Wu, L. (2010) Highly Sensitive Determination of Schisandrin and Schisandrin B in Plasma of Rats after Administration of Wurenchun (Fructus Schisandrae Chinensis Extracts) Preparations by LC-ESI-MS/MS. *Biomedical Chromatography*, **24**, 675-681.

[42] Sun, H., Wu, F., Zhang, A., Wei, W., Han, Y. and Wang, X. (2013) Pharmacokinetic Study of Schisandrin, Schisandrol B, Schisantherin A, Deoxyschisandrin, and Schisandrin B in Rat Plasma after Oral Administration of Shengmaisan Formula by UPLC-MS. *Journal of Separation Science*, **36**, 485-491. http://dx.doi.org/10.1002/jssc.201200887

[43] He, R., Tan, P., Han, J., Lin, H., Chen, X., Liu, Y. and Zhang, Y. (2013) ESI/MS Study on Fragmentation Pathways of Schisandrin B by the Discovery Studio, World Science and Technology/Modernization of Traditional Chinese Medicine and Materia. *Medica*, **15**, 527-530.

[44] Corveia, M.A. and Montellauo, P.O. (2005) Inhibition of Cytochrome P450 Enzymes. In: Ortiz de Montellano, P.R., Ed., *Cytochrome P450: Structure, Mechanism and Biochemistry*, Kluwer Academic, New York, 263-365.

[45] Iwata, H., Tezuka, Y., Kadota, S., Hiratsuka, A. and Watabe, T. (2004) Identification and Characterization of Potent CYP3A4 Inhibitors in Schisandra Fruit Extract. *Drug Metabolism and Disposition*, **32**, 1351-1358. http://dx.doi.org/10.1124/dmd.104.000646

[46] Donato, M.T. and Castell, J.V. (2003) Strategies and Molecular Probes to Investigate the Role of Cytochrome P450 in Drug Metabolism: Focus on *in Vitro* Studies. *Clinical Pharmacokinetics*, **42**, 153-178. http://dx.doi.org/10.2165/00003088-200342020-00004

[47] Erlank, H., Elmann, A., Kohen, R. and Kanner, J. (2011) Polyphenols Activate Nrf2 in Astrocytes via H_2O_2, Semiquinones, and Quinones. *Free Radical Biology and Medicine*, **51**, 2319-2327. http://dx.doi.org/10.1016/j.freeradbiomed.2011.09.033

[48] Rubiolo, J.A., Mithieux, G. and Vega, F.V. (2008) Resveratrol Protects Primary Rat Hepatocytes against Oxidative Stress Damage: Activation of the Nrf2 Transcription Factor and Augmented Activities of Antioxidant Enzymes. *European Journal of Pharmacology*, **591**, 66-72. http://dx.doi.org/10.1016/j.ejphar.2008.06.067

[49] D'Autreaux, B. and Toledano, M.B. (2007) ROS as Signalling Molecules: Mechanisms That Generate Specificity in ROS Homeostasis. *Nature Reviews Molecular Cell Biology*, **8**, 813-324. http://dx.doi.org/10.1038/nrm2256

22

In Vivo and *in Vitro* Evaluation of Anti Diabetic and Insulin Secretagogue Activities of *Capparis zeylanica*

Umamahesh Balekari, Ciddi Veeresham[*]

University College of Pharmaceutical Sciences, Kakatiya University, Warangal, India
Email: [*]ciddiveeresham@yahoo.co.in

Abstract

Since ancient times, traditional medicines have been in the usage for the treatment of Diabetes mellitus. An edible fruit from traditional medicinal plant *Capparis zeylanica* (CZ) was studied for its anti diabetic, insulin secretagogue activities and mechanisms involved in it. In Streptozotocin induced diabetes rats, oral administration of *Capparis zeylanica* methanolic extract (CZME) (200 mg/kg body weight) for 28 days showed a significant reduction in blood glucose levels by 35.53% and enhanced circulating insulin levels by 81.82% than the diabetic control rats. The insulin secretagogue activity mechanisms of the extract were evaluated by using mouse insulinoma beta cell line (MIN6-β). The extract stimulated insulin release in dependent manner of glucose concentration (3 - 16.7 mM) and extract dose (5 - 500 µg/mL). The insulin releasing effect of the extract was significantly enhanced by 3-isobutyl-1-methyl xanthine, glibenclamide, elevated extracellular calcium and K+ depolarized media. This insulin release was significantly reduced in calcium blocking conditions (by nifedipine and EGTA), in the presence of potassium channel opener (diazoxide). Hence, anti diabetic activity of CZME might be a result of its stimulatory effect on insulin release from pancreatic beta cells via K_{ATP} channel dependent and independent ways. These results indicate that CZ fruits have the potential to use in diabetes therapy.

Keywords

Anti Diabetic, Insulin Secretagogue, MIN6-β Cells, K_{ATP} Channel

1. Introduction

Diabetes mellitus is a chronic metabolic disorder manifested with elevated levels of glucose in the body, which

---

[*]Corresponding author.

is an effect of impaired insulin secretion, insulin effect, or both [1]. According to the latest reports, more than 382 million people are affected with diabetes in 2013 and estimated to reach a total of 592 million by 2035. The prevalence of global diabetes in 2013 was 8.3% and expected to reach 10.1% in the year 2035 [2].

The chronic metabolic disorders like diabetes necessitate long term management with oral hypoglycemic agents, which results into adverse effects and drug resistance [3] [4]. This signifies the necessity to focus on research and discovery of new anti diabetic drugs with improved safety and efficacy. From ancient system of medicine, drugs from natural sources were proven to be useful. Therefore, search for the advanced drugs from natural sources may prove to be useful.

Stimulation in insulin release from pancreatic beta cells is one of the major mechanisms of anti diabetic activity by natural products. In reported literature, the *in vitro* studies of *Ficus deltoidea* extracts on BRIN BD11 cells have provided pharmacological evidence for its anti diabetic activity. In the studies, the extracts reported insulin secretagogue activity is dependent on K^+-ATP channel and calcium [3]. In another study, aqueous extract of *Abutilon indicum* is also reported being effective in diabetes by enhancing insulin secretion in diabetic rats and also in INS-1E insulinoma cells [4].

Capparis zeylanica (CZ), Linn. (family: Capparidaceae), which is generally called as Indian caper, is a climbing shrub found throughout India, Bangladesh, Srilanka, Malaysia and some parts of Pakistan [5] [6]. In India, it has been used in the traditional Ayurvedic system of medicine as a cooling agent, cholagogue, bitter stomachic, sedative and anti-hydrotic and is also used in cholera, neuralgia, hemiplegia and rheumatism [7]. The plant also showed anti oxidant activity by aerial parts [8]; anti-microbial [9], anti-inflammatory [10] and analgesic activities [10] [11] were indicated by roots of the plant. Leaves of the plant have shown analgesic, antipyretic [12] and immunomodulatory effect [13]. CZ fruits are used as vegetables to prepare curry [14] and unripe fruits are pickled to eat [15]. These fruits are traditionally used as an antidote in snakebite [16] and ripened fruits are consumed for the treatment of diabetes [6]. So far, no scientific evidence is available on anti diabetic potential of the CZ fruits. Therefore, the present study was aimed to investigate the anti diabetic activity, mechanisms of activity of the methanolic extract of CZ fruits in *in vivo* by using STZ induced diabetes rats model and mouse insulinoma beta cells (MIN6-β) in *in vitro* conditions.

2. Materials and Methods

2.1. Plant Material and Extract Preparation

Ripened fruits of *Capparis zeylanca* were collected from the local market at Jangaon, Telangana, India. Fruits were identified and voucher specimens were deposited in the herbarium at Department of Botany, Kakatiya University, Warangal, India.

The dried and powdered plant material was extracted with methanol by cold percolation for 7 days. The extract was filtered and concentrated by using vacuum evaporation and freeze drying.

2.2. *In Vivo* Studies

2.2.1. Animals

Male Wister albino rats of weighing range 180 - 200 g were purchased from Sanzyme Ltd., Hyderabad, India. Animals were housed at standard laboratory conditions with free access to water and food. Institutional Animal Ethics Committee (IAEC) guidelines were followed for the study.

2.2.2 Acute Toxicity and Glucose Tolerance Test Studies

Acute toxicity studies were conducted on normal rats as previously described by Lorke [17]. The CZME treated four groups (n = 6) were administered with 0.25, 0.5, 1.0 and 2.0 g/kg body weight (bw) and vehicle alone (Carboxy methyl cellulose (CMC) 0.5%; 1 ml/kg bw) for control group. The acute toxicity resultant behavioral changes and mortality within the period of 24 hrs was observed.

The study dose of CZME was determined by oral glucose tolerance test (OGTT) in normal male Wister rats by the method of Gireesh *et al.* [18]. The rats were randomly divided in to five groups (n = 6). Rats in the group A received only glucose (2 g/kg bw); CZME at a dose of 50, 100 and 200 mg/kg was given respectively to the groups B, C and D. Group E received glibenclamide (5 mg/kg bw) alone as standard drug. The blood samples were collected at 0, 30, 60, 90 and 120 min after glucose loading and analyzed for glucose by glucose oxidase method [19].

2.2.3. Experimental Design and Treatment Schedule

For diabetes induction to overnight fasted rats, a fresh solution of Streptozotocin (STZ) in 0.1 M citrate buffer (pH 4.5) at a dose of 50 mg/kg bw was administered intra peritoneally. One week after STZ administration, rats with blood glucose above 250 mg/dL were used in study as diabetic animals.

A total of four groups (n = 8) of rats were used for 4 weeks study period. Group 1 (naïve animals *i.e.*, normal control) and group 2 (diabetic control) were received vehicle alone; group 3 and 4 received CZME (200 mg/kg bw) and glibenclamide (5 mg/kg bw), respectively. Rat blood samples were collected and plasma samples were separated and stored at −20°C until further analysis.

2.2.4. Determination of Body Weight, Plasma Glucose and Insulin Levels

During the study period of 4 weeks, body weight, plasma glucose and plasma insulin levels were determined on the 1st day and 28th day. Body weight and plasma glucose levels were determined on 7th and 15th days of treatment. Plasma glucose levels were estimated as mentioned above. Plasma insulin concentrations were determined by using insulin enzyme-linked immunosorbent assay (ELISA) kit.

2.3. *In Vitro* Studies on Insulin Secretory Activity

2.3.1. MIN6-β Cells Culture

MIN6-β cells were cultured at 37°C under atmosphere of 5% CO_2 in Dulbecco's modified Eagle's medium (DMEM) supplemented with 10% fetal calf serum, 2 mM glutamine, 10,000 units/mL of penicillin and 10 mg/mL of streptomycin. CZME stock solution was prepared by dissolving extract in Dimethyl sulphoxide (DMSO) and further diluted with Kreb's Ringer buffer (KRB) to prepare working solutions.

2.3.2. Cell Viability Assay (3-(4,5-Dimethylthiazol-2-yl)-2,5-Diphenyltetrazolium Bromide (MTT) Assay)

Cell viability assay was performed according to Adam *et al.* with brief modifications [3]. Briefly, 30,000 MIN6-β cells per well was seeded in 96 well plates and allowed to attach for overnight. Then the cells were treated with CZME at a concentration range of 5 - 1000 µg/ml and standard drug, glibenclamide (5 - 100 µM/ml), allowed for 72 hrs incubation. Followed by incubation, to each well a 20 µL solution of 3-(4,5-Dime-thylthia-zol-2-yl)-2,5-Diphenyltetrazolium Bromide (MTT) (5 mg/mL) was added and incubated for 4 hrs. After that, 100 µL of dimethylsulphoxide (DMSO) was added to each well and aspirated to dissolve the formazan crystals formed by reduction of MTT. Further, plates were shaken for 10 seconds for uniform mixing followed by read for absorbance at 570 nm by using Multiskan Ex microplate reader (Thermo scientific, USA).

2.3.3. Bioassay for Insulin secretion

The β-Cell insulin secretion assay was conducted as already described with brief modifications [20] [21] by seeding about 30,000 MIN6-β cells per well into 96-well plates. During study, cells were incubated for 60 min with only KRB (naïve), KRB containing glucose only at 3 mM (basal) and 11.1 mM (hyperglycemic) conditions. CZME at 5 - 1000 µg/mL dose range was used to evaluate dose dependent effect on insulin secretion. CZME sub maximal dose (500 µg/mL) and glibenclamide (10 µM) were used in the studies. Unless stated, the experiment was conducted at 11.1 mM glucose concentration.

The insulin secretagogue mechanisms of the extract were assessed by using insulin release modulators like diazoxide (β-cell K^+-ATP channel opener, 0.5 mM), 3-isobutyl-1-methylxanthine (IBMX) (phosphodiesterase inhibitor, 100 µM) and glibenclamide. Role of K^+-ATP channel and calcium on insulin secretion was evaluated by using calcium chloride ($CaCl_2$, 1.28 mM), ethylene glycol tetra acetic acid (EGTA, 1 mM), nifedipine (20 µM) and potassium chloride (KCl) at depolarizing concentration 30 mM.

After 60 min of incubation, aliquots from each well was collected and centrifuged (4000 g, 5 min, 4°C) and stored at −20°C until for further analysis of insulin by using ELISA.

2.4. Statistical Analysis

All the data were expressed as mean ± SD. One-way or two-way analysis of variance (ANOVA) was used upon suitability. The significance of difference was assessed by using the Dunnett's post hoc test or Bonferroni test. Values with P < 0.05 were considered to be significant. Graph Pad Prism (Graph Pad Software, San Diego, CA) was used for all statistical analysis.

3. Results

3.1. *In Vivo* Studies

3.1.1. Acute Toxicity and Glucose Tolerance Test Studies

CZME acute toxicity studies revealed that the extract at given doses did not showed any lethal or toxic effect on the animals. In 24 h observation period, no behavioral changes and mortality were observed as signs of acute toxicity.

In OGTT studies, CZME 200 mg/kg bw treatment significantly reduced blood glucose levels, where 50 and 100 mg/kg bw doses were not effective (**Table 1**). Therefore, CZME at 200 mg/kg bw dose was used in *in vivo* studies for anti diabetic and insulin secretagogue activity.

3.1.2. Body Weight, Blood Glucose and Insulin

After 28 days study period, a significant decrease (P < 0.001) was observed in the body weight (142.08 ± 1.33 g) of the STZ induced diabetic rats compared with naïve group (183.28 ± 1.34 g). However, treatment with CZME (200 mg/kg bw), glibenclamide (5 mg/kg bw) in diabetic rats prevented this significant loss in body weight and led to restoration in the body weights to near normal levels *i.e.* 174.71 ± 2.12 g (P < 0.001) and 179.79 ± 1.72 g (P < 0.001), respectively, when compared with diabetic control group (**Figure 1**).

Table 1. Oral glucose tolerance test of CZME at different doses.

	Time (min)				
	0 min	30 min	60 min	90 min	120 min
Naïve	75.26 ± 4.04	131.39 ± 6.11	101.26 ± 5.20	89.59 ± 4.43	83.97 ± 5.20
Glibenclamide (5 mg/kg)	70.35 ± 4.51	104.17 ± 4.34[#]	86.35 ± 3.38[#]	76.56 ± 3.79[#]	70.29 ± 3.23[#]
CZME (50 mg/kg)	81.67 ± 3.70	138.84 ± 4.38	101.35 ± 3.50	88.15 ± 4.36	85.38 ± 1.23
CZME (100 mg/kg)	80.92 ± 5.03	126.96 ± 4.42	96.95 ± 4.60	85.16 ± 4.72	83.98 ± 4.36
CZME (200 mg/kg)	81.49 ± 5.06	122.8 ± 4.70[*]	90.88 ± 4.31[#]	83.61 ± 4.63	81.23 ± 4.85

Values indicate mean ± SD. Data was analyzed by two-way ANOVA followed by Bonferroni test (n = 6); [#]P < 0.001, [*]P < 0.01 as compared to naïve animals at respective time points.

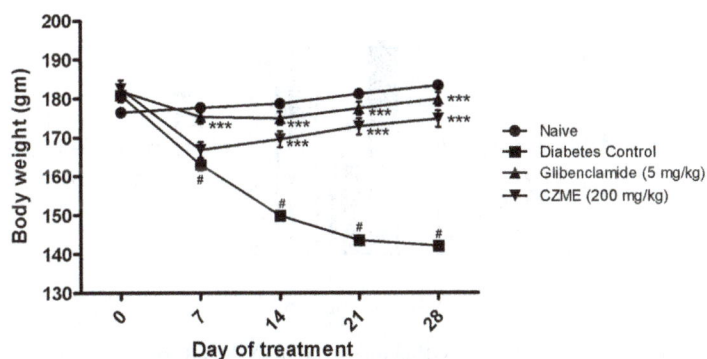

Figure 1. Effect of CZME extract (200 mg/kg) and standard drug glibenclamide (5 mg/kg) on body weight in STZ induced diabetes model in rats (Data was analyzed by two-way ANOVA followed by Bonferroni test (n = 6); [#]P < 0.001 as compared to naïve animals, [***]P < 0.001 as compared to diabetes control group at respective time points).

The effect of CZME on blood glucose and insulin levels in naïve and diabetic rats presented in **Figure 2**. In diabetic rats, administration of CZME (200 mg/kg bw) significantly (P < 0.01) reduced blood glucose levels by 35.53%, where as the standard drug glibenclamide reduced blood glucose levels by 35.51% (P < 0.01). In untreated diabetic rats, a significant rise (P < 0.01) 24.96% in the blood glucose levels was observed. However, a significant reduction in blood glucose levels were observed in treated animal groups.

The difference in plasma insulin levels in untreated diabetic animals group (0.34 ± 0.01 ng/mL) was significant (P < 0.001) in comparison with naïve animals (0.64 ± 0.01 ng/mL). Though, the plasma insulin levels were about same (0.33 ± 0.01 − 0.34 ± 0.01 ng/mL) on day 0 in groups 2, 3 and 4; the 28 days treatment with CZME (200 mg/kg bw) and glibenclamide (5 mg/kg bw) resulted insulin levels to 0.60 ± 0.01 ng/mL and 0.62 ± 0.02 ng/mL, respectively (**Figure 3**). This is a noteworthy (P < 0.001) difference in plasma insulin levels compared with untreated animals. Therefore, CZME administration restored decreased plasma insulin levels of diabetic rats.

3.2. *In Vitro* Studies on Insulin Secretory Activity

3.2.1. Cell Viability Assay

The effect of CZME on MIN6 β cells viability was shown in **Table 2**. Tested doses the extract and glibenclamide have not shown any significant reduction in the viability in comparison with control. Therefore, the standard drug and extract at studied doses were used in *in vitro* studies.

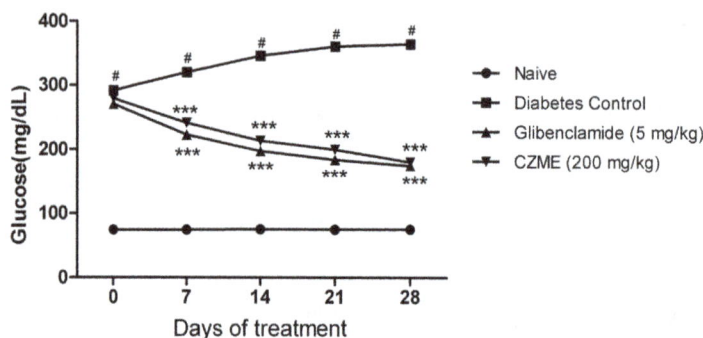

Figure 2. Effect of CZME extract (200 mg/kg) and standard drug glibenclamide (5 mg/kg) on blood glucose levels in STZ induced diabetes model in rats (Data was analyzed by two-way ANOVA followed by Bonferroni test (n = 6); [#]P < 0.001 as compared to naïve animals, [***]P < 0.001 as compared to diabetes control group at respective time points).

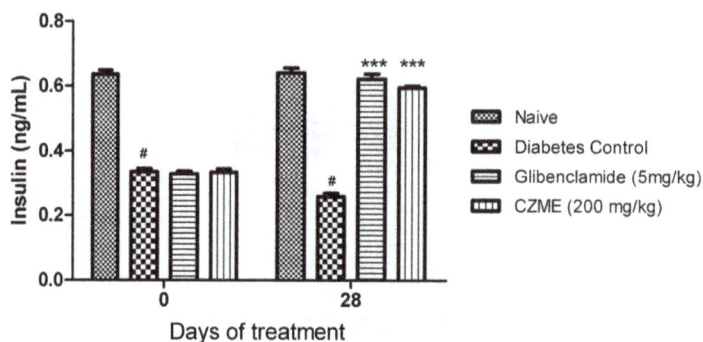

Figure 3. Effect of CZME extract (200 mg/kg) and standard drug glibenclamide (5 mg/kg) on plasma insulin levels in STZ induced diabetes rats on 0th and 28th day of treatment (Data was analyzed by two-way ANOVA followed by Bonferroni test (n = 6); [#]P < 0.001 as compared to naïve animals, [***]P < 0.001 as compared to diabetes control group at respective time points).

3.2.2. Effects of CZME on Insulin Secretion from MIN 6 Beta Cells

A dose dependent stimulation in insulin secretion was exhibited by CZME extract within the dose range of (5 - 1000 µg/mL) at 3 mM and 11.1 mM glucose, compared with respective glucose controls (**Figure 4**). The insulin release was about two folds at hyperglycemic conditions (11.1 mM) than basal concentration (3 mM). The maximum insulin secretion was observed at 500 µg/mL extract; therefore the same concentration was used in further studies. However, decline in insulin secretion was observed at extract concentration of 1000 µg/mL.

At 3 - 16.7 mM glucose concentration range, the MIN6 cells exhibited a glucose dependent rise in insulin secretion. The glucose dependent insulin release was significantly potentiated in the presence of CZME (500 µg/mL), compared with extract only (**Figure 5**). Glucose at sub-maximal dose of 11.1 mM was selected for further studies. The extract treatment alone led to an insignificant stimulation on insulin secretion (0.183 - 0.35 ng/mL) in comparison with insulin output ranges of 2.13 - 16.29 ng/mL and 5.30 - 35.24 ng/mL at basal and hyperglycemic conditions, respectively.

3.2.3. Insulin Secretion Mechanisms of CZME by Employing Insulin Release Modulators

Figure 6 presents the influence of insulin secretion modulators namely diazoxide, IBMX and glibenclamide on insulin secretion by CZME extract. The insulin output of 33.52 ± 1.38 ng/mL was significantly higher ($P < 0.05$) with extract treatment, than insulin secretion of 17.73 ± 0.57 ng/mL by extract in presence of diazoxide. This reduction in insulin enhancement specifies that the extract resulted insulin secretion was not an effect of MIN6 cells damage; K^+-ATP channel blockade directed depolarization led to elevated insulin levels. Extract treatment enhanced insulin release by MIN6 cells in the presence of IBMX (40.35 ± 1.09 ng/mL) than the absence. The glibenclamide significantly potentiated insulin output in the absence (31.98 ± 0.63 ng/mL, $P < 0.001$) and

Table 2. MIN6 β-Cell viability assay of Glibenclamide and CZME at different doses.

Glibenclamide (µM/mL)					
Concentration	1	5	50	100	Control
% Viability	97.84 ± 2.56	96.8 ± 1.45	96.32 ± 1.57	95.84 ± 1.18	100.05 ± 0.08
CZME (µg/mL)					
Concentration	5	50	500	1000	Control
% Viability	99.75 ± 2.24	98.79 ± 2.49	98.12 ± 2.71	96.78 ± 2.31	100.01 ± 0.02

Effect of glibenclamide and CZME on viability of MIN6 beta cells. (The values were expressed as Mean ± SD); (n = 6).

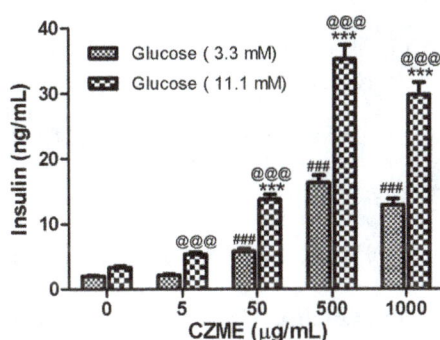

Figure 4. Effect of CZME extract (5 - 1000 µg/mL) on released insulin levels from MIN6 beta cells upon incubation for 60 minutes. All the values are the means ± SD (n = 5) of the insulin released as an effect of response to dose of extract at glucose basal (3.3 mM) and hyperglycemic (11.1 mM) conditions. ###P < 0.001 respective to control at basal condition. ***P < 0.001 relative to control at hyperglycemic condition. @@@P < 0.001 compared with insulin levels at basal and hyperglycemic conditions at same extract concentration.

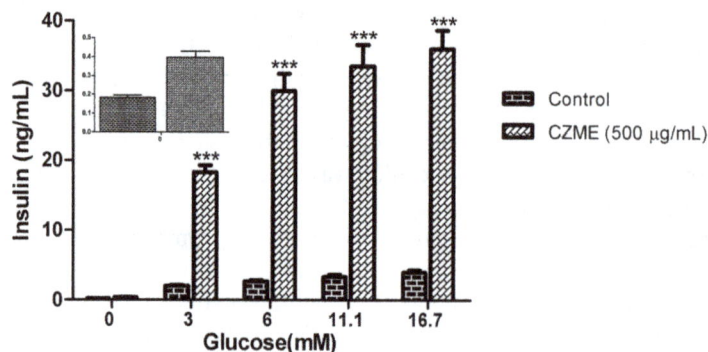

Figure 5. Effect of CZME extract (500 µg/mL) on released insulin levels) at different glucose levels (0 - 16.7 mM) from MIN6 beta cells upon incubation for 60 minutes. All the values are the means ± SD (n = 5) of the insulin released in response to glucose load. ***$P < 0.001$ relative to control condition. Graph insert shows insulin released at blank (0 mM glucose) with similar axes titles of main graph.

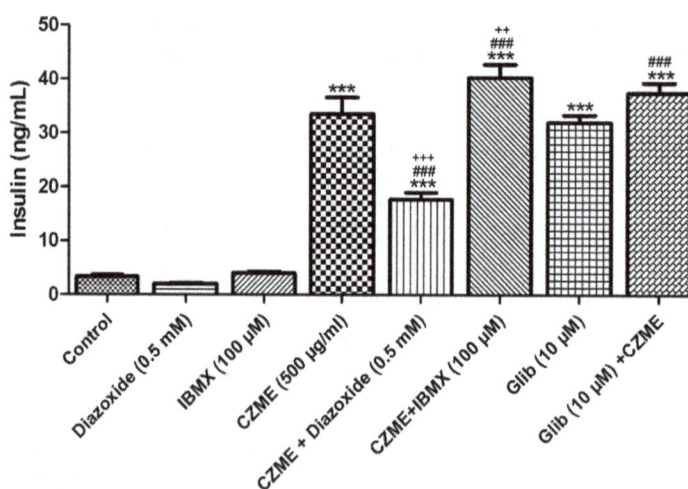

Figure 6. Effect of insulin release modulators (Diazoxide, IBMX and Glibenclamide) on insulin secretion from MIN6 beta cells upon incubation with 11.1 mM glucose for 60 minutes in the presence and absence of CZME (500 µg/mL). All the values are the means ± SD (n = 5). All the data was analyzed by one way ANOVA followed by Dunnet's test. ***$P < 0.001$ in comparison with control. +++$P < 0.001$, ++$P < 0.01$ in comparison with the extract. ###$P < 0.001$ in comparison with respective modulator in the absence of CZME.

presence (37.42 ± 0.86 ng/mL, $p < 0.001$) of extract compared with glucose control (3.33 ± 0.13 ng/mL).

3.2.4. Role of K⁺-ATP Channels and Calcium (Ca²⁺) on Insulin Secretion Effects of CZME

The extracts ability to enhance the insulin secretion from MIN6-β cells was retained even at depolarizing concentration of KCl (30 mM). In contrast, the CZME effect on insulin secretion was reduced in the presence of diazoxide. This signifies other than K⁺-ATP channel effect on insulin secretion by the extract. The Ca^{2+} dependency of the extract was displayed by stimulated insulin release in the presence of 1.28 mM calcium in incubation medium, compared with extract and glucose treated cells in basal medium. Under elevated extracellular Ca^{2+} conditions, the treatment of cells with nifedipine (calcium channel blocker), EGTA (Ca^{2+} chelator) led to significantly lowered insulin secretion (**Figure 7**). Therefore Ca^{2+} concentrations in extracellular environment and Ca^{2+} influxes affect the insulin release potential of CZME.

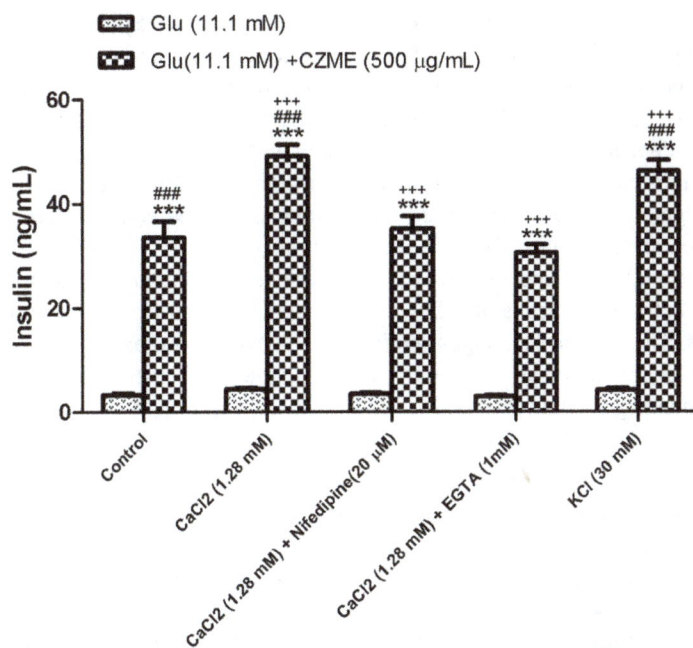

Figure 7. Role of K^+-ATP channels and calcium (Ca^{2+}) on insulin secretion from MIN6 beta cells upon incubation with 11.1 mM glucose in the presence and absence of CZME (500 µg/mL). All the values are the means ± SD (n = 5). All the data was analyzed by one-way ANOVA followed by Dunnet's test. ***P < 0.001 in comparison with control in the absence of extract. ###P < 0.001 in comparison with control in the presence of extract. +++P < 0.001 in comparison with respective control in the absence of CZME.

4. Discussion

The present study has demonstrated that the administration of *Capparis zeylanica* fruit methanolic extract (CZME) at a dose of 200 mg/kg bw reduces elevated blood glucose levels in STZ induced diabetic rats via enhancing insulin release. This is the first report on the anti hyperglycemic activity and insulin secretagogue effects of the edible fruit of *Capparis zeylanica*.

The treatment of diabetic rats with CZME leads to improved body weight, blood glucose and insulin levels in comparison with diabetic control group. Improved body weight in diabetic animals specifies the role of extract in protecting the body tissues from hyperglycemic damage [18] by enhancing glycemic control and structural protein synthesis [22]. CZME antihyperglycemic activity is comparable to the standard drug, glibenclamide. Enhanced circulating insulin levels in the extract treated diabetic animals are analogous to that of standard drug treated diabetic animals. Thus, CZME antihyperglycemic activity could be a result of insulin secretagogue effect [23].

In *in vitro* insulin secretion experiments on MIN6 beta cells, CZME stimulated insulin release in glucose and extract dose dependent manner. However, extract at higher dose (1000 µg/mL) did not show expected insulin secretion, which could be due to the interference from the other substances that were presented in it. Studies confirmed that CZME insulin secretagogue effect was significantly higher at hyperglycemic conditions, which indicated the role of β cell glucose metabolism in insulin secretagogue activity of the extract [24].

K_{ATP} channels in β cell membrane are pivotal in insulin exocytosis from β cell granules [25]. In distinction, K_{ATP} channel openers like diazoxide reduces insulin release. Therefore, present investigations evaluate the role of K_{ATP} channels in the insulin secretagogue effect of CZME. In the presence of Diazoxide, insulin secretion by CZME treatment is reduced significantly. This implies the role of K_{ATP} channels in the insulin release by CZME. However, the extract has also potentiated insulin secretion under depolarizing conditions (KCl 30 mM) which signifies K_{ATP} channel independent effects of the extract [26]. This may be an effect of intracellular actions on exocytosis. CZME treatment along with IBMX resulted increase in insulin secretion might be an effect of increase in intracellular cyclic adenosine monophosphate (cAMP) levels [25] [26].

The insulin secretagogue effect of the CZME was significantly dependent on the calcium. CZME administration significantly enhanced insulin release from beta cells in extracellular media (rich in calcium (1.28 mM)) than the normal media. Lowered insulin release by CZME from β cells in the presence of nifedipine (20 μM) and EGTA elucidates dependency on extracellular calcium and Ca^{2+} influx [25].

Limitation of the present study includes limited experimental sample size and studies in one species of animals. Further investigations have to be carried out to standardize the composition of extract and examine the adverse effects of the drug on large scale for longer duration.

In conclusion, present *in vivo* and *in vitro* studies revealed that *Capparis zeyalnica* fruit methanolic extract showed anti diabetic activity by means of influencing insulin secretion from pancreatic beta cells through physiological mechanisms. This insulin secretagogue effect of the extract was exerted by K_{ATP} channel dependent and independent ways. Hence, *Capparis zeyalnica* could be a natural remedy with anti hyperglycemic potential mainly through augmenting insulin secretion.

References

[1]   American Diabetes Association (2013) Diagnosis and Classification of Diabetes Mellitus. *Diabetes Care*, **36**, S67-S74. http://dx.doi.org/10.2337/dc13-s067

[2]   International Diabetes Federation (2013) International Diabetes Federation Diabetes Atlas. 6th Edition, International Diabetes Federation, Brussels.

[3]   Adam, Z., Khamis, S., Ismail, A. and Hamid, M. (2012) *Ficus deltoidea*: A Potential Alternative Medicine for Diabetes Mellitus. E*vidence-Based Complementary and Alternative Medicine*, **2012**, Article ID: 632763. http://dx.doi.org/10.1155/2012/632763

[4]   Krisanapun, C., Peungvicha, P., Temsiririrkkul, R. and Wongkrajang, Y. (2009) Aqueous Extract of *Abutilon indicum* Sweet Inhibits Glucose Absorption and Stimulates Insulin Secretion in Rodents. *Nutrition Research*, **29**, 579-587. http://dx.doi.org/10.1016/j.nutres.2009.07.006

[5]   Karanayil, R.S., Barij, N.S. and Aiyolu, R. (2011) Antidiarrheal Activity of *Capparis zeylanica* Leaf Extracts. *Journal of Advanced Pharmaceutical Technology & Research*, **2**, 39-42. http://dx.doi.org/10.4103/2231-4040.79803

[6]   Amit, L., Chaudary, A.K., Vikas, G., Bansal, P. and Renu, B. (2010) Phytochemistry and Pharmacological Activities of *Capparis zeylanica*: An Overview. *International Journal of Research in Ayurveda & Pharmacy*, **1**, 384-389.

[7]   Ruchi, S., Chaudhary, A.K. and Ranjit, S. (2012) Effect of Leaf Extract of *Capparis zeylanica* Linn. on Spatial Learning and Memory in Rats. *Journal of Natural Medicines*, **66**, 600-607. http://dx.doi.org/10.1007/s11418-012-0626-2

[8]   Agarwal, S.S. and Talele, G.S. (2009) Free Radical Scavenging Activity of *Capparis zeylanica*. *Medicinal Plants—International Journal of Phytomedicines and Related Industries*, **1**, 109-112. http://dx.doi.org/10.5958/j.0975-4261.1.2.014

[9]   Chopade, V.V., Tankar, A.N., Ganjiwale, R.O. and Yeole, P.G. (2008) Antimicrobial Activity of *Capparis zeylanica* Linn. Roots. *International Journal of Green Pharmacy*, **2**, 28-30. http://dx.doi.org/10.4103/0973-8258.39160

[10] Upaganlawar, A.B., Chopade, V.V., Ghule, B.V. and Yeole, P.G. (2008) Analgesic Effects of Methanolic Extract of *Capparis zeylanica* Linn. Roots. *Pharmacognosy Magazine*, **4**, 112-114.

[11] Chaudhary, S.R., Chavan, M.J. and Gaud, R.S. (2004) Anti-Inflammatory and Analgesic Activity of *Capparis zeylanica* Root Extracts. *Indian Journal of Natural Products*, **20**, 36-39.

[12] Ghule, B.V., Murugananthan, G. and Yeole, P.G. (2007) Analgesic Antipyretic Effects of *Capparis zeylanica* Leaves. *Fitoterapia*, **78**, 365-369. http://dx.doi.org/10.1016/j.fitote.2007.02.003

[13] Ghule, B.V., Murugananthan, G., Nakhat, P.D. and Yeole, P.G. (2006) Immunostimulant Effects of *Capparis zeylanica* leaves. *Journal of Ethnopharmacology*, **108**, 311-315. http://dx.doi.org/10.1016/j.jep.2006.03.041

[14] Reddy, K.N., Pattanaik, C., Reddy, C.S. and Raju, V.S. (2007) Traditional Knowledge on Wild Food Plants in India. *Indian Journal of Traditional Knowledge*, **6**, 223-229.

[15] Sharma, O.P. (2007) Plant Taxonomy. 17th Edition, Tata McGraw-Hill Education Private Ltd., New Delhi.

[16] Misra, S.N., Tomar, P.C. and Lakra, N. (2007) Medicinal and Food Value of *Capparis*—A Harsh Terrain Plant. *Indian Journal of Traditional Knowledge*, **6**, 230-238.

[17] Lorke, D. (1983) A New Approach to Practical Acute Toxicity Testing. *Archives of Toxicology*, **54**, 275-287. http://dx.doi.org/10.1007/BF01234480

[18] Gireesh, G., Thomas, S.K., Joseph, B. and Paulose, C.S. (2009) Antihyperglycemic and Insulin Secretory Activity of

Costus pictus Leaf Extract in Streptozotocin Induced Diabetic Rats and in *in Vitro* Pancreatic Islet Culture. *Journal of Ethnopharmacology*, **123**, 470-474. http://dx.doi.org/10.1016/j.jep.2009.03.026

[19] Huggett, A.S and Nixon, D.A. (1957) Use of Glucose Oxidase, Peroxidase, and O-Dianisidine in Determination of Blood and Urinary Glucose. *The Lancet*, **273**, 368-370. http://dx.doi.org/10.1016/S0140-6736(57)92595-3

[20] Keller, A.C., Ma, J., Kavalier, A., He, K., Brillantes, A.M. and Kennelly, E.J. (2011) Saponins from the Traditional Medicinal Plant *Momordica charantia* Stimulate Insulin Secretion *in Vitro*. *Phytomedicine*, **19**, 32-37. http://dx.doi.org/10.1016/j.phymed.2011.06.019

[21] Menichini, F., Tundis, R., Loizzo, M.R., Bonesi, M., Liu, B., Jones, P., *et al.* (2011) *C. medica cv Diamante* Peel Chemical Composition and Influence on Glucose Homeostasis and Metabolic Parameters. *Food Chemistry*, **124**, 1083-1089. http://dx.doi.org/10.1016/j.foodchem.2010.07.083

[22] Eliza, J., Daisy, P., Ignacimuthu, S. and Duraipandiyan, V. (2009) Antidiabetic and Antilipidemic Effect of Eremanthin from *Costus speciosus* (Koen.) Sm., in STZ-Induced Diabetic Rats. *Chemico-Biological Interactions*, **182**, 67-72. http://dx.doi.org/10.1016/j.cbi.2009.08.012

[23] Gandhi, G.R., Ignacimuthu, S. and Paulraj, M.G. (2012) Hypoglycemic and β-cells Regenerative Effects of *Aegle marmelos* (L.) Corr. Bark Extract in Streptozotocin-Induced Diabetic Rats. *Food and Chemical Toxicology*, **50**, 1667-1674. http://dx.doi.org/10.1016/j.fct.2012.01.030

[24] Latha, M., Pari, L., Sitasawad, S. and Bhonde, R. (2004) Insulin-Secretagogue Activity and Cytoprotective Role of the Traditional Antidiabetic Plant *Scoparia dulcis* (Sweet Broomweed). *Life Sciences*, **75**, 2003-2014. http://dx.doi.org/10.1016/j.lfs.2004.05.012

[25] Hannan, J.M., Marenah, L., Ali, L., Rokeya, B., Flatt, P.R. and Abdel-Wahab, Y.H. (2006) *Ocimum sanctum* Leaf Extracts Stimulate Insulin Secretion from Perfused Pancreas, Isolated Islets and Clonal Pancreatic β-Cells. *Journal of Endocrinology*, **189**, 127-136. http://dx.doi.org/10.1677/joe.1.06615

[26] Hannan, J.M., Marenah, L., Ali, L., Rokeya, B., Flatt, P.R. and Abdel-Wahab, Y.H. (2007) Insulin Secretory Actions of Extracts of *Asparagus racemosus* Root in Perfused Pancreas, Isolated Islets and Clonal Pancreatic B-Cells. *Journal of Endocrinology*, **192**, 159-168. http://dx.doi.org/10.1677/joe.1.07084

23

Drug Prescribing Trends among Consultants and General Practitioners in Sharjah-UAE

Suleiman I. Sharif*, Hoda Fazli, Yasamin Tajrobehkar, Zeinab Namvar, Laila M. T. Bugaighis

Department of Pharmacy Practice & Pharmacotherapeutics, College of Pharmacy, University of Sharjah, Sharjah, United Arab Emirates
Email: *sharifsi@sharjah.ac.ae

Abstract

Background: Inappropriate prescribing can lead to errors in dispensing medications and serious problems for patients. Objectives: Prescription analysis can identify such drawbacks of prescribing, increase awareness of prescribers of rational prescribing and consequently lead to proper delivery of pharmaceutical care and enhance therapeutic outcomes. Methods: In the present study, prescriptions issued by consultants from a hospital and by general practitioners from private practice in Sharjah-United Arab Emirates were analyzed using indicators suggested by World Health Organizations. These include information with regard to prescriber, patient and the medication prescribed. We also determined the average number of drugs/encounter and % of prescriptions with antibiotics and those with injections. Data were collected and analyzed using Microsoft Excel® and expressed in terms of both counts and percentages. Results: Almost all prescriptions were handwritten with easily readable ones being 65% for consultants and 46% for general practitioners. Average number of drugs/encounter was 2.1 and 2.8 for consultants and general practitioners, respectively. Antibiotics were prescribed in 27% and 44%; generic prescribing was 5% and 10% by consultants and general practitioners respectively and 8% of prescriptions by consultants contained injections. Variable results were obtained on information regarding the patient but consultants seem to be better in documenting patient's age and gender. Consultants and general practitioners tend to prescribe 3 drugs and more in 35% and 25% respectively. The most commonly prescribed therapeutic classes for both groups of prescribers were NSAIDs and antibiotics with ibuprofen and amoxicillin-clavulanic acid combination being the most commonly prescribed drugs of each class. Conclusion: To improve prescription writing, interventions must include, among others, incorporation of topics on prescription writing in medical curriculum and programs of continuing medical education.

*Corresponding author.

Keywords

Prescription Analysis, Trends, Consultants, General Practitioners

1. Introduction

Inappropriate use of medications in healthcare facilities is a common problem not only in developing but also in developed countries [1]-[4]. However, the situation is worse in developing countries as in addition to the deleterious effects on health care outcomes; it also exhausts the limited health budget. In the latter countries, the excessive and indiscriminate use of drugs significantly and advertently influences health care delivery as it increases the incidence and seriousness of adverse drug reactions and interactions and bacterial resistance [1]. The physician has to prescribe medicines that meet the patient clinical need at doses adequate to cover their individual requirements for adequate period of time and at affordable cost [5]. Dispensing errors can be dangerous [6]-[8]. This entails the dispenser to provide the patient with the appropriate strengths of the prescribed drugs and clearly indicating to the patient the appropriate dose and how to measure, administer and frequently use the medicine. Changing a medication to ensure affordability requires a consultation of the prescriber. The dispenser, the pharmacist, must also provide some instruction on proper storage of medicines. The role of the consumer requires strict adherence to the instruction given by both the prescriber and the dispenser to avoid over dosage, under treatment, drug interactions and degradation of active constituents of medicines due to bad storage conditions. Among the easiest ways to examine an aspect of drug misuse is prescription analysis. Such investigation examines the patterns of drug prescribing. Moreover, prescription analysis whether of private practice or that of health facilities can determine areas for improvement towards rational drug use. Moreover, feeding back results of prescription analysis to the actual prescribers and health authorities is a useful method of intervention [1]. In the present study, prescribing behavior, dispensing and use of medicines will be approached to pinpoint various factors that may influence rational drug use.

2. Methods

For studying the prescribing trends among consultants in a general hospital, and general practitioners, a total 1239 and 980 prescriptions were collected during the month of April, 2011 from a general hospital out-patients pharmacy and a community pharmacy in Emirate of Sharjah respectively. The prescriptions from the hospital were issued by consultants while those of the pharmacy represent general practitioners (GPs). Prescriptions were subjected to analysis using the World Health Organization (WHO) suggested indicators [9]. These include prescriber's information such as name, registration number and signature; patient's information including the name, age, sex, and address of patient plus brief diagnosis and history of allergy. All prescriptions were examined for eligibility. In addition information on the medicine were determined including dosage regimen, number of encounters per prescription, % generic drugs prescribed, most common therapeutic classes and the most common drug of each class. Prescriptions were also examined for medications prescribed as injections. In this study, names of patients were concealed in consideration of patients' privacy protection. Data were collected and analyzed using Microsoft Excel® and expressed in terms of both counts and percentages.

3. Results

In the present study, most prescriptions were hand written with 35% - 50% of them being difficult to read making dispensing at increased risk of errors. All prescriptions issued by consultants or general practitioners (GPs) were deficient in important information regarding the prescriber, the patient and the dosage regimen (**Table 1** and **Table 2**). The average number of drugs per prescription was 2.1 for consultants and 2.8 for general practitioners. Prescribing generic drugs was higher in the case of GPs (10%) as compared to consultants (5%). The trend for poly-pharmacy was more evident in prescriptions by consultants where prescriptions with 4 or more drugs totaled to 16% (**Table 3**). Prescriptions by consultants contained injections (8%) as compared to none of those issued by GPs. As shown in **Table 1**, prescribing two drugs of the same therapeutic class was more in case of GPs as it counted to 16% of all prescriptions while it was evident in only 3% of prescriptions by consultants.

Table 1. Comparison of % presence of prescriber's information, eligibility of prescription, average number of drugs/encounter, injections, antibiotics and medication information in prescriptions by consultants and general practitioners.

Information	Number (%) of prescriptions	
	Consultants (n = 1239)	General practitioners (n = 980)
Prescriber's		
Name	1090 (88%)	813 (83%)
Signature	1115 (90%)	941 (96%)
Specialty	991 (80%)	725 (74%)
License's number	558 (45%)	333 (34%)
Prescriptions		
Typed	0 (0%)	59 (6%)
Hand written	1090 (100%)	921 (94%)
Easily readable	805 (65%)	451 (46%)
Medication		
Average number of drugs/encounter	2.1	2.8
Dose	620 (50%)	892 (91%)
Route of administration	372 (30%)	186 (19%)
Duration of treatment	942 (76%)	608 (62%)
Generic drugs	62 (5%)	98 (10%)
Injections	37 (3%)	0 (0%)
Antibiotics	335 (27%)	431 (44%)
Two drugs of the same class	37 (3%)	431 (44%)
Possible drug-drug interaction	50 (4%)	44 (4.5%)

Table 2. Comparison of patient's information present in prescriptions by consultants and general practitioners.

Patient's information	Number (%) of prescriptions	
	Consultants (n = 1239)	General practitioners (n = 980)
Name	1202 (97%)	941 (96%)
Age	1115 (90%)	294 (30%)
Gender	1090 (88%)	353 (36%)
Address	0 (0%)	137 (14%)
Brief diagnosis	0 (0%)	7 (0.7%)
History of allergy	0 (0%)	0 (0%)

Table 3. Number and % of prescriptions with various numbers of medications issued by consultants and general practitioners.

Number of drugs	Number (%) of prescriptions	
	Consultants (n = 1239)	General practitioners (n = 980)
No drugs	25 (2%)	0 (0%)
One drugs	434 (35%)	470 (48%)
Two drugs	319 (28%)	265 (27%)
Three drugs	235 (19%)	157 (16%)
Four drugs	99 (8%)	59 (6%)
More than 4 drugs	99 (8%)	29 (3%)

Drug interactions were observed in 4% and 4.5% of encounters by consultants and GPs respectively (**Table 1**) counted to The most commonly prescribed class of drugs was the NSAIDs constituting 30% and 51% for consultants and general practitioners respectively (**Table 4**). In both cases ibuprofen was the most commonly prescribed of this class as more than 50% of prescriptions contained this drug. Antibiotics come second on the list. These drugs were prescribed in 27% and 44% of prescriptions by consultants and GPs respectively. The combination of amoxicillin and clavulanic acid was the favorite drug. The third class of drugs prescribed by consultants was gastrointestinal drugs (22%) and vitamins (36%) for general practitioners (**Table 4**).

4. Discussion

The present study aimed at comparing prescribing behavior of consultants in a hospital and GPs in private clinics. Prescription analysis can indicate areas of irrational drug use practice. Name of patient was deficient in very small % of prescriptions by both consultants and GPs. These results are similar to those reported for Saudi Arabia [2] [10]. Age of patient was not mentioned in 70% of prescriptions by GPs as compared to 10% of encounters by consultants. In the present study, lack of sex and age from prescriptions by consultants was within the ranges mentioned in the above Saudi studies.

Gender of patients was not mentioned in 64% of prescriptions by GPs as compared to 12% of those by consultants. Such information are essential for pharmacists dispensing these prescriptions to check on whether doses prescribed were appropriate or not and also in case of female patients to take precautions in cases of pregnancy and lactation. Similar to previous observations in Saudi Arabia [2], patient's address was present in only 14% of prescriptions by GPs and not mentioned at all in those by consultants. This is alarming since both the prescribing physician and the dispensing pharmacist need to immediately contact the patient in case of either prescription or dispensing error. In the present study diagnosis and history of allergy were completely omitted from all studied prescriptions. This is in contrast to results reported by others in Saudi Arabia [2] [10] [11] but similar to our previous observations in Sharjah [12].

In the present study, the name, signature, specialty and license number of the prescriber were not mentioned in small % of prescriptions. The percentage lack of such information was rather similar with both groups of prescribers. Most prescriptions analyzed were hand written with readability being of 65% and 46% for consultants and GPs respectively. Our results are less than those reported for Saudi Arabia [2] but far in excess of those reported in other studies [3] [10]. Poor legibility of handwriting can lead to misinterpretation by the pharmacist and result in errors in drug dispensing and administration [13] with consequent risks to the patient.

The average number of drugs per prescription for consultants was only slightly higher than that recommended by WHO [9]. However, in prescriptions by GPs the number of drugs/encounter was 2.8 which is similar to that described in India [14] [15]. In the present study, the % of encounters with more than 4 drugs for both consultants (8%) and GPS (6%) was markedly less than that observed in encounters by consultants (25%) in our earlier study in Sharjah [12].

Surprisingly, the dose of the drug was not mentioned in only 9% of GPs prescriptions as compared to 50% of prescriptions by consultants. These results on GPs patterns of prescribing seem, to some extent, better than those

Table 4. Most commonly prescribed therapeutic classes and drug of each class in prescriptions by consultants and general practitioners.

The most commonly prescribed therapeutic class and drug of each class Number (%) of prescriptions			
Consultants (n = 1239)		General practitioners (n = 980)	
NSAIDs	372 (30%)	NSAIDs	500 (51%)
Ibuprofen	644 (52%)	Ibuprofen	666 (68%)
Antibiotics	335 (27%)	Antibiotics	431 (44%)
Amoxicillin + clavulanic acid	818 (66%)	Amoxicillin + clavulanic acid	843 (86%)
GI drugs	273 (22%)	Vitamins	353 (36%)
Hyoscine-N-butylbromide	966 (78%)	Multi-vitamins	82 (84%)

of consultants. Reasons for such negligence could be attributed to overconfidence of consultants, ignorance, short consultation time or stressful conditions of work. None of these can be an accepted justification for such behavior. Route of administrations was lacking in about 70% and 80% of prescriptions by consultants and GPs respectively. On the other hand, duration of treatment was lacking in 24% and 38% of prescriptions by consultants and GPs respectively. Such prescribing trends of both consultants and GPs although it is not appropriate; it strongly emphasizes the role of pharmacists in providing rational pharmaceutical care through complementing the prescriber's deficiencies, if any, in dispensed prescriptions.

Generic prescribing was low in prescriptions by both groups of prescribers and even lower than that reported in our earlier study in Sharjah [12] and in some Western countries [3]-[5]. This is may be attributable to a more influential role of pharmaceutical promotional activities and medical insurance strategies in UAE. Inability of patients to purchase costly medications significantly contributes to the problem of noncompliance and prescribing generic drugs should be advocated among prescribers unless there is an issue of bioavailability.

None of the prescriptions by GPS included injections whereas 8% of those issued by consultants contained injections. This may increase the possibility of non-compliance in case of expensive injectable formulations that cannot be afforded by the patient. Analysis of the number of drugs per encounter demonstrated that the incidence of poly-pharmacy is also higher in prescriptions issued by consultants than those by GPS. Such trend increases the risk of adverse effects and drug interactions. The later was evident in about 4% of encounters by both groups of prescribers. In general, one would expect a better prescribing pattern by consultants. Unfortunately, in the present study, this was not always the case. Focus in programs of medical continuing education on prescription writing may help improving the patterns of prescribing of both groups of prescribers.

The most commonly prescribed drugs were NSAIDs followed by antibiotics. The latter were reasonably prescribed by consultants (27%). This is similar to our earlier findings in a hospital in Dubai [1]. On the other hand, GPs prescribed antibiotics in more than 40% of prescriptions. This is still far less than that prescribed in India [15]. The third common class was gastrointestinal drugs for consultants and multivitamins for GPs. No other medications were included in the prescriptions with multivitamins and the extensive use of multivitamins may be explained by the insistence of patients on receiving drugs to feel better.

Despite the fact that in some aspects of prescribing a more appropriate trend was shown by GPs than by consultants, prescribing by both groups still not ideal. Periodical monitoring of prescriptions can always be beneficial as it can pinpoint areas for improvement towards rational drug prescribing.

5. Limitations of the Study

The time constraint and difficulty in obtaining prescriptions did not allow us to analyze samples of prescriptions issued by consultants and GPs in other Emirates, therefore the results cannot be generalized to other Emirates than Dubai. Future studies will focus on prescriptions collected from various Emirates and hospitals.

6. Conclusion

A prescription should be wisely and appropriately written to include all the information that would be of help to the pharmacist who dispenses the medications and the patient who uses them. Periodical monitoring of prescriptions is useful as it can identify areas for improvement in prescription writing. Moreover, we suggest that interventions to improve prescribing behavior may include among others, feedback of results to the prescribers through personal interviews and incorporation of principles of rational prescription writing in medical curriculum and continuing medical education programs for both GPs and consultants.

References

[1]   Sharif, S.I., Al-Shaqra, M., Hajjar, H., Shamout, A. and Wess, L. (2008) Patterns of Drug Prescribing in a Hospital in Dubai, United Arab Emirates. *Libyan Journal of Medicine*, **3**, 10-12. http://dx.doi.org/10.4176/070928

[2]   Irshaid, Y.M., Al Homrany, M., Hamdi, A.A., Adjepon-Yamoah, K.K. and Mahfouz, A.A. (2005) Compliance with Good Practice in Prescription Writing at Outpatient Clinic in Saudi Arabia. *Eastern Mediterranean Health Journal*, **11**, 922-928.

[3]   Meyer, T.A. (2000) Improving the Quality of the Order-Writing Process for Inpatient Orders and Outpatient Prescriptions. *American Journal of Health-System Pharmacy*, **57**, S18-S12.

[4]   Montastruc, F., Gardette, V., Cantet, C., Piau, A., Lapeyre-Mestre, M., Vellas, B., Montastruc, J.-L. and Andrieu, S.

(2013) Potentially Inappropriate Medication Use among Patients with Alzheimer Disease in the REAL.FR Cohort: Be Aware of Atropinic and Benzodiazepine Drugs! *European Journal of Clinical Pharmacology*, **69**, 1589-1597. http://dx.doi.org/10.1007/s00228-013-1506-8

[5] DeVries, T.P., *et al.*, Eds. (1995) Guide to Good Prescribing: A Practical Manual. World Health Organization, Geneva, 51-5 (WHO/DAP/94.11).

[6] (1983) The Pharmaceutical Professions and Institutions. UAE Federal Law No: 4.

[7] Brahams, D. (1984) Legal Liability and the Negligent Prescription. *Practitioner*, **228**, 444-445.

[8] Yousif, E., Ahmed, A.M., Abdalla, M.E. and Abdelgadir, M.A. (2006) Deficiencies in Medical Prescriptions in a Sudanese Hospital. *Eastern Mediterranean Health Journal*, **12**, 915-918.

[9] WHO (1995) How to Investigate Drug Use in Health Facilities: Selected Drug Use Indicators. World Health Organization, Geneva, WHO/DAP/93.1.1995.

[10] Balbaid, O.M. and Al-Dawood, K.M. (1988) Assessment of Physician's Prescribing Practices at Ministry of Health Hospitals in Jeddah City, Saudi Arabia. *Saudi Medical Journal*, **19**, 28-35.

[11] Bawazir, S.A. (1992) Prescribing Patterns at Community Pharmacies in Saudi Arabia. *International Pharmacy Journal*, **6**, 222-224.

[12] Sharif, S.I., Alabdouli, A.H. and Sharif, R.S. (2013) Drug Prescribing Trends in a General Hospital in Sharjah-United Arab Emirates. *American Journal of Pharmacological Sciences*, **1**, 6-9. http://dx.doi.org/10.12691/ajps-1-1-2

[13] Velo, G.P. and Minuz, P. (2009) Medication Errors: Prescribing Faults and Prescription Errors. *British Journal of Clinical Pharmacology*, **67**, 624-628. http://dx.doi.org/10.1111/j.1365-2125.2009.03425.x

[14] Bapna, J.S., Tekur, U., Gitanjali, B., Shashindran, C.H., Pradhan, S.C., Thulasimani, M., *et al.* (1992) Drug Utilization at Primary Health Care Level in Southern India. *European Journal of Clinical Pharmacology*, **43**, 413-415. http://dx.doi.org/10.1007/BF02220618

[15] Kshirsagar, M.J., Langade, D., Patil, S. and Patki, P.S. (1998) Prescribing Patterns among Medical Practitioners in Pune. Bulletin World Health Organization, India.

24

Genomic Organization of Purinergic P2X Receptors

Raúl Loera-Valencia, Josué Obed Jaramillo-Polanco, Andrómeda Linan-Rico,
María Guadalupe Nieto Pescador, Juan Francisco Jiménez Bremont,
Carlos Barajas-López[*]

División de Biología Molecular, Instituto Potosino de Investigación Científica y Tecnológica, San Luís Potosí, México
Email: [*]cbarajas@ipicyt.edu.mx

Abstract

Purinergic P2X receptors are a family of ligand-gated cationic channels activated by extracellular ATP. P2X subunit protein sequences are highly conserved between vertebrate species. However, they can generate a great diversity of coding splicing variants to fulfill several roles in mammalian physiology. Despite intensive research in P2X expression in both central and peripheral nervous system, there is little information about their homology, genomic structure and other key features that can help to develop selective drugs or regulatory strategies of pharmacological value which are lacking today. In order to obtain clues on mammalian P2X diversity, we have performed a bio-informatics analysis of the coding regions and introns of the seven P2X subunits present in human, simian, dog, mouse, rat and zebrafish. Here we report the arrangements of exon and intron sequences, considering its number, size, phase and placement; proposing some ideas about the gain and loss of exons and retention of introns. Taken together, these evidences show traits that can be used to gain insight into the evolutionary history of vertebrate P2X receptors and better understand the diversity of subunits coding the purinergic signaling in mammals.

Keywords

Alternative Splicing, Intron, Genomic Organization, P2X, Purinergic Signalling

1. Introduction

Purinergic P2X receptors are a family of ligand-gated cationic channels activated by extracellular ATP [1].

---

[*]Corresponding author.

Seven subunits have been identified so far in mammalian species (P2X$_{1-7}$), and they are involved in numerous physiological roles like peristalsis, platelet aggregation, pain sensation, immune response and development [1]-[5]. To form a functional channel, P2X subunits assemble as homo or heteromeric trimers [6]. The pharmacological properties of the assembled P2X receptor vary in function to subunit composition [7] [8]. The subunit stoichiometry has a different arrangement among tissue in a given organism, and different composition among species, for example, the enteric nervous system of the rat, mouse and guinea pig expresses P2X$_2$/P2X$_3$ heteromeric receptors [6] [9] while sensory ganglia and heart of rodents and humans express homomeric P2X$_3$ receptors [10] [11]. In addition, P2X receptors can assemble from tissue specific splicing variants of its messenger RNA [1].

The physiological role of P2X receptors seems to be the same for different species of mammalians: purinergic neurotransmission. Even when the population of P2X subunits in a tissue between two species may vary [12] [13], the P2X subunit protein sequences are highly conserved between vertebrate species [14]. Sequences correspond to cysteine allowing disulfide bonds, and transmembrane domains I and II and a YXXXK motif in the c-terminus of each protein are specially conserved among species [1].

Despite the high conservation of P2X subunits between vertebrates, the analysis of completely sequenced genomes of non-vertebrate model organisms like *Drosophila melanogaster*, *Caenorhabditis elegans* and *Apis melifera* show no homologues to P2X receptors [14] [15]. Previous works have hypothesized that ATP is a very early neurotransmitter in evolution of vertebrates with a single P2X receptor as ancestor [16]. Phylogeny suggests that diversification of seven P2X subunits presented in mammalians is an evolutionary event subsequent to the split between vertebrates and invertebrates [17]. There are evidences showing that non-vertebrates like *Schistosoma mansoni* have P2X homologues [18], so it's been proposed that arthropods and nematodes lose their P2X homologues later in their own evolution [17].

The increase of genomic data is available from unicellular, and simple-celled organisms have substantially improved our knowledge about the evolutionary path of purinergic transmission and P2X receptors [14], however, to date there exist no selective agonist or modulator for the P2X family with few exceptions currently under testing [19]. Because of this, we have performed a bioinformatics analysis of the coding regions and introns of the seven P2X genes being presented in human, simian, dog, mouse, rat and zebrafish. Here we report the arrangements of exon and intron sequences, considering its number, size, phase and placement; proposing some ideas about the gain and loss of exons and retention of introns. We expect that these evidences show traits, which can be used to gain insight into the primary structure of vertebrate P2X receptors and help design selective pharmacological drugs and single-subunit regulatory strategies.

2. Materials and Methods

2.1. Analysis of Genomic Sequences of P2X Receptors

Several genomic cDNA sequences encoding P2X receptors of *Homo sapiens*, *Pan troglodytes*, *Rattus novergicus*, *Mus musculus*, *Canis lupus familiaris*, *Danio rerio* and *Anolis carolinensis* for P2X$_6$ (given the absence of *Danio rerio*'s P2X$_6$ receptor) were obtained from the NCBI (National Center for Biotechnology Information, Bethesda, MD, USA; http://www.ncbi.nlm.nih.gov) database and only a few of them from Ensembl database (www.ensembl.org). Each of the P2X receptors sequence and Gen Bank accession no. of each organism are shown in Supplementary **Table S1**.

All the P2X genes of the organisms mentioned above were analyzed for the determination of genomic organization, including the size, gain and loss of exons, as well as intron number, size, loss, retention, placement and phase. The exon-intron organization was obtained from the analysis of the information available in the NCBI database.

Pairwise alignments were conducted in order to establish exon and intron sequence identities among species using the Needleman-Wunsch (global) and Smith-Waterman (local) alignment programs at the EBI (European Bioinformatics Institute, Cambridge, UK; http://www.ebi.ac.uk) database. Microsynteny between P2X receptor genes from the different organisms was assembled using the information present in the NCBI database chromosome image (http://www.ncbi.nlm.nih.gov/gene). Prediction of possible transposable element sequences within the P2X genes was performed using Blastn algorithm of the NCBI database.

2.2. Molecular Phylogenetic Analysis

The aminoacid sequences of the P2X receptors were aligned and the respective phylogenetic tree constructed

Table 1. Gene information of P2X subunits used in the gene structure and phylogeny analyses.

P2X Gene	Gene lenght (bp)	Gene without UTR (bp)	mRNA (bp)	Messenger without UTR (bp)	Protein (aa)	mRNA Accession	Protein Accession	Status	Chromosome
P2X₁									
MUS	16,053	14,812	2441	1200	399	NM_008771.3	NP_032797.3	validated	11
RNO	15,053	13,782	2539	1200	399	NM_012997.2	NP_037129.1	provisional	10
HSA	20,076	18,412	2910	1200	399	NM_002558.2	NP_002549.1	reviewed	17
CAF	NE	13,559		1200	399	XM_548344.1	XP_548344.1	predicted	9
MMU	21,173	20,436	1937	1200	399	XM_001092205.2	XP_001092205.1	predicted	16
DAR	NE	27,735		1197	398	ENSDART00000011544	ENSDARP00000010823	provisional	5
P2X₂									
MUS	3224	2763	1712	1251	416	NM_001164833.1	NP_001158305.1	validated	5
RNO	3195	2782	1625	1212	403	Y10473	CAA71499.1	provisional	12
HSA	3570	3156	1629	1215	404	NM_174873.1	NP_777362.1	reviewed	12
CAF	NE	2757		1185	394	XM_851798.1	XP_856891.1	predicted	26
MMU	3485	3071	1626	1212	403	XM_001082602.2	XP_001082602.2	predicted	11
DAR	14,522	14,433	1292	1203	400	NM_198983.1	NP_945334.1	provisional	5
P2X₃									
MUS	39,283	36,287	4190	1194	397	NM_145526.2	NP_663501.2	validated	2
RNO	42,707	40,151	3773	1194	397	NM_031075.1	NP_112337.1	provisional	3
HSA	31,601	31,446	1349	1194	397	NM_002559.2	NP_002550.2	reviewed	11
CAF	NE	25,834		1194	397	XM_540614.1	XP_540614.1	predicted	18
PTR	33,271	32,483	1982	1194	397	XM_001136930.1	XP_001136930.1	predicted	11
DARa	15,454	14,977	1724	1233	410	NM_131623.1	NP_571698.1	provisional	14
DARb	12,235	10,544	2920	1239	412	NM_198986.2	NP_945337.2	provisional	1
P2X₄									
MUS	21,488	20,660	1995	1167	388	NM_011026.2	NP_035156.2	validated	5
RNO	17,652	16,846	1997	1167	388	NM_031594.1	NP_113782.1	provisional	12
HSA	24,246	23,385	2043	1167	388	NM_002560.2	NP_002551.2	reviewed	12
CAF	16,697	16,185	1679	1167	388	XM_543389.2	XP_543389.1	predicted	26
PTR	25,836	24,971	2032	1167	388	XM_509437.2	XP_509437.2	predicted	12
DARa	9193	9046	1330	1170	389	NM_153653.1	NP_705939.1	provisional	21
DARb	7918	7883	1243	1206	401	NM_198987.1	NP_945338.1	provisional	8
P2X₅									
MUS	12,158	11,238	2293	1368	455	NM_033321.3	NP_201578.2	validated	11
RNO	11,610	10,569	2436	1368	455	NM_080780.2	NP_542958.2	provisional	10
HSA	23,063	22,138	2206	1269	422	NM_002561.2	NP_002552.2	reviewed	17
CAF	13,312	12,894	1705	1287	428	XM_548343.2	XP_548343.2	predicted	9
PTR	26,312	20,930	2195	1269	422	XM_511272.2	XP_511272.2	predicted	17
DAR	23,322	22,426	2367	1443	481	NM_194413.1	NP_919394.1	provisional	5
P2X₆									
MUS	10,128	8952	2362	1170	389	NM_011028.2	NP_035158.2	validated	16
RNO	10,037	8919	2331	1170	389	NM_012721.2	NP_036853.2	validated	11
HSA	12,839	11,443	2754	1326	441	NM_005446.3	NP_005437.2	reviewed	22

Continued

CAF	NE	8980		1230	410	ENSECAFT00000023919	ENSCAFP00000022204	predicted	26
MMU	NE	12,957		1317	438	XM_001084368.2	XP_001084368.1	predicted	10
ACA	NE	4774		1167	389	ENSACAT00000011065	ENSACAP00000010841	predicted	NE
P2X$_7$									
MUS	40,374	37,231	4931	1788	595	NM_011027.2	NP_035157.2	validated	5
RNO	43,128	41,366	3540	1788	595	NM_019256.1	NP_062129.1	provisional	12
HSA	53,724	51,832	3680	1788	595	NM_002562.5	NP_002553.3	reviewed	12
CAF	NE	42,756		1788	595	NM_001113456.1	NP_001106927.1	provisional	26
MMU	55,453	54,038	3203	1788	595	XM_001092531.2	XP_001092531.1	predicted	11
DAR	20,914	20,847	1860	1791	596	NM_198984.1	NP_945335.1	provisional	8
P2X$_8$									
DAR	27,994	27,989	1178	1173	390	NM_198985.1	NP_945336.1	provisional	15

Table 2. Percent identity of mouse P2X paralogous (clustal W).

		1	2	3	4	5	6	7
1	**musP2X$_1$**	x	32.3	37.5	47.4	36.1	39.3	31.8
2	**musP2X$_2$**		x	41.3	39.4	40.1	35	28.1
3	**musP2X$_3$**			x	40.5	38.3	35.2	30.5
4	**musP2X$_4$**				x	45.9	41	40.5
5	**musP2X$_5$**					x	44.7	27.3
6	**musP2X$_6$**						x	29
7	**musP2X$_7$**							x

using the software MEGA version 4.0 with the maximum parsimonia method (500 bootstrap).

3. Results and Discussion

The seven P2X subunits (1 - 7) in mammals are diverse in size and gene organization. P2X$_2$ is the smallest of the subunits, with a 2.78 Kb transcript. The longest is P2X$_7$ with 37.23 Kb (see **Table 1**). However, the ORF size of the seven subunits from the species analyzed in this work has an average of 1.3 Kb without untranslated sequences—P2X4 has the smallest transcript with 1.16 Kb and P2X$_7$ possess the longest transcript of 1.78 Kb, their aminoacid sequences are 388 and 595 residues respectively. Mainly, the difference in size between P2X subunits is related to the size of their C-terminus domains.

3.1. Genomic Organization of P2X Genes of the Mouse

The P2X subunits of mouse consist of 12 to 13 exons and 11 to 12 introns according to the reported sequences of Gene Bank (**Figure 1(a)**). In detail, subunits P2X$_1$, P2X$_2$, P2X$_3$, P2X$_4$ and P2X$_6$ have 12 exons and 11 introns, whereas P2X$_5$ and P2X$_7$ have an arrangement of 13 exons and 12 introns.

Despite the differences of aminoacid sequences among P2X subunits (below 50% identity, **Table 2**), exon size trends to be conserved from Exons III to X, which is the middle portion of the ORF; with exons III and X as the most conserved (most of them are 72 and 66 nucleotides long respectively), whereas the last exons are the most variable in size (**Figure 1(a)**). In counterpart, the introns have a high variability in size and sequence, this could be the cause of identity differences at genomic DNA level between P2X genes in mice. The conservation of exon size and high variability of intron length has been previously described in other gene families in previous works [20], which are evidence of evolutionary mechanisms affecting their gene structure.

Exon III codes for 24 aminoacids located in the extracellular loop, and exon X forms the first half of the transmembrane region II, part of the channel pore [21]. In counterpart, the most variable regions of the exons of P2X subunits are those involved in traffic, receptor desensitization, cytoskeleton binding, receptor-receptor interaction and regulatory proteins, which contribute to the diversity of function of the assembled P2X receptors.

Intron size among P2X subunits in mouse is highly variable, with $P2X_2$ as the gen with the shortest introns (76 to 319 bp). Previous works showed shorter introns in constitutive genes compared to those of low expression [22] [23]. This is explained by the naturally selected gene compression since transcription and mRNA processing are slow and energetically costly processes [22] [24]. The small intron size of P2X2 correlates with its high prevalence in cells responsive to purinergic signaling like neurons of the peripheral nervous system [25]. On the other hand, subunits like $P2X_3$ seem to be present mostly at early stages of development and scarcely found in adult neurons according to other works [5] [26]-[28] and to our single cell PCR results performed in myenteric neurons of mice [29]. These results correlate with the longer size of $P2X_3$ introns in a gene that is not as widely expressed by neural cell types and does not need high efficiency transcription rates.

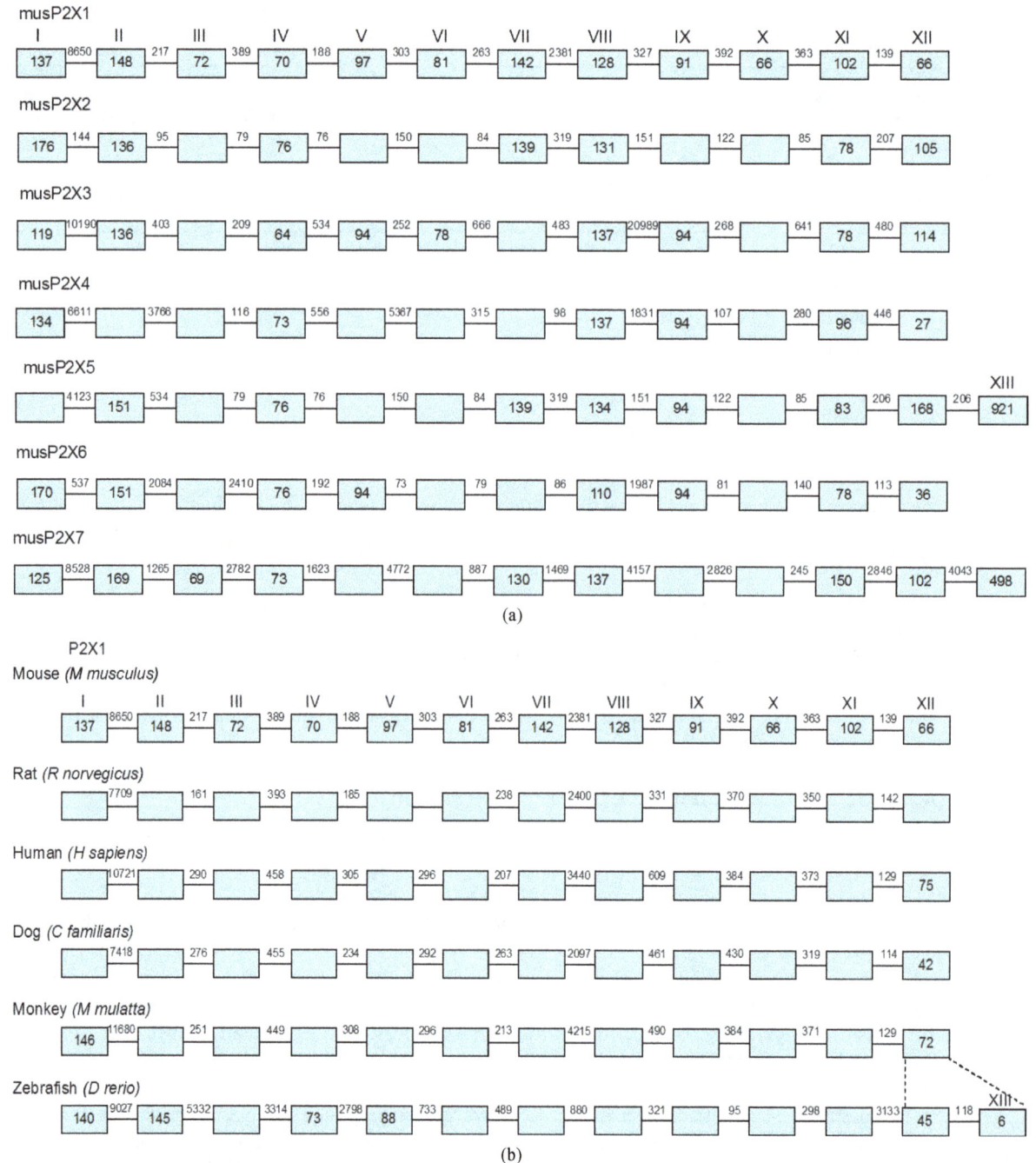

(a)

(b)

P2X2

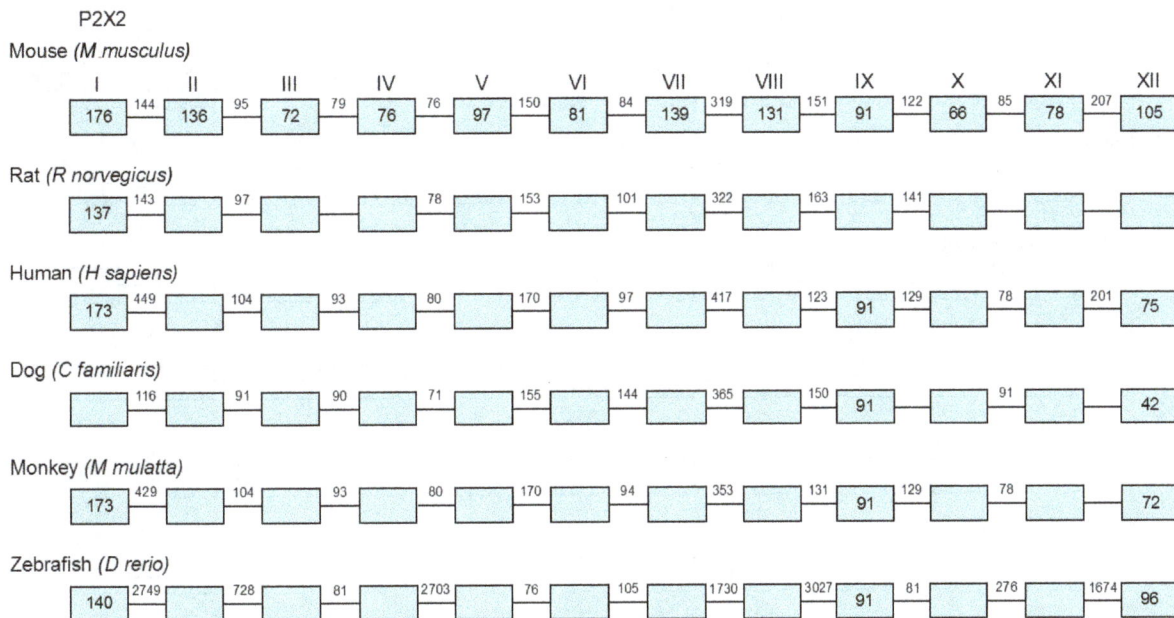

(c)

P2X3

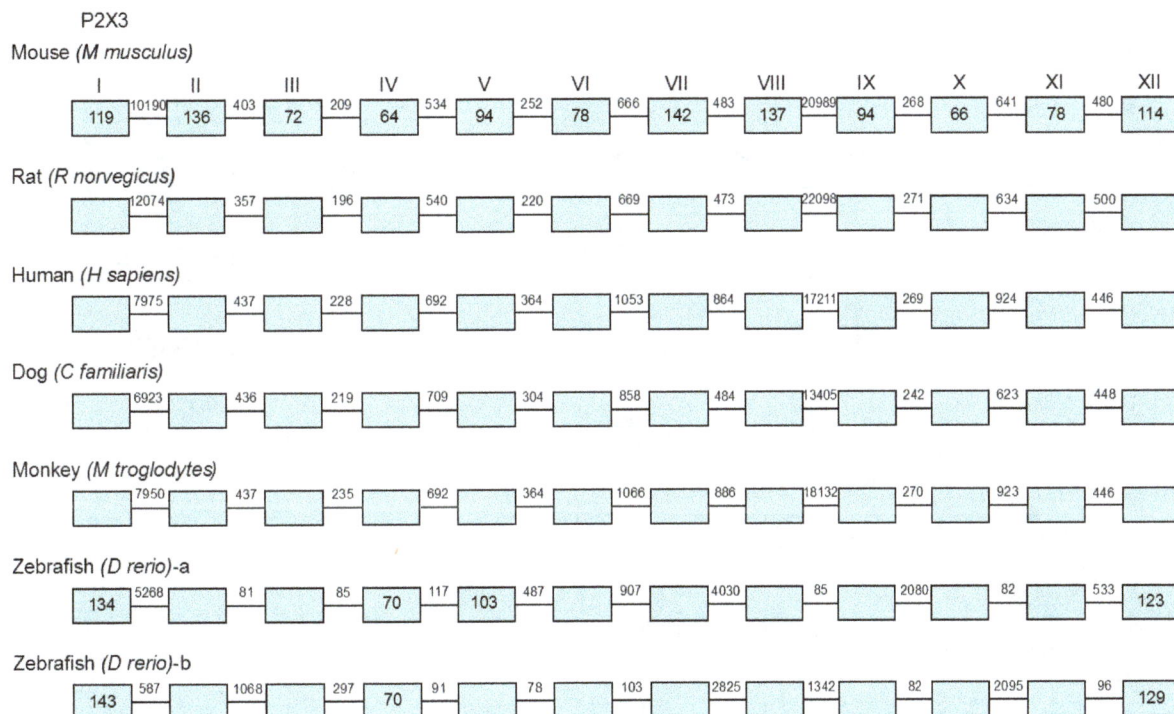

(d)

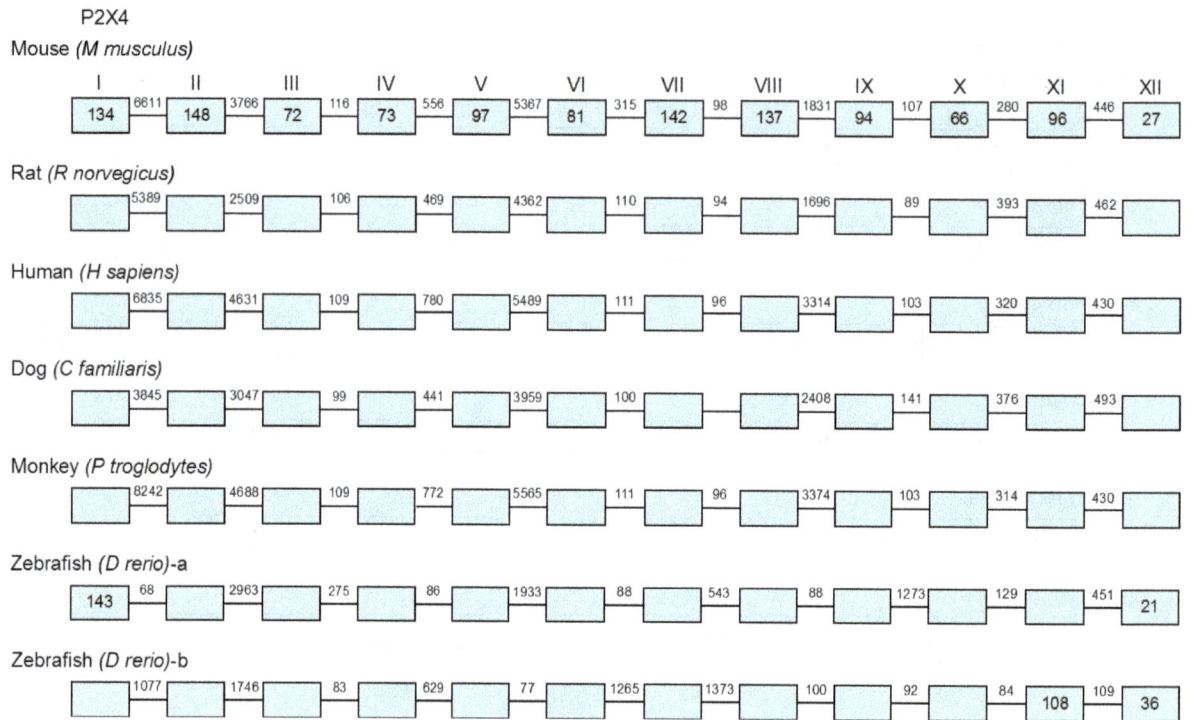

(e)

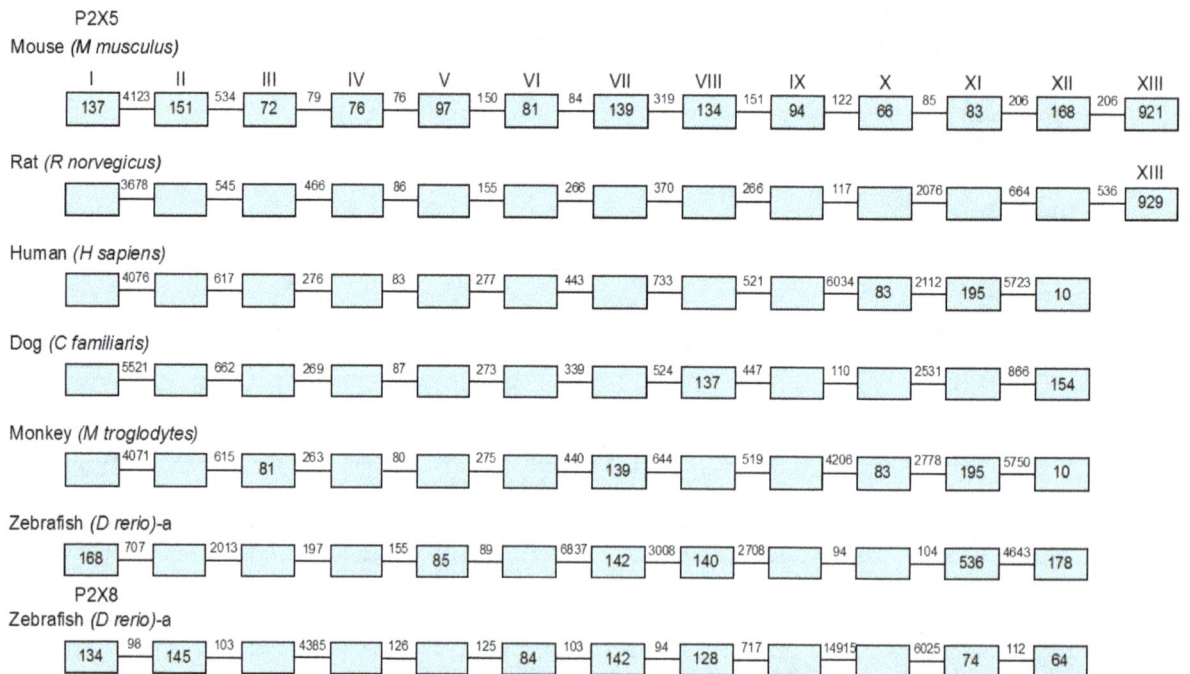

(f)

P2X6

Mouse (*M musculus*)

Rat (*R norvegicus*)

Human (*H sapiens*)

Dog (*C familiaris*)

Monkey (*M mulatta*)

Reptile (*A carolinensis*)

(g)

P2X7

Mouse (*M musculus*)

Rat (*R norvegicus*)

Human (*H sapiens*)

Dog (*C familiaris*)

Monkey (*M mulatta*)

Zebrafish (*D rerio*)

(h)

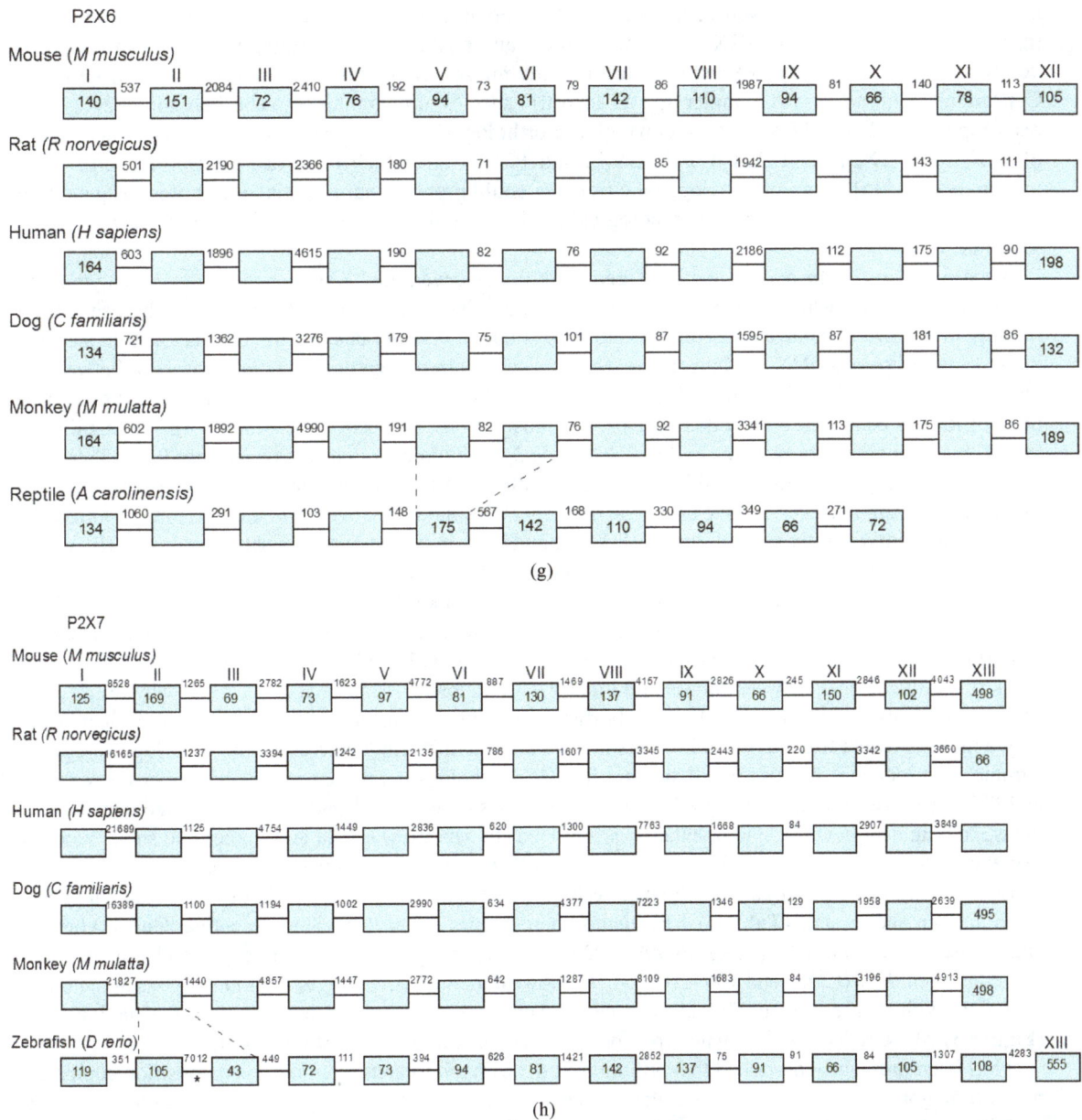

Figure 1. Schematic representation of the genomic organization of P2X receptors in several organisms. Exons are depicted as boxes with roman numbers on top, while introns are represented as solid lines. Numbers inside exons indicate the size in base pairs (bp) as well as number on top of the solid lines represent the intron size in bp. The first gene belongs to mouse in all cases and the lack of label below a given exon represents the conservation of size between homologous genes. (a) Genomic organization of the seven P2X subunits of mouse (Mus musculus); (b)-(h) Genomic organization of the P2X subunits compared between orthologous. When indicated, a dashed line points to exon fusion or exon separation between orthologous P2X genes.

Intron I is often referred to contain expression enhancers and other regulatory elements in mammals [30]-[32], this is the case of the purine nucleoside phosphorylase, where short portions of the intron 1 (around 170 bp) provided enhanced transcription in mammalian cell culture expression systems. In P2X orthologs (**Figures 1(b)-(h)**), intron I size and sequence it's also conserved, possibly pointing to unidentified regulatory elements in P2X genes.

3.2. Genomic Organization of P2X Orthologous Genes

To determine how P2X gene orthologous have been conserved in evolution among species, we analyzed the genomic organization of the seven P2X subunits of different mammalian species, including mouse (musP2X), rat (rnoP2X), primates (mmuP2X for Macacamulata and ptrP2X for Pan troglodytes), human (hsaP2X) and dog (cafP2X). Additionally, we included in this study the zebrafish (darP2X for *Dario rerio*) from the family Cyprinidae from the class Actinopterygii, as ancestral species of mammals. In zebrafish, nine P2X genes have been reported: $P2X_1$ to $P2X_5$ and $P2X_7$ which are orthologous to mammal subunits. Another two paralogous of $P2X_3$ and $P2X_4$ named $P2X_3b$ and $P2X_4b$, and $P2X_8$ from which there are no reported orthologous in mammals [33]-[35]. From our phylogenetic tree, we could propose that $P2X_8$ is an orthologous gene to $P2X_5$, although further functional and pharmacological evidence could uncover more similarities between these two subunits.

When we analyzed the exon size of P2X gene orthologous, we found a high conservation among the different species of mammals, whit some exceptions in the first and last exon (**Figure 1**). Also the zebrafish showed variability in the size of some exons compared to P2X subunits in mammals. On the contrary, intron size is variable in each ortholog of P2X subunits, however, the size of introns trend to be better conserved between the orthologous of a specific P2X subunit (**Figures 1(a)-(h)**). The zebrafish again presents the most variable arrangement of introns compared to the other species. For most introns, the identity percentage was not significant, but in rare events the identity rate was up to 70% (**Table 3**). Additionally, we discovered that P2X subunits have a conserved intron phase among musP2X paralogs (**Table 4**). Among orthologous, P2X genes conserve their intron phase as well, however, some changes do occur in $P2X_5$ and $P2X_7$, overall in the 3' region of introns (**Table 4**). Thus, we found that, in general, introns I, V, VI and VIII are in phase two, whereas exons II, III, VII, IX, X, XI and XII end up in phase zero. Only exon IV appear in phase one.

Some P2X paralogous are found in the same chromosome, like $P2X_1$ and $P2X_5$; $P2X_2$, $P2X_4$ and $P2X_7$ showing syntenic traits. On **Figure 2** we show the blocks of syntenic P2X genes in mouse and human. The comparison with all the analyzed species is shown in Supplementary **Table S1**. The genes $P2X_1$ and $P2X_5$ conform a block of syntenic genes between mouse and human with opposite orientation. In a similar way, $P2X_4$ and $P2X_7$ are syntenic between all orthologs. In the zebrafish case, with two different $P2X_4$ genes, only $P2X_4b$ keeps synteny with $P2X_7$ (Supplementary **Table S1**), and the $P2X_4a$ is different than b and other orthologous regarding its chromosome location. We also found synteny for $P2X_2$ orthologs but these are located further away from $P2X_4$ and $P2X_7$ (**Figure 2**). In the case of $P2X_3$, the genes in positions 1, 2, -1 and -2 are conserved completely in the mouse and human, however, the orientation is inversed. In zebrafish, $P2X_3a$ and b keep the same microsynteny than their orthologous. Genes that keep synteny with $P2X_6$ conserve order as well as orientation.

The ortholog genes $P2X_{1-7}$ are much conserved at the protein level, most of all between rat and mouse or between human and primate (**Table 3**). The identity percentages (Clustal W, Slow/Accurate, Gonnet) between rat and mouse range from 85% ($P2X_7$) to 99% ($P2X_3$). On a similar way, between human and primate, identities range between 97% ($P2X_4$) and 100% ($P2X_7$). The lowest identity percentages are found between mammals and zebrafish, with values around 50% in most cases. These results are in accordance with the phylogenetic tree (**Figure 3**) where rodents and primates are closer to each other and farthest from zebrafish.

It has been previously described that orthologous genes trend to conserve their intron position compared with non-orthologous genes, even when orthologous sequence identity is low [36]-[38]. We found low percentage of protein identity between $P2X_{1-7}$ from zebra fish regarding their respective mammalian orthologous. However, even when zebrafish is an evolutionary distant organism, it trended to conserve certain characteristics such as exon-intron organization and intron position with its mammalian counterparts, which makes evident the sharing of common ancestry in P2X evolution (**Figure 3**). The main difference between fish P2X genes and mammalian was centered in the size of introns, indicating some re-organization in exon-intron position after mammalian divergence.

In zebrafish, two paralogous genes for $P2X_3$ and $P2X_4$ have been reported with distinctive localization and genomic organization. Several lines of evidence have suggested that whole genome duplications occurred before the vertebrate/ascidian divergence [39] and, later on, in the lineage of teleostheus after tetrapod divergence where only one set of these duplicated genes were maintained [40]-[43]. This is supported by the existence of several duplicated segments in zebrafish chromosomes [44]. The two genes darP2X$_3$a and b seem to be the result of this duplication, since they are located in a cluster of duplicated genes found in different chromosomes and conserves synteny with their orthologous (Supplementary **Table S1**). In darP2X$_4$a and b there is no conservation of gene duplicates, each $P2X_4$ is located in a different chromosome near single copy genes. $P2X_4b$ is close in position to darP2X$_7$, but that is not the case of darP2X$_4$a, therefore, it is possible that $P2X_4a$ was origin-

Table 3. Global (needle) and local (water) alignments of P2X subunits gene orthologous in ebi's align software.

P2X₁	Mouse vs X (needle/water)				
	Rat	Human	Dog	Monkey	Zebrafish
Intron I	69.9/69.8	44.8/43.9	45.7/45.3	44.4/43.6	42.3/41.1
II	66.5/67	52.8/53.2	54/54	57.7/59.2	2.8/42.1
III	87.6/87.6	58.2/55.5	52.4/49.3	55.7/54.3	6.9/39.7
IV	86.8/86.8	44/44.4	47.8/47.3	42.9/43.7	4/42.9
V	78.3/78.3	56.9/57.4	57/56.3	57.1/57	21.2/40.2
VI	78/78.7	50.7/50.2	54.5/53.2	52/50.5	28.8/36.8
VII	81.5/80.9	40.9/40	42.3/42.3	33.4/34	21.2/41.1
VIII	81.3/83.7	33/50.2	46.2/48.3	21.7/47.1	40.9/44.7
IX	79.8/79.5	60/58.6	54.3/52.2	58.8/59.1	14.7/45.8
X	86.3/86.5	63.4/62.2	54.9/53.1	62.7/58.4	38.8/36
XI	84.5/84.5	54.5/59.1	54.4/53.6	57/57.2	2.7/46.3

P2X₂	Mouse vs X (needle/water)				
	Rat	Human	Dog	Monkey	Zebrafish
Intron I	89/90.3	21.3/46.5	54.8./57.8	22/53	3.6/30.5
II	92.9/94.8	55.9/55.9	48.7/49.6	56.8/57.8	7.2/48.1
III	87.7/89.9	53.9/50.9	51.1/48.1	51.9/50	43.5/48.6
IV	90/92.3	52.1/52.8	40.8/55.7	53.7/55.7	2.1/35.5
V	82.4/83.4	42.1/49.7	44.9/45.4	47.8/48.5	31/54.7
VI	67.6/68.9	43.1/49.1	36.2/44.4	43.9/49.5	37.5/51.8
VII	87.3/87.9	46/46.5	50.5/52.1	50.4/50.6	10.6/48.2
VIII	75.8/76.7	38.6/49.7	40.3/42.1	44.4/53.6	3.5/37.2
IX	75.5/76.6	47.2/47.2	37.4/52.6	49.3/49.3	33.6/43.2
X	82.8/84.7	57.6/58.8	55/57.1	58.5/61.2	21.1/46.5
XI	93.8/95.6	69.4/70.6	51.6/52.8	70.1/70.8	8/32.8

P2X₃	Mouse vs X (needle/water)					
	Rat	Human	Dog	Monkey	Zebrafishₐ	Zebrafish_b
Intron I	56.7/61	40.2/48.7	35.5/42.9	40.9/48.9	28.7/37.7	3.2/38.4
II	75.6/75.8	52.6/52.7	34.1/54.4	53.3/56.5	13.7/34.1	23.7/33.3
III	81.5/85.9	58.9/63.8	23.8/35.6	54.1/58.3	18.3/48.4	14.1/29.9
IV	79.7/80.4	49.1/49.4	44.6/44.6	49.6/49.9	13.2/46.2	8.8/36.7
V	78/78.3	48.9/48.9	44.5/49.2	48.9/48.9	26.4/40.1	20.5/47.8
VI	85.5/85.7	41.3/41.3	48.9/50.6	41.2/41.2	38.4/38.5	9.6/39.3
VII	80.1/80.3	36.2/52.5	45/47.4	38/48.6	7.9/38.8	10.8/40.1
VIII	68.7/68.8	43.7/48.2	39.4/43.7	40.8/44.8	0.3/58.2	4.1/38.6
IX	90.5/90.8	65.1/65.1	51.4/51.6	0.7/51.4	6.9/37.5	15.1/40
X	82.5/82.6	44.8/45.4	51.1/52.3	43.4/46.5	9.1/44.5	19.6/35.5
XI	74.6/74.8	55.5/55.5	50.2/50.2	55.1/55.1	40.9/44.5	12.5/45.5

P2X₄	Mouse vs X (needle/water)					
	Rat	Human	Dog	Monkey	Zebrafishₐ	Zebrafish_b
Intron I	55.2/54.6	40.4/46.1	34.5/43.7	41.2/40.3	0.7/46.7	9.7/43.3
II	41.1/41.6	29/40	42.7/44.1	30/39.7	43.3/43.5	39.7/41.6
III	71.2/71.2	63.9/63.6	55.6/56	59.3/55.8	25.7/39.6	41.9/48.4
IV	69.3/69.8	42.5/43.9	49.7/50.1	43.4/42.6	9.6/43.2	44.5/44.5
V	62.2/61.4	39.6/46.6	42.0/42.0	39.4/43.2	22.4/35.5	0.9/40.0
VI	24.9/30	23.9/45.9	22.9/37.4	22.7/46	16.6/39.6	17.3/33.6
VII	65.2/66.1	54.1/56.8	55.4/56.4	52.5/54.2	12.1/34.2	4.5/53.0

Continued

VIII	59.4/62.4	34.4/36.8	44.4/44.7	35.5/36.3	3.0/43.7	3.8/48.9
IX	72.5/72.5	51.9/49.6	46.6/48.6	53.2/51.9	6.0/42.7	50.5/50.9
X	54.7/54.6	50.3/50	45.6/45.9	52.9/50.1	27.3/39.3	18.0/42.6
XI	77.2/77	49.2/52.2	51.2/54.4	71.4/48.7	44.6/44.8	16.0/41.1

P2X$_5$	Mouse vs X (needle/water)					
	Rat	Human	Dog	Monkey	Zebrafish	P2X8 Zebrafish
Intron I	65.1/64.5	47/44.4	42.3/41.3	44.5/44.5	10.5/40	1.8/37.4
II	83.5/83.3	57.7/56.8	53.6/51.9	56.9/56.9	16.7/68.4	13.0/36.0
III	69.6/69	30.3/52.7	29.3/38.1	29.4/54.4	17.8/40.9	8.0/34.0
IV	84.9/84.9	68.5/68.5	63.2/64.2	68.5/68.5	27/66.7	28.6/38.4
V	80.7/80.7	38.9/42.8	40.5/50.2	43/42.8	32/35.8	27.0/35.7
VI	84.9/84.9	41.7/42.8	54.1/50.7	40.7/41.3	2.4/31.9	22.8/34.1
VII	71.5/74.1	42.2/42.3	50.8/48.3	47.2/46.1	9.1/37.3	13,1/36,8
VIII	76.4/76	33.5/53	30.8/41.3	33.5/46.6	20.2/45.5	21.5/37.2
IX	87.1/87.1	1.3/50.3	2.7/56.7	2.1/45.5	2.8/36.4	0.6/37.7
X	70.4/70.2	43.1/41	4.4/39.6	33.3/39.7	2.5/59.8	22.4/38.9
XI	68.5/68.7	7.0/38	43.3/45.8	6.9/38.1	10.8/48.1	10.2/43.9
XII	83.1/83.1	NA	NA	NA	6.6/40.5	

P2X$_6$	Mouse vs X (needle/water)					
	Rat	Human	Dog	Monkey	Zebrafish	Rat
Intron I	78.6/79.7	52.2/52.5	48/47.4	52.5/50.4	31.9/33.8	78.6/79.7
II	67.8/67.9	46.9/46.8	40.5/39.7	47.3/46.2	8.7/38	67.8/67.9
III	81/80.8	36.9/37.3	45.7/44.9	32.4/36.6	2.9/48.5	81/80.8
IV	77/78.9	66.5/64.1	50.5/57.1	62.6/58.7	50.5/46.4	77/78.9
V	86.5/86.5	55.1/54.7	46.7/56.6	53.4/54.1	-	86.5/86.5
VI	88.6/88.6	55.3/56.2	43.4/59.5	52.6/52.9	10/43	88.6/88.6
VII	86.2/86.2	65.6/70.5	64.1/65.1	64.9/70.5	29.1/50.6	86.2/86.2
VIII	63.8/63.6	46.6/42.3	44.8/42.8	39.4/38.6	10.2/42.8	63.8/63.6
IX	88.9/88.9	49.6/52.4	62.9/62.9	49.1/53.3	11.4/45.8	88.9/88.9
X	68.8/75.9	55.9/57.6	55.2/52.5	58.9/58.2	35.1/44.5	68.8/75.9
XI	81/80.5	57.3/72.2	53.8/54.7	55.6/70	-	81/80.5

P2X$_7$	Mouse vs X (needle/water)					
	Rat	Human	Dog	Monkey	Zebrafish	Rat
Intron I	-	-	54.2/60.2	-	2.8/41.8	-
II	83.1/83.3	56.2/62.4	25.5/48.9	47.4/50.8	20.8/39.4	83.1/83.3
III	63.7/63.9	35.8/45.3	39/39.7	35.7/46.9	2.6/53.9	63.7/63.9
IV	54.7/54.7	41.6/41.6	32.2/42.6	45.6/42.2	14.1/36.6	54.7/54.7
V	40.7/41.4	35.2/35.9	42.9/42.9	34.2/35.1	23.4/36.9	40.7/41.4
VI	70.2/70.2	45.9/45.9	22.4/33.6	47.6/43.5	36.5/38.4	70.2/70.2
VII	68.7/69	46.6/46.6	38/38	49.4/46.2	30.8/39.4	68.7/69
VIII	59.2/59.2	20.2/40	27.3/44.9	28.5/44.4	1.3/46.2	59.2/59.2
IX	59/59	29.2/45.9	25/43.8	29.3/45.4	2.1/39.3	59/59
X	69/69	21.1/60.4	38.1/40.1	23.8/52.8	18.4/46.6	69/69
XI	50.8/53.5	43/40.8	40/40.1	37/34.9	28.9/34.5	50.8/53.5
XII	64.1/63.8	44.6/41.9	39.9/41.6	43.7/41.7	22.2/36.7	64.1/63.8

Table 4. Intron phase of P2X paralogous of mouse.

Intron #	Intron Phase (at the end of intron)						
	$musP2X_1$	$musP2X_2$	$musP2X_3$	$musP2X_4$	$musP2X_5$	$musP2X_6$	$musP2X_7$
1	2	2	2	2	2/0[a]	2	2
2	0	0	0	0	0	0	0
3	0	0	0	0	0	0	0
4	1	1	1	1	1	1	1
5	2	2	2	2	2	2	2
6	2	2	2	2	2	2	2
7	0	0	0	0	0	0	0
8	2	2	2	2	2	2	2
9	0	0	0	0	0	0	
10	0	0	0	0	0/2[b]	0	0/1[c]
11	0	0	0	0	2	0	0/1[c]
12					2		

[a]Phase zero only in $darP2X_5$. [b]Phase two only in $hsaP2X_5$ and $ptrP2X_5$. Phase 1 in $darP2X_7$.

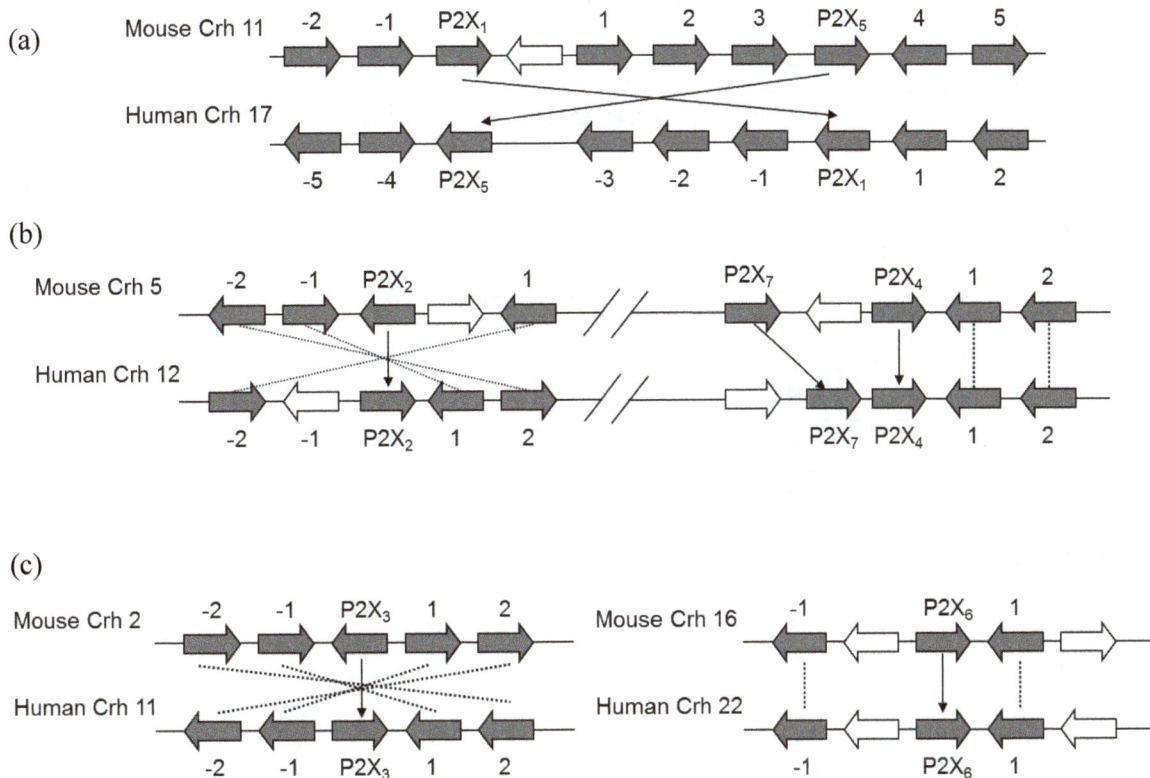

Figure 2. Microsynteny of P2X genes between mouse and human. The coding genes in chromosomes are depicted as filled arrows, while white filled arrows represent non-syntenic genes between mouse and human. The mouse was used as reference to catalog neighbor genes either upstream (negative numbers) or downstream (positive numbers) of the first P2X subunit found in the Watson DNA chain. Arrowhead lines represent the changes in P2X positions and dashed lines shows the changes in position of the neighbor genes. Gene Bank names for neighbor genes are shown in Supplementary **Table S1**. (a) Microsynteny of $P2X_1$ and $P2X_5$ genes. Schematic representation of the location of $P2X_1$ and $P2X_5$ in human and murine chromosomes respect to their chromosomic environment. Change in chromosome localization, sense of transcription and microsynteny of two genes for $P2X_1$ and five genes for $P2X_5$ can be observed; (b) Microsynteny of $P2X_2$, $P2X_4$ and $P2X_7$. Inversion of transcription sense and conservation of upstream genes -1 and -2 is shown, whereas genomic context is highly conserved for $P2X_4$ and $P2X_7$; (c) Microsynteny of $P2X_3$ and $P2X_6$. For $P2X_3$ inversion is observed in the whole chromosome context of the four neighbor genes. For $P2X_6$ genomic context is highly conserved for two genes on both sides.

nated in an independent duplication event explaining the lack of synteny in this gene.

We also analyzed the P2X orthologous intron phase to look for clues about the common ancestor of these genes as has been done elsewhere [45]. We found that intron phase is conserved in paralogous as well as in orthologous, with the zero phase as the most common, followed by phase two and phase one. Phase zero is the most common between mammalian orthologous and it's frequently found at the 3' region of a given gene [46]-[48]. Phase two is often referred as least common in gene arrangements; however P2X genes present this phase with a significant frequency. The implications of this phase conservation can be directly related to the allowance of functional variability. This is also correlated with the presence of phase zero in the conserved regions coding for transmembrane domains and C-terminus, which play significant roles in function and regulatory activity. Higher variability in exons coding for the extracellular domains could allow the evolution of regions affecting ligand affinity and gating.

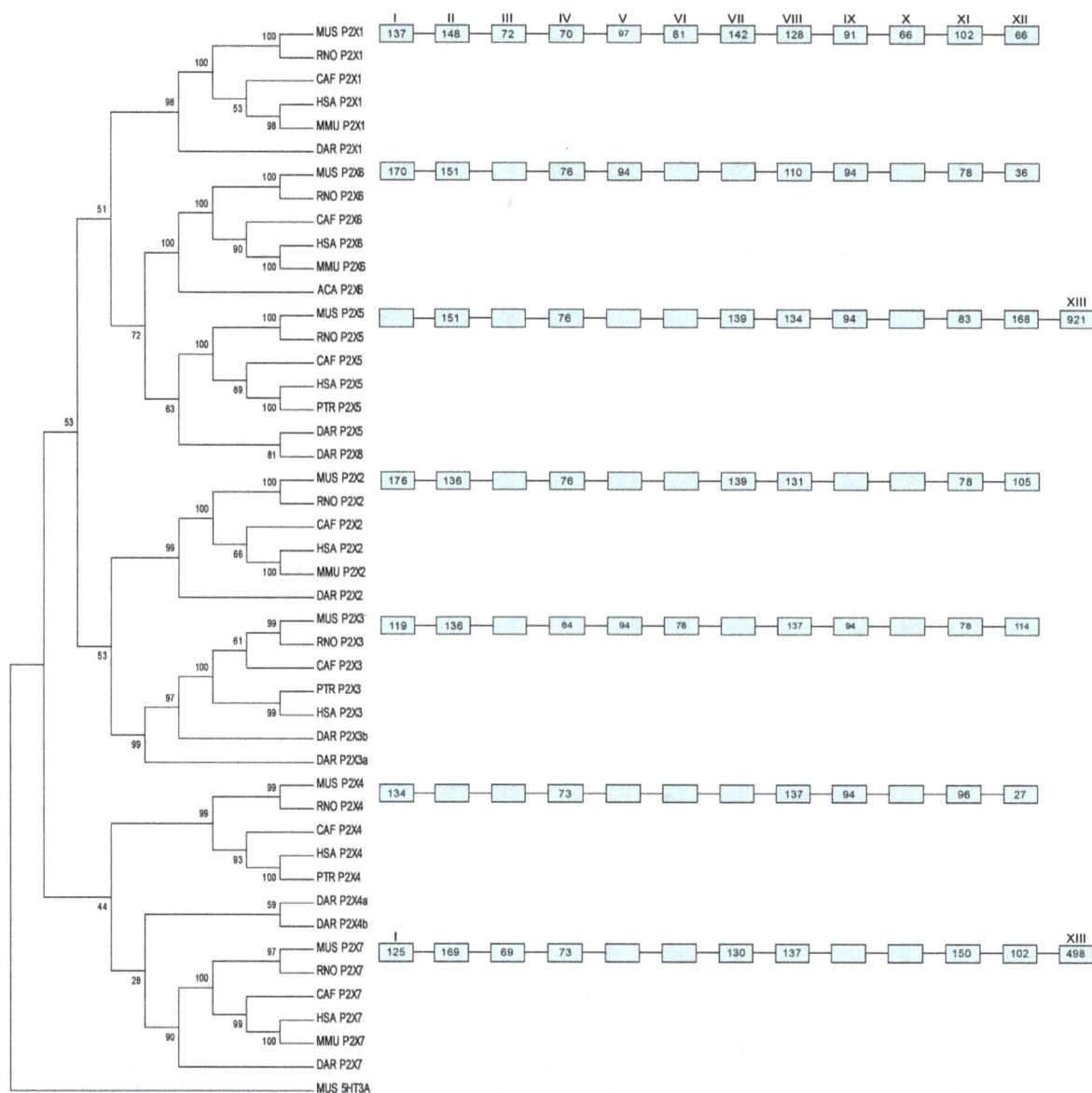

Figure 3. Phylogenetic tree representing P2X subunits from different organisms. Mus musculus (MUS), Rattusnorvegicus (RNO), Cannisfamiliaris (CAF), Homo sapiens (HSA), Macaccamulata (MMU), Danio rerio (DAR), Pan troglodytes (PTR). 5HT3 receptor from mouse was used as external gene to perform the alignment using the MEGA software version 4.0 with the maximum Parsimonia method (500 bootstrap). Numbers on the branches shows evolutionary distance represented as number of substitutions per residue. On the first branch of every clade the corresponding P2X subunit (1 to 7) gene is depicted.

In the next section, we describe particular characteristics of genomic organization for every P2X gene.

3.2.1. P2X$_1$

Mouse P2X$_1$ gene has a size of 16.05 Kb and mRNA of 1200 bp, which produces a protein of 399 aminoacids. The gen is organized in 12 exons and 11 introns. This organization is conserved among its mammals orthologous (rat, human, dog and primate) and differs with zebrafish organization, which has 13 exons and 12 introns (**Figure 1(b)**).

The size of P2X$_1$ exons is fully conserved in mammals, while conservations is sound only with exons III, VI, VII, IX and X of zebrafish (**Figure 1(b)**). An additional exon is present in darP2X$_1$ (exon XIII) with only 6 bp, from which only one aminoacid is coded together with the STOP codon.

P2X$_1$ introns are more divergent in size as well as in identity between the analyzed sequences. The first intron is the largest with >7400 bp in all the analyzed species. Using the Align algorithm (European Bioinformatics Institute) in its global (needle) and local (water) configuration we found identity values shown in **Table 3**. We showed that rat and mouse introns have the higher global identity (>66%) and intron IV has the highest unitary identity (87.6% in both needle/water modes). The zebrafish P2X$_1$ introns had the lower identity percentage (below 42.3% needle).

3.2.2. P2X$_2$

The P2X$_2$ gene of mouse is located in chromosome 5 and is characterized for being the shorter of mammal P2X genes (around 3 Kb, **Table 1**), mRNA without untranslated regions is 1248 bp long coding for a 416 aminoacid protein. P2X$_2$ gene was originally described by Brandle in 1997 with an organization of 11 exons and 10 introns, according to the NCBI reference P2X$_{2-1}$ (NM_053656). In previous work from our group we reported that P2X$_{2-2}$ isoform is actually the primary P2X$_2$ transcript and not the P2X$_{2-1}$ subunit as initially assumed. Based on this report we established the genomic arrangement of guinea pig P2X$_2$ as formed by 12 exons and 11 introns.

Since P2X$_{2-2}$ isoform is expressed in all mammals where splicing studies have been done (namely, mouse, rat and human), we have extrapolated the guinea pig model to the rest of species and confronted it with the genomic arrangement of zebrafish P2X$_2$ (**Figure 1(c)**). The addition of an exon in this 12 exon-11 intron arrangement is given by the separation of the last exon into two new exons (XI and XII) separated by an intron. To identify the donor and acceptor sites in this intron we use Net Gene2 algorithm (www.cbs.dtu.dk/services/NetGene2/) with all the analyzed P2X$_2$ gene sequences. In all genes we found a donor site with high confidence level at the beginning of the site where intron 11 is located. In the same way, we found an acceptor site in the same intron in human and guinea pig. For mouse and rat the site could be easily identified using the GT/AG rule. These sites support the existence of the intron 11 between exons XI and XII with a size of 91 or 206 bp, depending on the species (**Figure 1(c)**).

Phylogenetically, P2X$_2$ is closer to P2X$_3$ (**Figure 3**), which is reflected also in the conservation of the genomic arrangement of 12 exons and 11 introns between these paralogous. The same order is maintained among the orthologous of P2X$_2$, even with the more distant zebrafish (**Figure 1(c)**). With the exception of exons I, IX and XII, all exons conserve their size, including exon XI of 78 bp shared entirely by P2X$_3$ (**Figure 2**).

On its part, P2X$_2$ introns are less conserved and are characterized for their small size, however, introns size in zebrafish P2X$_2$ are variable, ranging from small (3, 5 and 9 of 81, 76 and 81 respectively) to large introns (intron 8 is 3027 bp). This contrasts with mammalian P2X$_2$ genes with no intron larger than 450 bp. In nucleotide sequence, the better conserved, both globally and locally regarding mouse is rat's introns 1 (89/90.3), intron 2 (92.9/94.8), intron 4 (90/92.3) and intron 11 (93.8/95.6). With the rest of orthologous the identity are equal or lower than 70%.

We have suggested that genomic organization of P2X$_2$ in mammals is composed of 12 exons and 11 introns, such as it's been displayed in Ensembl and fast DB databases. This model is based in the evidence that P2X$_{2-2}$ or P2X$_2$b is the only mammal homologous to zebrafish P2X$_2$, which have P2X duplications rather than reductions in gene number. Additionally we observed that P2X$_{2-2}$ genomic arrangement is conserved between mammalian orthologous and the distant zebrafish. In the same way, this isoform is more close to the paralogous P2X$_3$, indicating our proposed genomic organization has a better evolutionary meaning than the previously proposed model.

We also observed that mammalian P2X$_2$ size is smaller than zebrafish P2X$_2$, showing a large variation in intron size. This suggests that $P2X_2$ went over a shortening of introns that could have conferred a regulatory function in a similar way to some constitutive genes [22] [24]. All the intron phases are conserved in $P2X_2$ orthologous, suggesting that no major genomic re-arrangements have occurred. This is supported by functional evidence of our laboratory, where $P2X_2$ expression is sustained in myenteric neurons during embryonic development and to adulthood, implying the functionality of the subunit in a range of physiological events.

3.2.3. $P2X_3$

The murine $P2X_3$ receptor has a genomic size of 39.2 Kb and a mRNA of 1.4 Kb, coding for a 397 aminoacids protein. Its chromosomal localization is shown in **Table 1**. The genomic organization of $P2X_3$ is shown in Fig. 1D with an arrangement of 12 exons and 11 introns, which is conserved among orthologous.

The aminoacidic identities of $P2X_3$ between mouse and its orthologous were the highest of all P2X genes (higher than 93%). From the two $P2X_3$ genes in zebrafish, $darP2X_3b$ had the highest identity with mammalian $P2X_3$ (68% with Clustal W), while $darP2X_3a$ had 57% identity. When we compared $P2X_3a$ with $P2X_3b$, we found 58% of identity. These results are in agreement with the phylogenetic tree shown in **Figure 3**, where $darP2X_3b$ is closer to mammalian $P2X_3$ genes.

Figure 1(d) shows the high conservation between the mammalian orthologous, only some differences appear in exons I, IV, V and XII of zebrafish $P2X_3$ compared to mouse. Intron sequences between mouse and rat are highly identical; in intron 9 the conservation is 90.5/90.8% needle/water, intron 11 has a 74.6% needle identity, the same intron has up to 55.5% global identity compared to other mammals. As expected, the zebrafish has shorter and less conserved introns compared to other $P2X_3$ mammalian genes.

The evidence on $P2X_3$ suggests, together with other P2X subunits sequences, that zebrafish had a common ancestor with mammals. The divergence of these two lineages can be inferred with the accumulation of genetic material in mammal introns. In mammals, intron 8 has a larger size than zebrafish sequences. When we performed a PSI-BLAST analysis in this intron, we observed the presence of several elements similar to dSpmZea mays transposons, suggesting the increase in mammalian intronic sequences could be due to transposon insertion [37] [49] [50]. The phylogenetic analysis shows $darP2X_3a$ isoform diverging before the separation of mammalian clade (**Figure 3**), which leads us to propose that mammalian $P2X_3$ sequences are derived from $darP2X_3b$ found in the zebrafish ancestor.

3.2.4. $P2X_4$

Mouse $P2X_4$ receptor is located close to $P2X_7$ in chromosome 5, it has a 21.488 Kb size and mRNA of 1,995 bp, coding for a protein of 388 aminoacids (see **Table 1** and **Figure 2**). Analyzing genomic organization of $P2X_4$ (**Figure 1(e)**) we can see it's comprised of 12 exons and 11 introns. The phylogenetic tree shows it closer to $P2X_7$, however they do not share the same exon-intron arrangement. In zebrafish, $P2X_4$ paralogous (a and b) are kept in the same clade in the tree and have an identity of 57% between both proteins (**Figure 3**). Comparing $musP2X_4$ with the two zebrafish isoforms $darP2X_4a$ and $darP2X_4b$ using Clustal W, we encountered identities of 58% and 52% respectively (**Table 5**). Exon size is completely conserved among $P2X_4$ orthologous in mammals (**Figure 1(e)**). In zebrafish, the two $P2X_4$ genes conserve exon size compared to mouse; $darP2X_4a$ differs only in the first and last exon, whilst $darP2X_4b$ differs in the last two.

The size of introns is variable among $P2X_4$ orthologous; with sizes ranging from 99bp to 8 Kb. Introns 1 and 5 are the largest while intron 7 and 9 are the smallest. Comparing intron identity between orthologous we found the highest identities again between mouse and rat, particularly in introns 3, 4, 9 and 11, with 71/71%, 69/70%, 72/72% and 77/77% needle/water identity respectively (**Table 3**).

We observed that even when $darP2X_4a$ has a higher global identity with their orthologous than $darP2X_4b$, synteny occurs with $P2X_4b$ and $P2X_7$ suggesting that $P2X_4b$ was prior to genome duplication events that happened in zebrafish after mammalian divergence and therefore, originated the mammalian $P2X_4$ genes.

3.2.5. $P2X_5$

In mouse, $P2X_5$ receptor is located in chromosome 11 and has a size of 12.16 Kb with a mRNA of 2.293 Kb after the editing of their 13 exons and 12 introns. The $P2X_5$ subunit has 455 aminoacids. The genomic organization of mouse $P2X_5$ is quite unique, since it is conserved with the rat, but it's different to the other mammals analyzed, which present an organization of 12 exons and 11 introns.

Looking the phylogenetic tree on **Figure 2**, we can see that $darP2X_8$ is grouped in the same clade than $P2X_5$,

Table 5. Percent identity of mouse P2X orthologous genes (clustal W).

P2X$_1$	MUS	RNO	HSA	MMU	CAF	DAR	
MUS	***	97.5	89.5	90	89.2	55.2	
RNO		***	89	89.5	88.5	54.9	
HSA		12	***	97.5	90.7	54.4	
MMU				***	90.7	54.9	
CAF					***	56.2	
DAR						***	

P2X$_2$	MUS	RNO	HSA	MMU	CAF	DAR	
MUS	***	97.5	89.5	90	89.2	55.2	
RNO		***	89	89.5	88.5	54.9	
HSA		12	***	97.5	90.7	54.4	
MMU				***	90.7	54.9	
CAF					***	56.2	
DAR						***	

P2X$_3$	MUS	RNO	HSA	PTR	CAF	DARa	DARb
MUS	***	99	93.7	94	94.5	57.5	68
RNO		***	93.7	94	94.5	57.2	68
HSA			***	99.7	94.7	58	68.3
PTR				***	95	58	68.3
CAF					***	57.2	67.8
DARa						***	58.2
DARb							***

P2X$_4$	MUS	RNO	HSA	PTR	CAF	DARa	DARb
MUS	***	94.6	87.4	87.4	86.1	57.8	51.7
RNO		***	87.1	87.1	85.3	59.3	51.9
HSA			***	100	89.9	58.3	53.2
PTR				***	89.9	58.3	53.2
CAF					***	56.5	52.2
DARa						***	57.1
DARb							***

P2X$_5$	MUS	RNO	HSA	PTR	CAF	DAR	darP2X8
MUS	***	94.7	69.2	69	70	50.2	43.5
RNO		***	69	68.8	70.2	49.6	44
HSA			***	99.5	76.8	48.9	44
PTR				***	77	48.9	44
CAF					***	53	46.2
DAR						***	51

P2X$_6$	MUS	RNO	HSA	MMU	CAF	DAR	
MUS	***	94.7	69.2	69	70	60.2	
RNO		***	69	68.8	70.2	60.2	
HSA			***	99.5	76.8	58.5	
MMU				***	77	58	
CAF					***	59.6	
DAR						***	

P2X$_7$	MUS	RNO	HSA	MMU	CAF	DAR	
MUS	***	85	80.8	80.5	76.6	45.2	
RNO		***	80.3	80.2	76.4	44.5	
HSA			***	97.1	86.2	46.2	
MMU				***	85.5	46.2	
CAF					***	46.4	
DAR						***	

suggesting an evolutionary relationship between these two sequences. The gene darP2X$_8$ has 44% identity with musP2X$_5$, which is the same identity of darP2X$_5$. On the other hand the tree shows P2X$_5$ close to P2X$_6$ but their genomic organization is not conserved.

There is conservation in exon size between mammalian P2X$_5$ genes, overall among exons I to V (**Figure 1(g)**). With zebrafish orthologous P2X$_5$ and P2X$_8$ the size of exons is more variable. Intron sequence is the most similar between rat and mice with introns 3, 9 and 11, which have global identities superior to 70%.

As shown in **Figure 1(g)**, introns 2, 7, 8 and 11 are longer in zebrafish than in the other organisms analyzed, thus is probable that loss of genetic material could give some advantage in P2X$_5$ expression in mammals [51] [52].

The receptor darP2X$_8$ is grouped with P2X$_5$ in the phylogenetic tree; therefore we compared the nucleotide sequence and observed certain similarity between them. For example, the highest identity of 66.3% occurred for Exon VI (needle, data not shown). This is evidence of distant divergence between P2X$_5$ and P2X$_8$. However this is the only case where zebrafish has the same intron phase than the mammalian P2X$_5$ genes. This is additional evidence to the previously suggested evolutionary relationship between P2X$_5$ and P2X$_8$ in chicken (Gallus gallus) [53].

3.2.6. P2X$_6$

The murine P2X$_6$ gene has a size of 10.13 Kb and a mRNA of 1170 bp, generating a product of 389 aminoacids. The P2X$_6$ is organized in 12 exons and 11 introns; this organization is conserved among mammalian orthologous. Since zebrafish seems to lack P2X$_6$, we choose a reptile (*Anolis carolinensis*) as a possible distant species to compare gene sequences. In the case of *A. carolinensis* P2X$_6$ gene (acaP2X$_6$), its organization has 11 exons and 10 introns (**Figure 1(g)**).

Comparing exon size of mouse P2X$_6$ with its orthologous we observed that is conserved in all the mammalian species, with the exception of the first and last exons, as with other P2X analyzed. However, exon V of acaP2X$_6$ is 175 bp long, which is equivalent to the sum of the individual size of exons V (94 bp) and VI (81 bp) from mouse P2X$_6$. Reptilian exons from VI to X conserve the size with exons VII to XI of musP2X$_6$, respectively.

Introns present the higher divergence in size and identity among the analyzed sequences. Introns 2, 3 and 8 are the largest (more than 1200 bp) in mammals; while in reptile intron 1 had the larger size with 1060 bp (**Figure 1(g)**). Comparing intron sequence of mouse P2X$_6$ against its orthologs, as observed in **Table 3**, we found that rat and mouse have the highest identity (above 63%), with intron 9 the highest in score (88.9/88.9% needle/water). Introns from reptile P2X$_6$ had the lower identity percentage (below 50.5%).

Our analysis of P2X$_6$ sequences between mammals and reptile suggest that P2X genes were present in a common ancestor. We encountered the accumulation of genetic material in the case of some mammalian P2X$_6$ introns, including the presence of an intron between exons V and VI of mammals that is not observed in reptile. Mammalian exons V and VI match exactly in size with reptilian exon V, with identities of 60.8 and 73.2% respectively when aligned locally (data not shown). This explains the presence of only 11 exons in the reptile compared to the 12 exons in mammalian P2X$_6$. The presence of the same genetic structure in all of mammalians points that the intron present between exons V and VI was acquired more recently after reptilian and mammalian divergence through insertion. It has been proposed recently that the increased number of introns in an organism is related to less efficient expression. The insertion of this intron can contribute, along with other multiple regulatory mechanisms, to the in vivo behavior of P2X$_6$ receptors.

3.2.7. P2X$_7$

The murine gene coding for P2X$_7$ is the largest of the P2X family. In mice it has 37.2 Kb with a transcript of 1785 bp, giving a protein of 595 aminoacids. The gene organization of P2X$_7$ consists of 13 exons and 12 introns in mammalians and 14 exons and 13 introns in zebrafish (dar P2X$_7$, **Figure 1(h)**). This genomic organization is different to what is seen for other P2X genes (**Figure 1(a)**).

The P2X$_7$ subunit is notable for its longer C-terminus, with 230 aminoacids for mouse, compared to the shorter C-terminus of musP2X$_6$ with only 25 aminoacids and musP2X$_5$ with 94 aminoacids (second largest). Protein size is identical in the five mammalian species (**Table 1**), which is also reflected in the high conservation of the exon size. The only differences we found were in exons VII and XII of dog (**Figure 1(h)**).

The introns of P2X$_7$ are in general long, overall intron 1 which has more than 21000 bp in both human and mouse, contrasting with intron 10 with 84 to 245 bp. Intron 2 is very well conserved among species, with identities as high as 83% local/global between rat and mouse. Intron phase is conserved among mammalian species, however, darP2X$_7$ (fish) have a shift in phases due to an insertion of an intron in exon II. Also the last three introns of the zebrafish uses phase one instead the phase zero of mammals.

The main difference between the P2X$_7$ of mammalians is their large size compared to the one of zebrafish (**Table 1**). Also exon-intron organization of the zebrafish is different to the mammalian genes, since it consists of a large intron of 7012 bp with a translated sequence corresponding to the reverse transcriptase of a retrotrasposon (Accession No.: XP_694080). This evidence suggests the insertion of the intronic sequence in exon 2 after the divergence of mammalian and fish lineages, generating the new exons II and III in darP2X$_7$ only. This suggests an evolutionary story where several insertions occurred in the lineage of zebrafish, elongating the introns of P2X$_7$ and conserved until know possibly to an advantage in expression regulation.

4. Concluding Remarks

The evolutionary origin of P2X receptors is still unclear; however, ancestral organisms diverging as far as 1 billion years ago have a single P2X receptor that has pharmacological and biophysical properties that resemble those of the seven P2X subunits in vertebrates [14] [17] [18] [54] [55]. As we have shown in this work, there is a high conservation of the gene structure among P2X receptors in the different organisms analyzed, even in the distant species of fish and reptile. This is additional evidence pairs with previous reports proposing that a single gene in a common ancestor very recently originates the current diversity of P2X subunits in vertebrates [14] [17]. After vertebrate divergence, P2X genes underwent duplications, gain of intron sequences and exon rearrangements that give the seven genes coding for P2X subunits a complexity underlying an important portion of the purinergic signaling in mammals.

Our phylogenic tree shows P2X$_4$ and P2X$_7$ as members of a more related clade. This is in agreement with previous hypothesis suggesting their origin from gene duplication [56]. Their joint evolution can be driven by the selective pressure generated by their functional role in the central nervous system, where these two subunits are mainly responsible for the activation of the inflammasome after injury [57]. In a similar way, the localization of P2X$_2$ and P2X3 in a clade with a recent common ancestor correlates with their high rate of appearance as heteromers in sensory neurons [9]. More importantly, an increasing amount of works have proven that P2X represents important therapeutic targets in pathologies as important as chronic pain in cancer and inflammation [58] [59]. With only few selective antagonists available [19], new strategies such as gene therapy can be the more effective choice when it comes to selectively regulate heteromeric P2X activation in cells [60]. In this work we provide a comprehensive depiction of the genomic organization of P2X receptors in the major model species of mammals. We expect our results will help to better understand phenomena at the transcription level such as splicing variants of P2X receptors and also to provide easy to access reference about the differences of P2X subunits at the nucleotide level, thus allowing to better design future strategies in basic science and therapeutics of P2X physiology.

Acknowledgements

This work is funded by the National Council of Science and Technology in Mexico (CONACYT). We thank Dr. Yair Cárdenas-Conejo for his valuable inputs and comments to this work.

References

[1] North, R.A. (2002) Molecular physiology of P2X receptors. *Physiological Reviews*, **82** 1013-1067. http://dx.doi.org/10.1152/physrev.00015.2002

[2] Cockayne, D.A., Dunn, P.M., Zhong, Y., Rong, W., Hamilton, S.G., Knight, G.E., Ruan, H.Z., Ma, B., Yip, P., Nunn, P., McMahon, S.B., Burnstock, G. and Ford, A.P. (2005) P2X$_2$ Knockout Mice and P2X$_2$/P2X$_3$ Double Knockout Mice Reveal a Role for the P2X$_2$ Receptor Subunit in Mediating Multiple Sensory Effects of ATP. *The Journal of Physiology*, **567**, 621-639. http://dx.doi.org/10.1113/jphysiol.2005.088435

[3] Burnstock, G. (2007) Physiology and Pathophysiology of Purinergic Neurotransmission. *Physiological Reviews*, **87**, 659-797. http://dx.doi.org/10.1152/physrev.00043.2006

[4] Coutinho-Silva, R., Knight, G.E. and Burnstock, G. (2005) Impairment of the Splenic Immune System in P2X$_2$/P2X$_3$ Knockout Mice. *Immunobiology*, **209**, 661-668. http://dx.doi.org/10.1016/j.imbio.2004.09.007

[5] Huang, L.C., Greenwood, D., Thorne, P.R. and Housley, G.D. (2005) Developmental Regulation of Neuron-Specific P2X$_3$ Receptor Expression in the Rat Cochlea. *Journal of Comparative Neurology*, **484**, 133-143.

http://dx.doi.org/10.1002/cne.20442

[6]   Torres, G.E., Egan, T.M. and Voigt, M.M. (1999) Hetero-Oligomeric Assembly of P2X Receptor Subunits. Specificities Exist with Regard to Possible Partners. *The Journal of Biological Chemistry*, **274**, 6653-6659.
        http://dx.doi.org/10.1074/jbc.274.10.6653

[7]   Valera, S., Hussy, N., Evans, R.J., Adami, N., North, R.A., Surprenant, A. and Buell, G. (1994) A New Class of Ligand-Gated Ion Channel Defined by P2X Receptor for Extracellular ATP. *Nature*, **371**, 516-519.
        http://dx.doi.org/10.1038/371516a0

[8]   Surprenant, A., Buell, G. and North, R.A. (1995) P_{2X} Receptors Bring New Structure to Ligand-Gated Ion Channels. *Trends in Neurosciences*, **18**, 224-229. http://dx.doi.org/10.1016/0166-2236(95)93907-F

[9]   Xiang, Z. and Burnstock, G. (2004) $P2X_2$ and $P2X_3$ Purinoceptors in the Rat Enteric Nervous System. *Histochemistry and Cell Biology*, **121**, 169-179. http://dx.doi.org/10.1007/s00418-004-0620-1

[10]   Chen, C.C., Akopian, A.N., Sivilotti, L., Colquhoun, D., Burnstock, G. and Wood, J.N. (1995) A P2X Purinoceptor Expressed by a Subset of Sensory Neurons. *Nature*, **377**, 428-431. http://dx.doi.org/10.1038/377428a0

[11]   Garcia-Guzman, M., Stuhmer, W. and Soto, F. (1997) Molecular Characterization and Pharmacological Properties of the Human $P2X_3$ Purinoceptor. *Molecular Brain Research*, **47**, 59-66.
        http://dx.doi.org/10.1016/S0169-328X(97)00036-3

[12]   Ren, J., Bian, X., DeVries, M., Schnegelsberg, B., Cockayne, D.A., Ford, A.P. and Galligan, J.J. (2003) $P2X_2$ Subunits Contribute to Fast Synaptic Excitation in Myenteric Neurons of the Mouse Small Intestine. *The Journal of Physiology*, **552**, 809-821. http://dx.doi.org/10.1113/jphysiol.2003.047944

[13]   Ruan, H.Z. and Burnstock, G. (2005) The Distribution of $P2X_5$ Purinergic Receptors in the Enteric Nervous System of Mouse. *Cell and Tissue Research*, **319**, 191-200. http://dx.doi.org/10.1007/s00441-004-1002-7

[14]   Fountain, S.J. and Burnstock, G. (2009) An Evolutionary History of P2X Receptors. *Purinergic Signalling*, **5**, 269-272.
        http://dx.doi.org/10.1007/s11302-008-9127-x

[15]   Burnstock, G. and Verkhratsky, A. (2009) Evolutionary Origins of the Purinergic Signalling System. *Acta Physiologica*, **195**, 415-447. http://dx.doi.org/10.1111/j.1748-1716.2009.01957.x

[16]   Trams, E.G. (1981) On the Evolution of Neurochemical Transmission. *Differentiation*, **19**, 125-133.
        http://dx.doi.org/10.1111/j.1432-0436.1981.tb01140.x

[17]   Bavan, S., Straub, V.A., Blaxter, M.L. and Ennion, S.J. (2009) A P2X Receptor from the Tardigrade Species *Hypsibius dujardini* with Fast Kinetics and Sensitivity to Zinc and Copper. *BMC Evolutionary Biology*, **9**, 17.
        http://dx.doi.org/10.1186/1471-2148-9-17

[18]   Agboh, K.C., Webb, T.E., Evans, R.J. and Ennion, S.J. (2004) Functional Characterization of a P2X Receptor from *Schistosoma mansoni. The Journal of Biological Chemistry*, **279**, 41650-41657.
        http://dx.doi.org/10.1074/jbc.M408203200

[19]   Muller, C.E. (2015) Medicinal Chemistry of P2X Receptors: Allosteric Modulators. *Current Medicinal Chemistry*, **22**, 929-941. http://dx.doi.org/10.2174/0929867322666141210155610

[20]   Rodriguez-Kessler, M., Delgado-Sanchez, P., Rodriguez-Kessler, G.T., Moriguchi, T. and Jimenez-Bremont, J.F. (2010) Genomic Organization of Plant Aminopropyl Transferases. *Plant Physiology and Biochemistry*, **48**, 574-590.
        http://dx.doi.org/10.1016/j.plaphy.2010.03.004

[21]   Li, M., Chang, T.H., Silberberg, S.D. and Swartz, K.J. (2008) Gating the Pore of P2X Receptor Channels. *Nature Neuroscience*, **11**, 883-887. http://dx.doi.org/10.1038/nn.2151

[22]   Castillo-Davis, C.I., Mekhedov, S.L., Hartl, D.L., Koonin, E.V. and Kondrashov, F.A. (2002) Selection for Short Introns in Highly Expressed Genes. *Nature Genetics*, **31**, 415-418. http://dx.doi.org/10.1038/ng940

[23]   Eisenberg, E. and Levanon, E.Y. (2003) Human Housekeeping Genes Are Compact. *Trends in Genetics*, **19**, 362-365.
        http://dx.doi.org/10.1016/S0168-9525(03)00140-9

[24]   Rao, Y.S., Wang, Z.F., Chai, X.W., Wu, G.Z., Zhou, M., Nie, Q.H. and Zhang, X.Q. (2010) Selection for the Compactness of Highly Expressed Genes in *Gallus gallus. Biology Direct*, **5**, 35.
        http://dx.doi.org/10.1186/1745-6150-5-35

[25]   Linan-Rico, A., Jaramillo-Polanco, J., Espinosa-Luna, R., Jimenez-Bremont, J.F., Linan-Rico, L., Montano, L.M. and Barajas-Lopez, C. (2012) Retention of a New-Defined Intron Changes Pharmacology and Kinetics of the Full-Length $P2X_2$ Receptor Found in Myenteric Neurons of the Guinea Pig. *Neuropharmacology*, **63**, 394-404.
        http://dx.doi.org/10.1016/j.neuropharm.2012.04.002

[26]   Brosenitsch, T.A., Adachi, T., Lipski, J., Housley, G.D. and Funk, G.D. (2005) Developmental Downregulation of $P2X_3$ Receptors in Motoneurons of the Compact Formation of the Nucleus Ambiguus. *European Journal of Neuroscience*, **22**, 809-824. http://dx.doi.org/10.1111/j.1460-9568.2005.04261.x

[27] Ruan, H.Z., Moules, E. and Burnstock, G. (2004) Changes in P2X$_3$ Purinoceptors in Sensory Ganglia of the Mouse during Embryonic and Postnatal Development. *Histochemistry and Cell Biology*, **122**, 539-551. http://dx.doi.org/10.1007/s00418-004-0714-9

[28] Xiang, Z. and Burnstock, G. (2004) Development of Nerves Expressing P2X$_3$ Receptors in the Myenteric Plexus of Rat Stomach. *Histochemistry and Cell Biology*, **122**, 111-119. http://dx.doi.org/10.1007/s00418-004-0680-2

[29] Loera-Valencia, R., Jimenez-Vargas, N.N., Villalobos, E.C., Juarez, E.H., Lomas-Ramos, T.L., Espinosa-Luna, R., Montano, L.M., Huizinga, J.D. and Barajas-Lopez, C. (2014) Expression of P2X$_3$ and P2X$_5$ Myenteric Receptors Varies during the Intestinal Postnatal Development in the Guinea Pig. *Cellular and Molecular Neurobiology*, **34**, 727-736. http://dx.doi.org/10.1007/s10571-014-0055-8

[30] Majewski, J. and Ott, J. (2002) Distribution and Characterization of Regulatory Elements in the Human Genome. *Genome Research*, **12**, 1827-1836. http://dx.doi.org/10.1101/gr.606402

[31] Kalari, K.R., Casavant, M., Bair, T.B., Keen, H.L., Comeron, J.M., Casavant, T.L. and Scheetz, T.E. (2006) First Exons and Introns—A Survey of GC Content and Gene Structure in the Human Genome. *In Silico Biology*, **6**, 237-242.

[32] Zhu, L., Zhang, Y., Zhang, W., Yang, S., Chen, J.Q. and Tian, D. (2009) Patterns of Exon-Intron Architecture Variation of Genes in Eukaryotic Genomes. *BMC Genomics*, **10**, 47. http://dx.doi.org/10.1186/1471-2164-10-47

[33] Egan, T.M., Cox, J.A. and Voigt, M.M. (2000) Molecular Cloning and Functional Characterization of the Zebrafish ATP-Gated Ionotropic Receptor P2X$_3$ Subunit. *FEBS Letters*, **475**, 287-290. http://dx.doi.org/10.1016/S0014-5793(00)01685-9

[34] Diaz-Hernandez, M., Cox, J.A., Migita, K., Haines, W., Egan, T.M. and Voigt, M.M. (2002) Cloning and Characterization of Two Novel Zebrafish P2X Receptor Subunits. *Biochemical and Biophysical Research Communications*, **295**, 849-853. http://dx.doi.org/10.1016/S0006-291X(02)00760-X

[35] Kucenas, S., Li, Z., Cox, J.A., Egan, T.M. and Voigt, M.M. (2003) Molecular Characterization of the Zebrafish P2X Receptor Subunit Gene Family. *Neuroscience*, **121**, 935-945. http://dx.doi.org/10.1016/S0306-4522(03)00566-9

[36] Babenko, V.N., Rogozin, I.B., Mekhedov, S.L. and Koonin, E.V. (2004) Prevalence of Intron Gain Over Intron Loss in the Evolution of Paralogous Gene Families. *Nucleic Acids Research*, **32**, 3724-3733. http://dx.doi.org/10.1093/nar/gkh686

[37] Carmel, L., Rogozin, I.B., Wolf, Y.I. and Koonin, E.V. (2007) Patterns of Intron Gain and Conservation in Eukaryotic Genes. *BMC Evolutionary Biology*, **7**, 192. http://dx.doi.org/10.1186/1471-2148-7-192

[38] Rogozin, I.B., Wolf, Y.I., Sorokin, A.V., Mirkin, B.G. and Koonin, E.V. (2003) Remarkable Interkingdom Conservation of Intron Positions and Massive, Lineage-Specific Intron Loss and Gain in Eukaryotic Evolution. *Current Biology*, **13**, 1512-1517. http://dx.doi.org/10.1016/S0960-9822(03)00558-X

[39] Okamura, Y., Nishino, A., Murata, Y., Nakajo, K., Iwasaki, H., Ohtsuka, Y., Tanaka-Kunishima, M., Takahashi, N., Hara, Y., Yoshida, T., Nishida, M., Okado, H., Watari, H., Meinertzhagen, I.A., Satoh, N., Takahashi, K., Satou, Y., Okada, Y. and Mori, Y. (2005) Comprehensive Analysis of the Ascidian Genome Reveals Novel Insights into the Molecular Evolution of Ion Channel Genes. *Physiological Genomics*, **22**, 269-282. http://dx.doi.org/10.1152/physiolgenomics.00229.2004

[40] Amores, A., Force, A., Yan, Y.L., Joly, L., Amemiya, C., Fritz, A., Ho, R.K., Langeland, J., Prince, V., Wang, Y.L., Westerfield, M., Ekker, M. and Postlethwait, J.H. (1998) Zebrafish Hox Clusters and Vertebrate Genome Evolution. *Science*, **282**, 1711-1714. http://dx.doi.org/10.1126/science.282.5394.1711

[41] Postlethwait, J.H., Yan, Y.L., Gates, M.A., Horne, S., Amores, A., Brownlie, A., Donovan, A., Egan, E.S., Force, A., Gong, Z., Goutel, C., Fritz, A., Kelsh, R., Knapik, E., Liao, E., Paw, B., Ransom, D., Singer, A., Thomson, M., Abduljabbar, T.S., Yelick, P., Beier, D., Joly, J.S., Larhammar, D., Rosa, F., Westerfield, M., Zon, L.I., Johnson, S.L. and Talbot, W.S. (1998) Vertebrate Genome Evolution and the Zebrafish Gene Map. *Nature Genetics*, **18**, 345-349. http://dx.doi.org/10.1038/ng0498-345

[42] Woods, I.G., Kelly, P.D., Chu, F., Ngo-Hazelett, P., Yan, Y.L., Huang, H., Postlethwait, J.H. and Talbot, W.S. (2000) A Comparative Map of the Zebrafish Genome. *Genome Research*, **10**, 1903-1914. http://dx.doi.org/10.1101/gr.10.12.1903

[43] Taylor, J.S., Braasch, I., Frickey, T., Meyer, A. and Van de Peer, Y. (2003) Genome Duplication, a Trait Shared by 22000 Species of Ray-Finned Fish. *Genome Research*, **13**, 382-390. http://dx.doi.org/10.1101/gr.640303

[44] Woods, I.G., Wilson, C., Friedlander, B., Chang, P., Reyes, D.K., Nix, R., Kelly, P.D., Chu, F., Postlethwait, J.H. and Talbot, W.S. (2005) The Zebrafish Gene Map Defines Ancestral Vertebrate Chromosomes. *Genome Research*, **15**, 1307-1314. http://dx.doi.org/10.1101/gr.4134305

[45] Ruvinsky, A. and Watson, C. (2007) Intron Phase Patterns in Genes: Preservation and Evolutionary Changes. *The Open Evolution Journal*, **1**, 1-14. http://dx.doi.org/10.2174/1874404400701010001

[46] Fedorov, A., Suboch, G., Bujakov, M. and Fedorova, L. (1992) Analysis of Nonuniformity in Intron Phase Distribution.

Nucleic Acids Research, **20**, 2553-2557. http://dx.doi.org/10.1093/nar/20.10.2553

[47] Artamonova, I.I. and Gelfand, M.S. (2007) Comparative Genomics and Evolution of Alternative Splicing: The Pessimists' Science. *Chemical Reviews*, **107**, 3407-3430. http://dx.doi.org/10.1021/cr068304c

[48] Ruvinsky, A. and Ward, W. (2006) A Gradient in the Distribution of Introns in Eukaryotic Genes. *Journal of Molecular Evolution*, **63**, 136-141. http://dx.doi.org/10.1007/s00239-005-0261-6

[49] Fedorov, A., Roy, S., Fedorova, L. and Gilbert, W. (2003) Mystery of Intron Gain. *Genome Research*, **13**, 2236-2241. http://dx.doi.org/10.1101/gr.1029803

[50] Roy, S.W. (2004) The Origin of Recent Introns: Transposons? Genome Biology, **5**, 251. http://dx.doi.org/10.1186/gb-2004-5-12-251

[51] Ogino, K., Tsuneki, K. and Furuya, H. (2010) Unique Genome of Dicyemid Mesozoan: Highly Shortened Spliceosomal Introns in Conservative Exon/Intron Structure. *Gene*, **449**, 70-76. http://dx.doi.org/10.1016/j.gene.2009.09.002

[52] Collins, L. and Penny, D. (2006) Investigating the Intron Recognition Mechanism in Eukaryotes. *Molecular Biology and Evolution*, **23**, 901-910. http://dx.doi.org/10.1093/molbev/msj084

[53] Bo, X., Schoepfer, R. and Burnstock, G. (2000) Molecular Cloning and Characterization of a Novel ATP P2X Receptor Subtype from Embryonic Chick Skeletal Muscle. *The Journal of Biological Chemistry*, **275**, 14401-14407. http://dx.doi.org/10.1074/jbc.275.19.14401

[54] Fountain, S.J., Cao, L., Young, M.T. and North, R.A. (2008) Permeation Properties of a P2X Receptor in the Green Algae *Ostreococcus tauri*. *The Journal of Biological Chemistry*, **283**, 15122-15126. http://dx.doi.org/10.1074/jbc.M801512200

[55] Fountain, S.J., Parkinson, K., Young, M.T., Cao, L., Thompson, C.R. and North, R.A. (2007) An Intracellular P2X Receptor Required for Osmoregulation in *Dictyostelium discoideum*. *Nature*, **448**, 200-203. http://dx.doi.org/10.1038/nature05926

[56] Dubyak, G.R. (2007) Go It Alone No More—$P2X_7$ Joins the Society of Heteromeric ATP-Gated Receptor Channels. *Molecular Pharmacology*, **72**, 1402-1405. http://dx.doi.org/10.1124/mol.107.042077

[57] Bernier, L.P. (2012) Purinergic Regulation of Inflammasome Activation after Central Nervous System Injury. *The Journal of General Physiology*, **140**, 571-575. http://dx.doi.org/10.1085/jgp.201210875

[58] Kaan, T.K., Yip, P.K., Patel, S., Davies, M., Marchand, F., Cockayne, D.A., Nunn, P.A., Dickenson, A.H., Ford, A.P., Zhong, Y., Malcangio, M. and McMahon, S.B. (2010) Systemic Blockade of $P2X_3$ and $P2X_{2/3}$ Receptors Attenuates Bone Cancer Pain Behaviour in Rats. *Brain*, **133**, 2549-2564. http://dx.doi.org/10.1093/brain/awq194

[59] Sperlagh, B. and Illes, P. (2014) $P2X_7$ Receptor: An Emerging Target in Central Nervous System Diseases. *Trends in Pharmacological Sciences*, **35**, 537-547. http://dx.doi.org/10.1016/j.tips.2014.08.002

[60] Tsuchihara, T., Ogata, S., Nemoto, K., Okabayashi, T., Nakanishi, K., Kato, N., Morishita, R., Kaneda, Y., Uenoyama, M., Suzuki, S., Amako, M., Kawai, T. and Arino, H. (2009) Nonviral Retrograde Gene Transfer of Human Hepatocyte Growth Factor Improves Neuropathic Pain-Related Phenomena in Rats. *Molecular Therapy*, **17**, 42-50. http://dx.doi.org/10.1038/mt.2008.214

Supplementary

Table S1. Microsynteny of P2X subunit genes between mouse and human.

Mouse				Human	
	-2 Zzef1	zinc finger, ZZ-type with EF hand domain 1		Zzef1	2
	-1 Atp2a3	ATPase, Ca++ transporting, ubiquitous		Atp2a3	1
p2x1	P2rx1	purinergic receptor P2X, ligand-gated ion channel, 1		P2rx1	
	1 Camkk1	calcium/calmodulin-dependent protein kinase kinase 1, alpha		Camkk1	-1
	><			><	
	2 Itgae	integrin alpha E, epithelial-associated		Itgae	-2
p2x5	P2rx5	purinergic receptor P2X, ligand-gated ion channel, 5		P2rx5	
	4 Tmem93	transmembrane protein 93		Tmem93	-4
	5 Tax1bp3	Tax1 (human T-cell leukemia virus type I) binding protein 3		Tax1bp3	-5
	-2 Pxmp2	peroxisomal membrane protein 2		Pxmp2	2
	-1 Pole	polymerase (DNA directed), epsilon		Pole	1
p2x2	P2rx2	purinergic receptor P2X, ligand-gated ion channel, 2		P2rx2	
	><			><	
	1 Fbrsl1	fibrosin-like 1		Fbrsl1	-1
//					
	><			><	
p2x7	P2rx7	purinergic receptor P2X, ligand-gated ion channel, 7		P2rx7	
	><			><	
p2x4	P2rx4	purinergic receptor P2X, ligand-gated ion channel, 4		P2rx4	
	1 Camkk2	calcium/calmodulin-dependent protein kinase kinase 2, beta		Camkk2	1
	2 Anapc5	anaphase-promoting complex subunit 5		Anapc5	2
	-2 Prg2	proteoglycan 2, bone marrow		Prg2	2
	-1 Prg3	proteoglycan 3		Prg3	1
p2x3	P2rx3	purinergic receptor P2X, ligand-gated ion channel, 3		P2rx3	
	1 Ssrp1	structure specific recognition protein 1		Ssrp1	-1
	2 Tnks1bp1	tankyrase 1 binding protein 1		Tnks1bp1	-2
	-1 Thap7	THAP domain containing 7		Thap7	-1
	><			><	
p2x6	P2rx6	purinergic receptor P2X, ligand-gated ion channel, 1		P2rx6	
	1 Slc7a4	solute carrier family 7 (cationic amino acid transporter, y+ system), member 4		Slc7a4	1
	><			><	

Permissions

All chapters in this book were first published in PP, by Scientific Research Publishing; hereby published with permission under the Creative Commons Attribution License or equivalent. Every chapter published in this book has been scrutinized by our experts. Their significance has been extensively debated. The topics covered herein carry significant findings which will fuel the growth of the discipline. They may even be implemented as practical applications or may be referred to as a beginning point for another development.

The contributors of this book come from diverse backgrounds, making this book a truly international effort. This book will bring forth new frontiers with its revolutionizing research information and detailed analysis of the nascent developments around the world.

We would like to thank all the contributing authors for lending their expertise to make the book truly unique. They have played a crucial role in the development of this book. Without their invaluable contributions this book wouldn't have been possible. They have made vital efforts to compile up to date information on the varied aspects of this subject to make this book a valuable addition to the collection of many professionals and students.

This book was conceptualized with the vision of imparting up-to-date information and advanced data in this field. To ensure the same, a matchless editorial board was set up. Every individual on the board went through rigorous rounds of assessment to prove their worth. After which they invested a large part of their time researching and compiling the most relevant data for our readers.

The editorial board has been involved in producing this book since its inception. They have spent rigorous hours researching and exploring the diverse topics which have resulted in the successful publishing of this book. They have passed on their knowledge of decades through this book. To expedite this challenging task, the publisher supported the team at every step. A small team of assistant editors was also appointed to further simplify the editing procedure and attain best results for the readers.

Apart from the editorial board, the designing team has also invested a significant amount of their time in understanding the subject and creating the most relevant covers. They scrutinized every image to scout for the most suitable representation of the subject and create an appropriate cover for the book.

The publishing team has been an ardent support to the editorial, designing and production team. Their endless efforts to recruit the best for this project, has resulted in the accomplishment of this book. They are a veteran in the field of academics and their pool of knowledge is as vast as their experience in printing. Their expertise and guidance has proved useful at every step. Their uncompromising quality standards have made this book an exceptional effort. Their encouragement from time to time has been an inspiration for everyone.

The publisher and the editorial board hope that this book will prove to be a valuable piece of knowledge for researchers, students, practitioners and scholars across the globe.

List of Contributors

Hafsa Tayyab Mustafa
AME GLOBAL FZE, Sharjah, United Arab Emirates

Abduelmula R. Abduelkarem
College of Pharmacy, University of Sharjah, Sharjah, United Arab Emirates

Prosper Obunikem Uchechukwu Adogu
Consultant Public Health Physician (MBBS, FWACP, FMCPH), Department of Community Medicine, NAU/NAUTH, Nnewi, Nigeria

Ifeoma A. Njelita
Consultant Public Health Physician, (MBBS, MPH, FWACP), Department of Community Medicine, NAUTH, Nnewi, Nigeria

Nonye Bibiana Egenti
Consultant Public Health Physician (MBBS, MPH, FMCPH), Department of Community Medicine, University of Abuja, Abuja, Nigeria

Chika Florence Ubajaka
Consultant Public Health Physician (MBBS, FMCPH), Department of Community Medicine, NAU/NAUTH, Nnewi, Nigeria

Ifeoma A. Modebe
Consultant Public Health Physician (MBBS, FWACP), Department of Community Medicine, NAU/NAUTH, Nnewi, Nigeria

Tinashe Mudzviti
School of Pharmacy, University of Zimbabwe, Harare, Zimbabwe
Newlands Clinic, Harare, Zimbabwe

Nyasha T. Mudzongo
School of Pharmacy, University of Zimbabwe, Harare, Zimbabwe

Samuel Gavi
Department of Clinical Pharmacology, College of Health Sciences, Harare, Zimbabwe

Cleophas Chimbetete
Newlands Clinic, Harare, Zimbabwe

Charles C. Maponga
School of Pharmacy, University of Zimbabwe, Harare, Zimbabwe
Center of Excellence in Bioinformatics and Life Sciences and The School of Pharmacy and Pharmaceutical Sciences, University at Buffalo, SUNY, Buffalo, NY, USA

Gene D. Morse
Center of Excellence in Bioinformatics and Life Sciences and The School of Pharmacy and Pharmaceutical Sciences, University at Buffalo, SUNY, Buffalo, NY, USA

Masoud Behzadifar
Department of Health, Yazd University of Medical Sciences, Yazd, Iran
Health Management and Economics Research Center, Iran University of Medical Sciences, Tehran, Iran

Hamidreza Dehghan and Abouzar Keshavarzi
Department of Health, Yazd University of Medical Sciences, Yazd, Iran

Korush Saki
Department of Medicine, Shahid Beheshti University of Medical Sciences, Tehran, Iran

Meysam Behzadifar
Department of Medicine, Ilam University of Medical Sciences, Ilam, Iran

Maryam Saran
Department of Medicine, Tehran University of Medical Sciences, Tehran, Iran

Ali Akbari Sari
Department of Health Management and Economics, Tehran University of Medical Sciences, Tehran, Iran

Vijay Saradhi Mettu and A. Ravinder Nath
Department of Pharmacy, University College of Technology, Osmania University, Hyderabad, India

P. Yadagiri Swami and P. Abigna
Department of Chemistry, University College of Science, Osmania University, Hyderabad, India

Geeta Sharma
Forma Therapeutics Singapore, Singapore City, Singapore

Froylán Ibarra-Velarde, Yolanda Vera-Montenegro and Karla Sánchez-Peralta
Departamento de Parasitología, Facultad de Medicina Veterinaria y Zootecnia, Universidad Nacional Autónoma de México, México, D.F., México

Joaquín Ambía Medina
Laboratorio Salud Animal, México, D.F., México

Pedro Ochoa Galván
Departamento de Génetica, Facultad de Medicina Veterinaria y Zootecnia, Universidad Nacional Autónoma de México, México, D.F., México

Patrick Rutendo Matowa
Pharmaceutical Technology Department, Harare Institute of Technology, Harare, Zimbabwe

Mohammed Hassanein, Mohammed Shamssain and Nageeb Hassan
Clinical Pharmacy Department, College of Pharmacy and Health Science, Ajman University of Science and Technology, Ajman, United Arab Emirates

Christopher Oswald Migoha
Tanzania Food and Drugs Authority, Dar es Salaam, Tanzania
Pharm R&D Lab, School of Pharmacy, Muhimbili University of Health and Allied Sciences, Dar es Salaam, Tanzania

Eliangiringa Kaale
Pharm R&D Lab, School of Pharmacy, Muhimbili University of Health and Allied Sciences, Dar es Salaam, Tanzania

Godliver Kagashe
Department of Pharmaceutics, School of Pharmacy, Muhimbili University of Health and Allied Sciences, Dar es Salaam, Tanzania

Theophilus C. Onyekaba
Department of Pharmaceutical Chemistry, Faculty of Pharmaceutical Sciences, Delta State University, Abraka, Nigeria

Chukwudinma C. Achilefu and Chika J. Mbah
Department of Pharmaceutical and Medicinal Chemistry, Faculty of Pharmaceutical Sciences, University of Nigeria, Nsukka, Nigeria

Safaa Yehia Eid
Department of Biochemistry, Faculty of Medicine, Umm Al-Qura University, Makkah, Kingdom of Saudi Arabia
Institute of Pharmacy and Molecular Biotechnology, Heidelberg University, Heidelberg, Germany

Mahmoud Zaki El-Readi
Department of Biochemistry, Faculty of Medicine, Umm Al-Qura University, Makkah, Kingdom of Saudi Arabia
Institute of Pharmacy and Molecular Biotechnology, Heidelberg University, Heidelberg, Germany
Department of Biochemistry, Faculty of Pharmacy, Al-Azhar University, Assiut, Egypt

Sameer Hassan Fatani and Essam Eldin Mohamed Nour Eldin
Department of Biochemistry, Faculty of Medicine, Umm Al-Qura University, Makkah, Kingdom of Saudi Arabia

Michael Wink
Institute of Pharmacy and Molecular Biotechnology, Heidelberg University, Heidelberg, Germany
Xiaohui Yin, Xiuxia Gu, Yun He, Di Zhu, Jie Chen, Jue Wu, Xueqin Feng, Jinhao Li and Caiping Mao

Institute for Fetology & Reproductive Medicine Center, First Hospital of Soochow University, Suzhou, China

Zhice Xu
Center for Prenatal Biology, Loma Linda University, Loma Linda, CA, USA

Kalyani Chimajirao Patil, Laura McPherson and Craig James Daly
College of Medical, Veterinary & Life Sciences, School of Life Sciences, University of Glasgow, Glasgow, UK

Muhammad Ahmed
Department of Pharmacology and Toxicology, Faculty of Pharmacy, Umm Al-Qura University, Makkah, Kingdom of Saudi Arabia

Yoshifumi Murata and Kyoko Kofuji
Faculty of Pharmaceutical Science, Hokuriku University, Kanazawa, Japan

Shushin Nakano and Ryosei Kamaguchi
Morishita Jintan Co. Osaka Technocenter, Hirakata, Japan

Yuko Iwase, Noriyasu Kamei and Mariko Takeda-Morishita
Laboratory of Drug Delivery Systems, Faculty of Pharmaceutical Sciences, Kobe Gakuin University, Kobe, Japan

Yoshiyuki Hattori, Shohei Arai, Takuto Kikuchi, Megumi Hamada, Ryou Okamoto, Yoko Machida and Kumi Kawano
Department of Drug Delivery Research, Hoshi University, Tokyo, Japan

Hermine Boukeng Jatsa
Laboratory of Animal Physiology, Department of Animal Biology and Physiology, Faculty of Science, University of Yaoundé I, Yaoundé, Cameroon
Laboratory of Schistosomiasis, Department of Parasitology, Institute of Biological Sciences, Federal University of Minas Gerais, Belo Horizonte, Brazil
Laboratory of Immunopharmacology, Department of Biochemistry and Immunology, Institute of Biological Sciences, Federal University of Minas Gerais, Belo Horizonte, Brazil

Cintia Aparecida de Jesus Pereira and Deborah Aparecida Negrão-Corrêa
Laboratory of Schistosomiasis, Department of Parasitology, Institute of Biological Sciences, Federal University of Minas Gerais, Belo Horizonte, Brazil

Ana Bárbara Dias Pereira and Fernão Castro Braga
Laboratory of Phytochemistry, Department of Pharmaceutical Products, Faculty of Pharmacy, Federal University of Minas Gerais, Belo Horizonte, Brazil

Glauber Meireles Maciel and Rachel Oliviera Castilho
Laboratory of Pharmacognosy, Department of Pharmaceutical Products, Faculty of Pharmacy, Federal University of Minas Gerais, Belo Horizonte, Brazil

Pierre Kamtchouing
Laboratory of Animal Physiology, Department of Animal Biology and Physiology, Faculty of Science, University of Yaoundé I, Yaoundé, Cameroon

Mauro Martins Teixeira
Laboratory of Immunopharmacology, Department of Biochemistry and Immunology, Institute of Biological Sciences, Federal University of Minas Gerais, Belo Horizonte, Brazil

Melappa Govindappa, Kavya C. Hemmanur, Shrikanta Nithin, Chandrappa Chinna Poojari and Channabasava
Endophytic Natural Product Laboratory, Department of Biotechnology, Shridevi Institute of Engineering & Technology, Tumkur, India

Gopalakrishna Bhat Kakunje
Madhuca, Srinivasa Nagara, Chitpady, Udupi, India

Tomoya Sasahara, Natsumi Ohkura, Mariko Shin, Akira Onodera and Katsutoshi Yayama
Laboratory of Cardiovascular Pharmacology, Department of Biopharmaceutical Sciences, Kobe Gakuin University, Kobe, Japan

Tianxiu Qian
Department of Chemistry, The Hong Kong University of Science and Technology, Hong Kong SAR, China
Institute of Medicinal Plant Development, Chinese Academy of Medical Sciences & Peking Union Medical College, Beijing, China

Pou Kuan Leong and Kam Ming Ko
Division of Life Science, The Hong Kong University of Science and Technology, Hong Kong SAR, China

Wan Chan
Department of Chemistry, The Hong Kong University of Science and Technology, Hong Kong SAR, China

Umamahesh Balekari and Ciddi Veeresham
University College of Pharmaceutical Sciences, Kakatiya University, Warangal, India

Suleiman I. Sharif, Hoda Fazli, Yasamin Tajrobehkar, Zeinab Namvar and Laila M. T. Bugaighis
Department of Pharmacy Practice & Pharmacotherapeutics, College of Pharmacy, University of Sharjah, Sharjah, United Arab Emirates

Raúl Loera-Valencia, Josué Obed Jaramillo-Polanco, Andrómeda Linan-Rico, María Guadalupe Nieto Pescador, Juan Francisco Jiménez Bremont and Carlos Barajas-López
División de Biología Molecular, Instituto Potosino de Investigación Científica y Tecnológica, San Luís Potosí, México